WORKPLACE HEALTH PROMOTION PROGRAMS

WORKPLACE HEALTH PROMOTION PROGRAMS

PLANNING, IMPLEMENTATION, AND EVALUATION

Carl I. Fertman

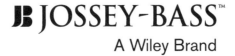

JB JOSSEY-BASS™
A Wiley Brand

Published by Jossey-Bass
A Wiley Brand
One Montgomery Street, Suite 1000, San Francisco, CA 94104-4594—www.josseybass.com

Limit of Liability/Disclaimer of Warranty: While the publisher and author have used their best efforts in preparing this book, they make no representations or warranties with respect to the accuracy or completeness of the contents of this book and specifically disclaim any implied warranties of merchantability or fitness for a particular purpose. No warranty may be created or extended by sales representatives or written sales materials. The advice and strategies contained herein may not be suitable for your situation. You should consult with a professional where appropriate. Neither the publisher nor author shall be liable for any loss of profit or any other commercial damages, including but not limited to special, incidental, consequential, or other damages. Readers should be aware that Internet Web sites offered as citations and/or sources for further information may have changed or disappeared between the time this was written and when it is read. This publication is designed to provide accurate and authoritative information in regard to the subject matter covered. It is sold with the understanding that the publisher is not engaged in rendering professional services. If legal, accounting, medical, psychological or any other expert assistance is required, the services of a competent professional person should be sought.

Jossey-Bass books and products are available through most bookstores. To contact Jossey-Bass directly call our Customer Care Department within the U.S. at 800-956-7739, outside the U.S. at 317-572-3986, or fax 317-572-4002.

Wiley publishes in a variety of print and electronic formats and by print-on-demand. Some material included with standard print versions of this book may not be included in e-books or in print-on-demand. If this book refers to media such as a CD or DVD that is not included in the version you purchased, you may download this material at http://booksupport.wiley.com. For more information about Wiley products, visit www.wiley.com. Wiley publishes in a variety of print and electronic formats and by print-on-demand. Some material included with standard print versions of this book may not be included in e-books or in print-on-demand. If this book refers to media such as a CD or DVD that is not included in the version you purchased, you may download this material at http://booksupport.wiley.com. For more information about Wiley products, visit www.wiley.com.

Library of Congress Cataloging-in-Publication Data:
Fertman, Carl I., 1950- author.
  Workplace health promotion programs : planning, implementation, and evaluation / Carl I. Fertman.
    pages cm
  Includes bibliographical references and index.
  ISBN 978-1-118-66942-6 (pbk.), 978-1-118-66668-5 (ePDF), (978-1-118-66932-7) (epub)
  1. Employee health promotion. 2. Work environment. 3. Quality of work life. I. Title.
  RC969.H43F47 2015
  658.3′82—dc23
                                                                        2015018218

Cover image: ©iStock/malija;
Background Texture ©iStock/studiocasper

Cover design: Wiley

Printed in the United States of America
10 9 8 7 6 5 4 3 2 1

For Irving Fertman, Amaia Rose Kapenga, and Samuel Francis Kapenga, generation to generation with gratitude and love

CONTENTS

FIGURES, TABLES, BOXES, AND EXHIBITS

Figures

Tables

Boxes

Exhibits

Employers and employees are committed to improving and promoting employees' health and well-being. Healthy employees are productive employees. Sick employees do not come to work, and if they do come to work, it is not good for them, work colleagues, and production. Employers and employees also think a lot about how expensive health care is in the United States and that workplace health promotion programs can contribute to controlling and lowering the cost of health care for the employer and employee. At first, the concept of a program to improve or promote the health of employees as well as contribute to lowering health care cost may sound a little intimidating. It becomes clear, however, that the idea of such a program to improve employee health and lower health care expenses is appealing and seems worthwhile, although turning the idea into reality demands work and expertise. In other words, it is easy to say that something should be done or needs to be done. It is very different to know how to plan, implement, and evaluate a program to actually achieve a specific health outcome, improve the health status of employees, and lower health care expenses. It is a complex process.

Opportunities to promote health of individuals and lower health care costs at the workplaces are abundant. Promoting employees' health helps individuals to lead socially and economically productive lives. It makes economic sense as part of an overall business plan to control and lower health care costs for employers and employees. The goal of *Workplace Health Promotion Programs: Planning, Implementation, and Evaluation* is to provide a comprehensive introduction to workplace health promotion programs by combining theory and practice. Each of the chapters in this text corresponds to a key step identified through research and practice to promote the health of individuals at their place of work. The chapters can help you to achieve a specific health outcome or an improvement in the overall health status of employees while addressing health care cost concerns.

Overview of the Book

The book provides the insights and tools to plan, implement, and evaluate evidence-based workplace health promotion policies, interventions, practices, and services. The book gives you a tangible sense of how programs should work, and when they work best, so you will know how to champion and advocate for programs and to work with teams, partnerships, and collaborations to successfully plan, implement, and evaluate programs. This comprehensive book includes everything you need to know about health promotion theory, strategic human resource management, worker health and safety, priority health program areas, and evaluation strategies, and it provides examples of how to work with small and midsized employers, hospitals, larger employers, and schools and colleges to promote employee health. I have divided the book into five parts. In Part One I present the foundations of workplace health promotion programs. In Parts Two (planning), Three (implementation) and Four (evaluation) I provide a step-by-step guide to each phase of a workplace health promotion program. Practical tips, tools, and specific examples aim to facilitate readers' understanding of these phases and also help to build technical skills in planning and leading evidence-based workplace health promotion programs. In Part Five I present workplace health promotion programs across four arenas: in small and midsized employers, within the federal government (the largest U.S. employer), in hospitals, and in schools (elementary to college). All of the chapters present key points for effective workplace programs to promote worker health and safety.

1. Chapter 1: I discuss the nature and definition of workplace health promotion programs, the history of workplace health and safety programs, the impact of the Patient Protection and Affordable Care Act on workplace health promotion programs, and the controversies and pitfalls for such programs.

2. Chapter 2: I apply the major health promotion program approaches, theories, and models to workplace health promotion programs with practical guidelines to their selection and use in creating evidence-based programs.

3. Chapter 3: I explain how human resource management makes employee health promotion a priority and describes actions to facilitate high quality workplace health promotion programs.

4. Chapter 4: I discuss workplace health promotion programs in terms of planning, management, and initial actions with a focus on needs assessment, workplace health readiness, and capacity for health.

5. Chapter 5: I provide tools to assess workplace health champions, advocates, culture, and climate as well as important workplace policies and legal requirements.

6. Chapter 6: I explain how to assess workplace health promotion teams, partnerships, and collaborations that strengthen program planning, implementation, and evaluation.

7. Chapter 7: I detail how to assess employee needs to support and make program decisions. You learn what to expect to have and to know at the end of the planning process.

8. Chapter 8: In this chapter I explain why employee physical health is not just about primary care. I also consider how to give the employees opportunities and encouragement to improve their current physical health by utilizing workplace primary care centers and other health advocates (e.g., concierges) disease management, absence management, pharmacy benefit management, as well as medical-second opinions and value-based benefit design.

9. Chapter 9: I describe employers' concerns for employees' mental health, especially considering that organizational performance is directly related to the mental health of their workers. I present common and effective mental and behavioral health workplace programs to address employee mental health and behavioral disorders that have a direct impact on workplace absenteeism, presenteeism (attending work when sick), accidents, turnover, and productivity.

10. Chapter 10: In this chapter I describe workplace physical activity spanning the workplace and community. I discuss how small and midsized workplaces and many large workplaces do not have physical activity space or facilities (e.g., fitness center, gym, pool, walking trails, bike path, showers, changing area, equipment storage and maintenance) but rather use existing facilities in the surrounding workplace communities and employee neighborhoods.

11. Chapter 11: I describe in this chapter how to engage and support employees to eat well for good nutrition with healthy dietetic practices and dietary habits within a supportive environment that is respectful of workers' family, ethnic, economic, and community influences. I discuss as well how programs increasingly are raising awareness to challenge employers and employees to think critically about issues and dilemmas involving food production, food consumption behaviors, and nutritional outcomes as controversies in contemporary society.

12. Chapter 12: My focus in this chapter is how to create physically healthy and safe workplace environments, and how to prevent hazards in the workplace that cause accident, injury, disability, or illness. Employers have a legal requirement and incentive to implement

physically healthy and safe workplace environments as a means to control workers' compensation expenses (e.g., insurance premium rate increases) and costs (e.g., lost production, fines, and legal expenses related to unsafe conditions).

13. Chapter 13: In this chapter I explain how employers create and sustain psychologically healthy and safe workplace environments to promote employees' psychological well-being—environments that do not harm employee mental health in negligent, reckless, or intentional ways. I emphasize that psychologically unhealthy and unsafe work environments have a pervasive impact upon a workplace culture and climate, with potentially serious negative impacts on workplace production, product quality, and consumer satisfaction and service.

14. Chapter 14: My focus here is health education delivered through individual (one-to-one) or group instruction, as well as through interactive electronic media, in order to promote changes in individuals, groups of individuals, or the general worker population. I discuss social media (media for social interaction, using highly accessible and scalable publishing techniques and web-based platforms) as an eHealth tool to promote health, with the options to communicate health and safety information in the workplace as it changes with each new technological advance.

15. Chapter 15: I present in this chapter a discussion of best practices for the improvement and accountability of workplace health promotion programs, including economic evaluations, one of which is return on investment (ROI). Explained is how to provide a continuous feedback cycle for program decision making with employers, employees, program staff, and program providers (vendors). Presented are tools for evaluations that are feasible, scalable, sustainable, and scientific, built on a foundation supported by a strategic organizational commitment and shared vision for innovation.

16. Chapter 16: I describe the use of big data in the evaluation of workplace health promotion programs, explaining data mining and three levels of analytics with increasing functionality and value (descriptive, predictive, and prescriptive). Analyzing and using the data is seen as a means to maximize resources and improve worker health outcomes by designing health promotion programs and benefits matched to the needs of employees.

17. Chapter 17: In this chapter I explain how small and midsized employers plan, implement, and evaluate workplace health promotion

programs is to balance their (employers') value on the well-being of employees with their (employers') concerns about workplace health promotion programs. I discuss as well how to work with coalitions, partnerships, and collaborations to leverage resources, and public and voluntary health agencies to create modest but effective strategies to meet specific employee health needs of small and midsized employers.

18. Chapter 18: I present in this chapter ways to create well-supported and active hospital employee health promotion programs with a strong focus on employee and family wellness. I emphasize the need to attend to hospital workers' physical and psychological safety. Hospitals record work-related injuries and illnesses at a rate of almost twice the rate for private industry as a whole.

19. Chapter 19: In this chapter I explain how the largest U.S. employer, the federal government, promotes employee health. Information and tools are provided to work the U.S. Office of Personnel Management and Federal Occupational Health, the largest provider of occupational health and safety services in the federal government, serving more than 360 federal agencies and reaching 1.8 million federal employees.

20. Chapter 20: In the final chapter I identify opportunities for schools and universities to promote employee health. I present required tools and skills needed to network and build support across all of the school levels and units with emphasis on tailoring and fitting program to school employees' health needs.

At the beginning of each chapter the Learning Objectives give a framework and guide to the chapter topics. The key terms at the end of each chapter can be used as a reference while reading this book as well as a way to recap key definitions in planning, implementation, and evaluation of workplace health promotion programs.

Practical examples I provide throughout the book reinforce the need for workplace health promotion programs to be based on in-depth understanding of the intended audiences' perceptions, beliefs, attitudes, behaviors, and barriers to change as well as the cultural, social, and environmental context in which they live. By referring to current theories and models of health promotion, I also reinforce the need for workplace health promotion practitioners to base their programs on theories, models, and approaches that guide and inform workplace health promotion program planning, implementation, and evaluation.

Each chapter ends with practice and discussion questions to help the reader to reflect upon as well as utilize key concepts. A chapter case study asks what would you do to build practical and real life skills to plan, implement, and evaluate programs. Finally, all chapters are interconnected but are also designed to stand alone, and to provide a comprehensive overview of the topic they cover.

Each chapter of this textbook is designed to engage you in thought, discussion, and action. Where possible, I used examples about real programs that relate to common elements of life, practical questions, and a conversational tone to engage you in a personal way. A number of special features will help you explore ideas, test recommended approaches, and develop knowledge and competencies that will inform your workplace health promotion efforts. These features include:

- Learning Objectives at the beginning of each chapter focus on the most important concepts to be covered. They help you highlight and organize your reading and notes around the learning objectives. The chapter content is designed to help you understand those concepts as they are applied in real-world settings.

- Extensive information on networking with human resources, business, health, educational, and human services professionals will help to develop a larger framework of support for workplace health promotion.

- Information on teams, partnerships, and collaborations.

- Useful tools as you seek additional information and expand your knowledge about a variety of workplace health promotion-related organizations and information sources.

- Chapter summaries at the end of each chapter are a one- or two-paragraph review of the major concepts covered in the chapter.

- The "What Would You Do?" case study at the end of each chapter is a fictionalized composite of an individual in the field presenting real-life scenarios to inspire discussion and further thought on the practical aspects of workplace health promotion. The cases are designed to engage you in discussion and application of the knowledge and competencies described in that chapter.

- The "For Practice and Discussion" topics and questions at the end of each chapter contain instructions for recommended activities that can be undertaken on your own if an instructor hasn't already assigned them. Some activities can occur totally within the confines of a classroom. Others may require you to visit a local employer, neighborhood, or community organization for a strong real-world experience. Moreover, some activities can reinforce your work on a course project if one is assigned, or further develop your professional resume or portfolio.

- Key Terms are listed at the end of the chapter. The chapters are designed to help you understand those concepts as they are applied in real-world settings.

- Web links are included throughout the book to encourage further exploration to support planning, implementing, and evaluating workplace health promotion programs.

Workplace Health Promotion Programs: Planning, Implementation, and Evaluation examines how to promote health at the workplace. I hope that the guidance and resources in this book leave you feeling competent to make a difference in the lives of individuals at their places of employment. I wish you success as you apply your knowledge, tools, and skills. I hope that this book helps guide and inspire a healthier world for all individuals.

To the Instructor

Workplace Health Promotion Programs: Planning, Implementation, and Evaluation provides a comprehensive introduction to workplace health promotion programs by combining theory and practice. Chapters correspond to a key step identified through research and practice to promote the health of individuals at their place of work. Using the book, your students will have a tangible sense of how evidence-based programs should work, when they work best, and how to champion and advocate for programs to achieve specific health outcomes or an improvement in the overall health status of employees while addressing health care cost concerns. The design includes:

- Text and resources draw from real-world experience of professionals who work to create healthy workplaces.

- Course material currently used in workplace health promotion.

- An emphasis on developing individual responsibility through active involvement with diverse communities.

- Evidence-based policies, practices, interventions, and services.

- A focus on practical application and simple, clear, relatable tools and language.

- Content that is easily adaptable for both undergraduate and graduate students and experienced professionals.

- The Student Course Workplace Program Project Guide at the website can be used for a term-long student project (completed individually or as a team) that encourages creativity and practical experience working with schools and communities. You will find that many of the For Practice and Discussion Questions activities throughout each chapter are components of such a project.

- The Book Companion website includes chapter objectives, practice quizzes, Responsibilities and Competencies boxes, web links, examples of Student Course Workplace Program Projects created by former students, the Glossary and flashcards, and instructor resources (e.g., Instructor Manual, TestGen Computerized Test Banks compatible with Blackboard and other eLearning platforms, and PowerPoint presentations).

- All electronic instructor resources are available for download on the Wiley Instructor Resource Center. Go to www.wiley.com/go/whpp to download the materials. Students will also be able to purchase the e-book version of this test from this page.

Students will find this book easy to understand and use. I am confident that if the chapters are carefully read and an honest effort is put into completing the activities and visiting the web links, students will gain the essential knowledge and skills for workplace health promotion program planning, implementation, and evaluation.

ACKNOWLEDGMENTS

My friend and Jossey-Bass senior editor Andy Pasternack (1955–2013) fought cancer with the intelligence, passion, and humor that he brought to everything he did. He was a remarkable and talented man and a wonderful colleague. It is an honor that during the final year of his life he worked with me to develop and bring life to this book. He was kind, warm, funny, and always collaborative. I miss him.

Workplace Health Promotion Programs: Planning, Implementation, and Evaluation is a team effort. I thank the multitude of students preparing for careers in health education, public health, business, counseling, social work, community health, psychology, allied health, medicine, and nursing whose input identified the need for and shaped the content of this book. My graduate students who work with me to design, implement, and evaluate workplace health promotion programs are thanked for their time and energy. I acknowledge the workplaces, health and medical institutions, government offices, health care providers, and health insurance companies, brokers, and agents that open their doors to me and my students each year as partners in cocreating healthy workplaces for employers and employees. We get to know their organizations. . . and they get to know us too. The Pittsburgh Business Group on Health and its members are recognized for their years of ongoing support and generosity. Diane McClune and Jessica Brooks from the Business Group are thanked for their guidance and time. Carolyn Kontos from Highmark is thanked for her encouragement and insight. Judy Trawick and Karen Kuroda from Federal Occupational Health are thanked for their support and energy. My University of Pittsburgh Health and Physical Activity Department colleagues Dr. John Jakicic, Department Chair, Dr. Carma Rae Sprowls Repcheck, Internship Clinical Coordinator, and Dr. Robert Robertson, Professor Emeritus, are thanked for their support and partnership with me to create healthy workplaces.

I want to thank proposal reviewers Danielle Robinson Fastring, Debra L. Fetherman, Rick Petosa, and Jeff Schlicht, who provided valuable feedback on the original book proposal. Bob LeFavi, Melinda Moore, and Jennifer Thomas provided thoughtful and constructive comments on the complete draft manuscript.

Acknowledged and thanked are Melissa Schwenk and Lisa Belloli for their editing and preparation of the figures, tables, and manuscript. I acknowledge and thank Seth Schwartz, Wiley/Jossey-Bass editor, for his time, energy, and support.

I thank Barb Murock, my wife, for her love and support—and for biking with me on the Pittsburgh hills and the many places our bikes take us.

Carl I. Fertman, Pittsburgh, Pennsylvania
August 2015

ABOUT THE AUTHOR

Carl I. Fertman, PhD, MBA, MCHES, is associate professor of Health and Physical Activity in the School of Education at the University of Pittsburgh. He teaches courses in evidence-based health promotion program design and health theories. Dr. Fertman works extensively in the planning, implementation, and evaluation of workplace health promotion programs that include large, midsized, and small businesses, hospitals, schools and colleges, community organizations, government offices, and sole proprietorships. Dr. Fertman is an expert at evidence-based programs that link and balance workplace, community, and family resources to be reflective and unique to a workplace and its employees. Dr. Fertman has worked with the British and Turkish governments to promote the health of their citizens. He has authored numerous health promotion program and service evaluations for federal and state departments of education, health, human services, welfare, and labor. Dr. Fertman has authored six books in the field of health promotion. He is the coeditor of the Society for Public Health Education (SOPHE) textbook published by Wiley/Jossey-Bass, *Health Promotion Programs: From Theory to Practice*. In addition, Dr. Fertman has published more than 80 articles, monographs, and book chapters on the prevention of alcohol and drug problems, mental health promotion, and health promotion programs and services. In 2015 he was elected to the National SOPHE Board of Directors as National Trustee for Professional Development.

PART ONE

FOUNDATION

CHAPTER 1

WORKPLACE HEALTH PROMOTION PROGRAM FOUNDATIONS

What Are Workplace Health Promotion Programs?

Workplace health promotion programs are designed to promote physical and mental health and well-being in the workplace. *Workplaces* are defined as organizations that employ people to produce products, services, arts, care, and goods. The organizations can comprise a single person or many; they can be small, midsized, or large and range from employing a few people at one shop to employing thousands of people at many locations around the world. Workplace health promotion programs have their roots in the socioecological model of health, which spans the individual, family, workplace, community, and larger environment and health advocacy to create and impact public policy at the organizational, local, regional, and national levels.

Workplace health promotion programs can improve physical, psychological, educational, and work outcomes for individuals and help control or reduce overall health care costs by emphasizing prevention of health problems, promoting healthy lifestyles, improving individual compliance with occupational safety and health regulations, and facilitating access to health services and care. Such programs play a role in creating healthier workers and workplaces but also healthier families and communities. Workplace health promotion programs contribute to an environment that promotes and supports the health of individuals and the overall public. Workplace health promotion programs take advantage of their pivotal position

LEARNING OBJECTIVES

- Define *workplace health promotion programs*
- Summarize the historical context for workplace health promotion
- Discuss the impact of the Affordable Care Act on workplace health promotion
- Identify workplace health promotion controversies and pitfalls

in peoples' jobs and places of employment to provide individual employees as well as their family members with the knowledge and skills they need to make informed decisions about their health. They foster good health, work performance, work quality, and quality of life (Fertman, Allensworth, & Auld, 2010). Workplace health promotion programs depend on the combined efforts and commitment of employers, employees, and society to improve the health and well-being of people at work (Centers for Disease Control and Prevention [CDC], 2013a).

Workplace health promotion programs are a coordinated and comprehensive set of health promotion and protection strategies implemented in the workplace; these strategies include programs, policies, and benefits as well as safety, health, and environmental support systems (and links to the surrounding community and larger society) designed to encourage the health and safety of all employees and their families. Workplace health promotion programs involve (CDC, 2013b):

- Having an organizational commitment to improving the health of the workforce

- Providing employees with appropriate information and establishing comprehensive communication strategies

- Involving employees in decision-making processes

- Developing a working culture that is based on partnership

- Organizing work tasks and processes so that they contribute to, rather than damage, health

- Implementing policies and practices that enhance employee health by making the healthy choices the easy choices

- Recognizing that organizations have an impact on people and that this is not always conducive to their health and well-being

The federal government's Healthy People 2010 initiative (U.S. Department of Health and Human Services [USDHHS], 2000) proposed a definition of comprehensive workplace health promotion programs as those that incorporated five key elements: (1) health education (i.e., skill development and lifestyle behavior change, along with information dissemination and awareness building), (2) supportive social and physical work environment (i.e., support of healthy behaviors and implementation of policies promoting health and reducing risk of disease), (3) integration (i.e., incorporating the program into the organization's structure), (4) linkage (i.e., connecting to related programs such as employee assistance programs), and (5) worksite screening and education (i.e., programs linked to appropriate medical care) (Soto Mas, Allensworth, & Carnara, 2010).

Workplace health promotion programs address occupational health and safety, organization and conditions of work, leave policies and benefits, and workplace wellness initiatives that are integrated to maximize resources and ensure success. The most promising programs feature a strong employer commitment and are responsive to employees' needs. The workplace is viewed as a health-promoting environment that connects employee health and the health of the organization, community, and society (Polanyi, Frank, Shannon, Sullivan, & Lavis, 2000). The most effective programs feature advocacy strategies that create and impact health policy at the workplace, community, regional, state, and national levels (Fertman et al., 2010).

Finally, workplace health promotion programs are part of strategic human resource management: integrating strategies and systems to achieve an overall mission to ensure the success of an organization while meeting the needs of the organization's clients, customers, consumers, stockholders, and other stakeholders as well as the employees. The personnel office of the 1980s processed paperwork; verified and rekeyed data; answered routine inquiries; monitored compliance; hired, suspended, and fired employees; and kept track of vacation and sick days. Today the personnel office is called the department of human resources, and charged with the following tasks: growing and retaining staff, increasing employee engagement, recruiting and hiring the best people, controlling costs, focusing on "best practices," deciding employees benefit offerings (including health insurance coverage, workers' compensation, and disability management), and being a proactive and creative force to address emerging and changing conditions. The human resource department is recognized as contributing to an organization's bottom line whether it is profits, services, goods, or products. And it is true for all organizations regardless of their size: large, midsized, or small. Workplace health promotion programs as part of strategic human resource management make organizations successful (Schwind, Das, Wagar, Fassina, & Bulmash, 2013).

Historical Context for Workplace Health Promotion

Workplace health promotion reflects three major revolutionary steps or phases in the quest to promote healthy individuals and healthy communities (Kickbusch & Payne, 2003). The three phases parallel the transformation of the company personnel office from a paper-processing operation to the modern-day human resource department directed by a chief human capital officer who leads, contributes, improves, and advances the organization's mission and goals. Personnel offices dealt with problems with little perceived corporate value beyond doing what was required by the law, and were often portrayed as overwhelmed and unavailable. Strategic human resources is a corporate partner, expert counsel, and an effective presence within the organization (ADP, 2008). And workplace health promotion is key to an organization's strategic human resources.

First Phase

The first workplace health promotion program phase, which focused on addressing sanitary conditions, infectious diseases, and unsafe conditions, occurred in the mid-19th century. Occupational safety and health, primarily to *protect* health, was the concern in this phase. The first American industries to employ company doctors—railroads, mining companies, lumber companies, iron works, steel mills, and other heavy manufacturing companies—had several things in common, including dangerous work conditions, high accident rates, and often remote locations with little access to health care outside the company. Railroad work conditions were particularly dangerous (Figure 1.1). In 1900 there were more than 1 million railroad workers in the United States. According to the Interstate Commerce Commission, 1 of every 28 employees was injured and 1 of every 99 was killed on the job in the year ending June 1900 (Aldrich, 1997; Drudi, 2007). Other industries did not have it much better. The National Safety Council estimates that, in 1912, work-related injuries resulted in between 18,000 and 21,000 deaths across the United States. In 1913 the Bureau of Labor Statistics documented appropriately 23,000 industrial deaths among a workforce of 38 million, a rate of 61 deaths per 100,000 workers (CDC, 2015). The combination of frequent accidents and generally distant locations from

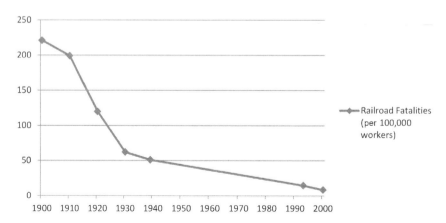

Figure 1.1   Railroad Fatalities 1900 to 2000
Source: Aldrich, 1997; Drudi, 2007.

preexisting medical systems made creating company-owned health clinics necessary for both the employees and their families. Thus, in many places, industrial medicine became the community's medicine as well a precursor to today's full-service primary care and the pharmacy health centers offered by some large employers (Schoenleber, 1933).

The focus of workplace health care slowly began to shift from injury response to preventive medicine (Starr, 1982). A prime example of this shift is Kaiser Steel. During World War II the corporation and its foundation formed a group practice called *Kaiser Permanente*. Using hospitals located on company property near shipyards, Kaiser operated a full-service medical program to treat employees and their dependents. Kaiser was one of the first large companies to make health care part of its organizational philosophy (Draper, 2005). Many other companies hired doctors and developed variations of the Kaiser model of company medicine; these include New York Bell's primary-care clinics for employees and their family members and the in-house wellness programs operated by Tenneco and Uniroyal (Draper, 2005).

Over time minimal occupational safety standards and regulations were established to ensure safer working conditions for the U.S. workforce. They culminated in the Occupational Safety and Health Act of 1970, which was passed to ensure "so far as possible every working man and woman in the nation safe and healthful working conditions and to preserve our human resources." In spite of such measures, work-related injuries and fatalities remain a considerable threat to public health.

A modern-day example of engaging employers and employees in workplace health and safety concerns is the Occupational Safety & Health Administration (OSHA)'s Voluntary Protection Program (VPP; U.S. Department of Labor, n.d.). VPP establishes a cooperative relationship among employees, management, and government to achieve safety and health excellence. Participants develop and implement systems to identify, evaluate, prevent, and control occupational hazards to prevent employee injuries and illnesses. More than 270 federal and private-sector industries participate in VPP. Sites vary in size from three employees to over 18,000 employees (U.S. Department of Labor, n.d.).

Second Phase

The second health promotion program phase occurred in the 1970s with the release of the Lalonde report (Lalonde, 1974), produced in Canada and formally titled *A New Perspective on the Health of Canadians*. It proposed the concept of the "health field," identifying two main health-related objectives: improvement of the health care system, and the prevention of health problems and promotion of good health. The report is considered the "first modern government document in the Western world to acknowledge that our emphasis upon a biomedical health care system is wrong, and that we need to look beyond the traditional health care (sick care) system if we wish to improve the health of the public." The report is considered to have led to the development and evolution of health promotion, recognizing both the need for people to take more responsibility in changing their behaviors to improve their own health, and also the contribution of healthy communities and environments to health. The Lalonde report set the stage for health promotion efforts. Workplace health promotion in this phase emphasized a healthy lifestyle to encourage healthier individual behaviors through the provision of support and information and the development of skills.

In the second phase of workplace health promotion programs, health promotion, medical benefits, short- and long-term disability, workers' compensation, disease management, case management programs, primary care, pharmacy, and other health programs were combined into a single process that emphasized improving outcomes, measurement and bench-marking, coordination of services, and creating synergy between program and services. Workplace-based health and wellness services were broadly categorized into risk management, medical management, and population management, although some types of services may fall into more than one category. The overall goal was to help manage costs and improve outcomes for the employee by reducing duplication of services, to help ensure that quality health care providers were selected, and to help employees navigate the often confusing medical system so they could return to full health and functionality as soon as possible (Fabius & Frazee, 2009).

Major companies made major investments in workplace health and health promotion for their employees during the 1980s. One example is Johnson & Johnson (http://www.jnj.com/about-jnj), who strove to create a culture of wellness at its many operations. The programs in this phase emphasized healthy lifestyle to encourage healthier individuals' behaviors through the provision of support and information, and the development of skills (Table 1.1). They utilized strategies such as a health risk assessment (HRA), blood screenings to identify biological health indicators and determine health risks, preventive services, education to improve self-management of acute and chronic conditions, and wellness education in the areas of nutrition, fitness, smoking cessation, and stress management (offered on- and off-site). The latter was the most visible sign of an organization's commitment to employee wellness and promotion by offering outreach to employees and commitment from top management, usually with highly visible leadership and participation by managers and directors.

Table 1.1   Phase Two—Examples of Programs and Services to Encourage Healthier Individual Behavior

1. Clinical preventive services based on U.S. Preventive Services Guidelines available to employees' organization health care plans. Well baby, well child, and adult preventive visits covered by all health care plan options. Preventive screenings, lab tests, and immunizations are covered.

2. Self-care and health consumerism education to improve self-management of acute and chronic conditions, communication with primary physicians, and appropriate use of health services. Interventions include introductory meeting on self-care and health consumerism, the distribution of information, and continuous message reinforcement through corporate communications and local education programs.

3. Wellness education in the areas of nutrition, fitness, smoking cessation, and stress management is offered on-site with links to community resources such as nonprofit health associations, hospitals, or fitness facilities. These efforts often focus on support for individual self-improvement, while avoiding controversial areas, including organizational dynamics and management behavior that may unwittingly have a negative impact on outcomes related to health, safety, diversity, competition (internal and external), or family.

4. Partnerships with other program areas such as employee assistance, work and family, and occupational medicine are developed. Over time the partnerships will be enhanced by greater attention to organizational- and community-level interventions designed to address the full range of public health, nutrition, safety, fitness, social actions, and family support issues.

5. Employees, pensioners, and spouses are encouraged to complete a lifestyle assessment to identify areas for which programs and services, geared to improving lifestyle and health behaviors, may be recommended to help control cancer and cardiovascular risk factors.

Partnerships with health care providers and community groups focused on health promotion appeared during this phase. (In the next, or third, phase these early partnerships will blossom in size, impact, and complexity.) Additional organizational strategies in phase two included integrated health care benefits with employee health services, a preventive health orientation in all programs, improved employee health communication, and development of systems and metrics to make informed decisions on program design and resource allocation.

In the second phase, leaders and advocates for workplace programs needed to justify the economic value of health promotion efforts to employers. While it may make intuitive sense that investing in employee health promotion is worthwhile, employee health is also viewed as ones' personal responsibility and as something private, beyond the scope and responsibility of the employer. At the heart of the matter is the basic question: Are corporations (workplaces) responsible for more than generating profits and jobs? If so, how far should this line of reasoning be taken (Carroll, Lipartito, Post, & Werhane, 2012)? In this phase the argument was made that employee health and health status was integral to an organization's performance and profits (however defined, such as in dollars, shareholder dividends, service contracts, grants, hours of services, or student achievement). Economic analysis of health promotion was introduced, and it indicated that promoting employee health was not only cost-effective but also a good return on investment (ROI). This encouraged organizations to make investments in health promotion. What followed were studies that showed that workplace wellness programs reduced tobacco use among participants, lowered high blood pressure, decreased work absences due to illness or disability, and improved other general measures of worker productivity (Table 1.2). A growing body of evidence indicated that health promotion programs are cost-effective.

The pinnacle of the second phase of workplace health promotion programs is the Healthy People 2010 initiative goal to increase the proportion of workplaces that offer an employee health promotion program

Table 1.2   Early (1990s) Return on Investment (ROI) Studies

Du Pont saw that each dollar invested in workplace health promotion yielded $1.42 over 2 years in lower absenteeism costs. Absences from illness unrelated to the job among 45,000 blue-collar workers dropped 14% at 41 industrial sites where the health promotion program was offered, compared with a 5.8% decline at 19 sites where it was not (Bertera, 1990).

The Travelers Corporation claims a $3.40 return for every dollar invested in health promotion, yielding total corporate savings of $146 million in benefits costs. Sick leave was reduced 19% during the 4-year study. In addition, the overall health of 36,000 employees and retirees improved by reducing poor health habits and increasing good ones (Golaszewski, Snow, Lynch, Yen, & Solomita, 1992).

The Stay Alive & Well program at Reynolds Electrical & Engineering Company, based in Las Vegas, cost $76.24 per employee during the 2 years of its operation. Over half of the 1,600 employees participated (with up to 80% participation rates in the intervention program). Participants significantly lowered cholesterol levels, blood pressure, and weight, and experienced 21% lower lifestyle-related claim costs than nonparticipants. Resulting savings: $127.89 per participant with a benefit to cost ratio of 1.68 to 1 (Anthem Health Systems, 1993).

Superior Coffee and Foods, a subsidiary of Sara Lee Corporation based in Bensenville, Illinois, attributes impressive results to the success of the company's comprehensive wellness program. Superior showed 22% fewer admissions to a hospital, 29% shorter hospital stays, and 42% lower expenses per admission when comparing costs for this division's 1,200 employees with costs for other divisions (Ahsmann, 1994).

Average medical costs of high-risk Steelcase employees—those whose lifestyles include two to four health risks such as smoking, little exercise, being overweight—were 75% higher than those of low-risk employees. High-risk employees at one factory site who participated in a health promotion program became low-risk, cutting their average medical claims in half and thus lowering their medical insurance costs by an average of $618 per year. If all high-risk employees (20% of the total employee population) in one location changed their lifestyles to become low-risk, the projected savings could total $20 million over 3 years (Tze-ching Yen, Edington, & Witting, 1994).

With savings estimated to be as high as $8 million, the California Public Employees' Retirement System sent its 55,000 retirees a health risk appraisal form, which they followed (in some cases) with individualized reports and letters and self-care materials to encourage change and help reduce health risks among retirees, and at the same time reduce the health care claim costs (Fries, Harrington, Edwards, Kent, & Richardson, 1994).

(through the eighth level of educational and community-based programs, or ECBP-8) and to increase the proportion of employees who participate in employer-sponsored health promotion activities of ECBP-9 (USDHHS, 2015b). Health promotion programs were now viewed as having many benefits. They led to improvements in lifestyle habits that reduce the likelihood of health problems arising over time. Furthermore if such programs are well integrated into the overall health and productivity management system of the organization, they can spur additional savings by complementing the goals of other programs and can create an environment of wellness that supports and maintains health. While occupational safety and health are dedicated to the prevention of injury and treatment of illness (in phase 1), workplace health promotion (in phase 2) can touch the lives of all employees. And this was now believed to be at least equally important to caring for the injured and ill, because the well workers are the ones doing the majority of the work.

Third Phase

In the third and current phase of workplace health promotion, emphasis is on workplace determinants of health. Although genes, behavior, and medical care play a role in how well we feel and how long we live, such factors as economics, social conditions, and the culture in which we are born, live, learn, work, and play have the most significant impact on our mental and physical health. These are called determinants of health. Differences (disparities) in health status in the workplace and wider community results from the determinants (USDHHS, 2000, 2015a). Disparities occur in physical health (e.g., higher rates of obesity, asthma, tooth decay, sexually transmitted infections), mental health (e.g., higher rates of depression, anxiety, stress, substance use), and built environments (e.g., higher rates of violence, crime, inadequate housing, recreation facilities). In the workplace, health determinants (Figure 1.2) are categorized as originating in the job itself (job strain, fatigue, anxiety, depression, musculoskeletal disorders, and physical illness), the organization (remuneration, benefits, and worker participation in decision making), and society at large (gender, economics, education, disability, geographic location, culture, ethnicity, social conditions, and sexual orientation) (Polanyi et al., 2000; Soto Mas et al., 2010).

In the third phase, organizational policy and procedures are prominent in addressing health determinants at the workplace. For example, 41% of civilian workers receive paid personal days, but this percentage varies by occupation—from 58% in management, professional, and related fields

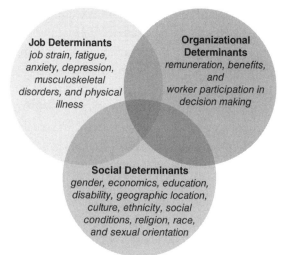

Figure 1.2 Workplace Health Determinants
Source: Polanyi et al., 2000; Soto Mas et al., 2010.

to 30% in service fields. The argument is that policies need to recognize employee differences and provide enough flexibility for employees to attend to their own health needs and those of their families. For example, paid sick days help workers recover from illnesses and provide care for sick family members, potentially preventing more severe illness and use of expensive hospital care (U.S. Bureau of Labor Statistics, 2013). The CDC recommends that workers who are ill stay home from work to prevent spreading disease at the workplace (CDC, 2013a).

In the third phase there are a growing number of tools and resources for workplace health promotion. These include the CDC's Successful Business Strategies to Prevent Heart Disease and Stroke Toolkit (http://www.cdc .gov/dhdsp/pubs/employers_toolkit.htm), the CDC/National Business Group on Health Employer Guide to Clinical Prevention Services (http:// www.businessgrouphealth.org/preventive/background.cfm), CDC Lean for Life Employer Toolkit (http://www.cdc.gov/Features/LEANforLife/), and the New York City Department of Health and Mental Hygiene Workplace Food Initiative (http://www.nyc.gov/html/doh/html/living/cdp-pan-hwp .shtml). These tools enable employers to prepare business cases for health promotion programs, identify competent partners from the private and public sectors, and evaluate both health-related and financial outcomes from their programs. In the third phase some state governments have taken the lead to develop and implement programs. Noteworthy examples are King County, Washington (http://www.kingcounty.gov/healthservices /health.aspx), and the state of Delaware (http://dhss.delaware.gov/dhss/), where extensive health promotion programs are implemented and evaluated.

In the third phase attention turns to the small employers and health promotion. Slightly more than half of the private-sector workforce in the United States is employed by smaller businesses—those with fewer than 50 employees. Workers in small businesses typically have less flexibility in the workplace, enjoy fewer employer-sponsored benefits, and are less likely to have access to workplace wellness initiatives than other workers. Strategies for increasing the offering of health-promoting benefits by small employers include creating a consortium of small employers, using health care insurers to provide wellness services, and partnering with community organizations such as YMCAs and recreation centers to provide exercise facilities and classes.

One example of a local collaborative effort to extend health promotion to small businesses is the Harlem Business Wellness Initiative (HBWI), which involves the Mailman School of Public Health at Columbia University, Harlem Hospital Center, and the Harlem (New York City) business community. The goal of the project is to translate principles from workplace health promotion programs that are successful in large business to the small business environment found in inner-city settings. Through the HBWI, the services of a team of health educators are offered free of charge to small businesses. Services include conducting computerized health appraisals, creating personalized counseling sessions, and collaboratively developing health action plans that may include lifestyle changes and/or referrals to preventive services (Conova, 2007).

Impact of the Patient Protection and Affordable Care Act on Workplace Health Promotion

The Patient Protection and Affordable Care Act, commonly known as the Affordable Care Act (ACA) and passed in 2010, is aimed primarily at decreasing the number of uninsured Americans and reducing the overall costs of health care. It provides a number of mechanisms—including mandates, subsidies, and tax credits—to employers and individuals (employees) in order to increase the coverage rate. Additional reforms are aimed at improving health care outcomes, reducing hospital readmissions, and coordinating the delivery of health care, leading to reductions in the overall cost of health care in the United States. The ACA requires insurance companies to cover all applicants and to offer the same rates regardless of preexisting conditions or gender.

Medicaid expansion under the ACA helps low-wage workers employed in jobs we rely on every day—from child care aide to bus driver to waitress—who lack access to affordable health insurance and health promotion programs. These low-wage uninsured workers can gain health coverage if their states accepted federal dollars to expand Medicaid under the ACA. As of 2015, 27 states (and the District of Columbia) have chosen this option and expanded health coverage to adults with incomes up to 138% of poverty (in 2015, that amounts to an annual income of $27,310 for a family of three). More than half of residents in these states who benefit from Medicaid expansion are working adults (Mahan, 2015).

A significant element of the ACA is the creation and participation of accountable care organizations (ACOs), which relates to how we will pay for health care in the future. An ACO is a health care organization characterized by a payment and coordinated care delivery model that seeks to tie provider reimbursements to quality metrics and reductions in the total cost of care for an assigned population of individuals. A group of coordinated health care providers forms an ACO, which then provides care to a group of individuals (i.e., employees). The ACO is accountable to the individuals and the third-party payer for the quality, appropriateness, and efficiency of the health care provided (McClellan, McKethan, Lewis, Roski, & Fisher, 2010).

Historically, health care was paid for on a fee-for-service basis. This means that individual doctors, hospitals, and other providers are paid for each service they furnish to an individual. Critics of this system have long contended that it creates incentives for providers to furnish or order more services. And different providers who see the same individual (employee) often fail to coordinate their activities, leading to duplicative or conflicting treatments.

The significance of ACOs for workplace health promotion programs is a higher degree of accountability for program quality, appropriateness, and efficiency, as well a focus on improved program outcomes. The expectations are now for workplace health promotion programs (as well as all health care providers and services) to: use evidence-based interventions and practices; reduce variability in strategies, methods, and resource use that cannot be clinically justified; increase coordination of programs through the use of information technology and team-based initiatives, while emphasizing prevention and disease management; and give individuals (employees) a stronger voice in their own health and health care and in defining what matters (McClellan et al., 2014). The ACO's utilization of case management and care stratification lend further support to fitting and tailoring workplace programs to different populations of employees at a workplace (Peels et al., 2014).

The ACOs, with their raised expectations for workplace health promotion programs, are not the only significant element of the ACA for employee health promotion. For example there are provisions intended to expand health promotion and prevention activities and programs such as workplace health promotion programs. A total of $200 million has been dedicated to wellness program start-up grants for businesses with fewer than 100 employees (Section 10408). Another provision established a technical assistance role for the CDC to provide resources for evaluating employer wellness programs (Section 4303). In addition, the Department of Health and Human Services was awarded $10 million from the ACA Prevention and Public Health Fund to distribute to organizations with expertise in working with employers to develop and expand workplace wellness activities, such as tobacco-free policies, flextime for physical activity, and healthier food choices in the workplace.

Section 1302 of the ACA provides for the establishment of an essential health benefit (EHB) package. The law directs that EHB be equal in scope to the benefits covered by a typical employer plan and cover at least the following 10 general categories: ambulatory patient services; emergency services; hospitalization; maternity and newborn care; mental health and substance use disorder services, including behavioral health treatment; prescription drugs; rehabilitative and habilitative services and devices; laboratory services; preventive and wellness services and chronic disease management; and pediatric services, including oral and vision care.

Finally, the ACA raises the limit on incentives that employers are allowed to offer through a group health plan for participating in a wellness program (health promotion program) that requires meeting health-related standards. This provision gives employers greater latitude in rewarding group health plan participants and beneficiaries for healthy lifestyles. The ACA outlaws health status underwriting in group health benefit programs and allows group health plans to offer incentives to employees for participation, or penalties for nonparticipation, in health promotion programs that meet certain requirements.

The ACA recognizes three different types of health promotion programs. Participatory programs either do not offer a reward or do not make a reward contingent on an individual satisfying a condition related to a health status factor. A participatory program might simply pay for a gym membership or a smoking cessation program or reward an employee who completes a health risk assessment. Participatory programs must be offered to all similarly situated employees on a nondiscriminatory basis.

Activity-only programs require an employee to perform or complete an activity related to a health factor to obtain an award. Outcome-based programs further require a participant to achieve a certain health-based outcome, such as cessation of smoking or achieving a certain biometric measure, to obtain a reward.

Activity-only or outcome-based programs must meet five requirements under the ACA rules. First, all eligible individuals must be given the opportunity to qualify for the reward at least once per year. Second, the total reward offered under the programs cannot exceed 30% of the total cost of employee-only coverage under the plan (50% for tobacco prevention and reduction programs), including both employer and employee contributions.

Third, programs must be reasonably designed to promote health or prevent disease. Fourth, the full reward must be available to all similarly situated individuals. Activity-only programs must thus allow a reasonable alternative standard or waiver of an otherwise applicable standard for individuals for whom it is unreasonably difficult or medically inadvisable to achieve a program standard. An outcome-based program must allow a reasonable alternative standard (or waiver of the otherwise applicable standard) for obtaining the reward to any individual who does not meet the initial standard based on a measurement, test, or screening.

Fifth, plans and issuers must disclose the availability of reasonable alternatives for meeting standards in any plan materials and at the time that individuals are notified that they did not achieve program standards (Jost, 2015).

Workplace Health Promotion Controversies and Pitfalls

Workplace health promotion programs are controversial. Employers believe that they improve employee health, reduce absenteeism, and cut the cost of employee health benefit programs. They are encouraged in this belief by health promotion program vendors, who aggressively tout the benefits of their programs. Disability advocates, on the other hand, are concerned that workplace health promotion programs are perpetuating discrimination against the disabled and health status underwriting. Privacy advocates worry about who has access to the sensitive medical information that programs demand of participants. Others worry about the control that employers assert over their employees' lives through health promotion programs, as employees spend hours of off-the-clock time every week meeting the demands of programs while wearable devices track their footsteps.

Going forward, the controversies about workplace health promotion programs can be expected to impact programs operating across workplaces (small, midsized, and large) in all sectors of the economy (public, private, government, and nonprofit). And while programs hold great promise for better health for all, four pitfalls exist to challenge them: socioeconomic factors, structure and cost, access, and adherence to best practices for health outcomes. The four pitfalls exist in concert with the ongoing program controversies and are part of the larger context within which programs exist and operate.

Socioeconomic factors require organizations to carefully and continuously monitor economic, social, and labor market trends and—noting changes in governmental policies, legislation, and public policy statements—to identify environmental threats and opportunities that in turn help formulate new action guidelines. Some of the strongest environmental forces facing organizations today are listed in Figure 1.3. These forces are economic (e.g., recession), technological (e.g., automation), political (e.g., new government policies), social (e.g., concern for our environment), demographic (e.g., changing composition of our workforce), legal (e.g., changes in minimum wage laws), and cultural (e.g., ethnic diversity).

Today's health care system is dominated by large commercial interests driven by investors' demand for profit, by nonprofits almost equally focused on revenues, and by government policy decisions that are sometimes shaped

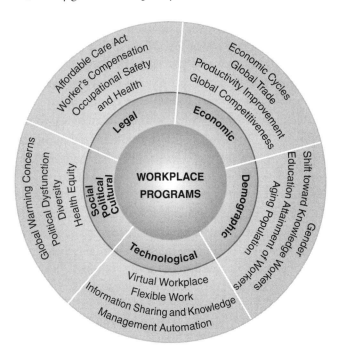

Figure 1.3   Socioeconomic Factors and Challenges
Source: Schwind et al., 2013.

by larger ideological, political, and budgetary concerns. For better or worse, health care has become big money and big politics. As a result for the foreseeable future, the structure and cost of health care in the United States will continue to be a problem. The health care system is overwhelming for even the most sophisticated consumer. For example, Figure 1.4 shows the market a consumer in Pittsburgh, Pennsylvania, faces when selecting health care. It is typical of the market anyone would face making health care decisions. In the illustration, two large hospital systems dominate the hospitals and medical facilities, while two large competing medical insurance companies associated with the systems fund the services. A number of large national insurance companies have recently entered the market, further complicating service and access to care. Health care in the United States is the most expensive in the world, with only moderate outcomes when compared with other countries. Over the last few decades health care spending has risen at rapid rates for both the government and the private sector. In 1970, it accounted for 7.2% of the nation's gross domestic product; by 2010, that had increased to 17.9% (Centers for Medicare & Medicaid Services, 2013). Fueling the boom are expensive new drugs and technologies, plus an increase in chronic conditions such as diabetes, asthma, and heart disease, which are costly to treat. Experts also cite unnecessary spending, with some estimating that 20% or more of total spending is tied to forms of waste, including overtreatment, failure to coordinate a patient's care among providers, and fraud. The consequences are higher costs and lower quality (Berwick & Hackbarth, 2012).

Unfortunately, not all health promotion programs are created equal. Some program designs can be harmful to consumers. Particularly for people with health problems or those with lower incomes, certain kinds of programs can actually make health coverage unaffordable and can result in compromised access to health care. Going forward, some health promotion programs can pose problems for consumers' access to care if the programs use certain kinds of rewards or penalties. The role of workplace health promotion programs in the health care system could change in the coming years, as could the potential effects these changes have on achieving the goal of the ACA, which is to bring quality, affordable health coverage to all. We want to ensure, in the designing of workplace health promotion programs, that they do not harm consumers' (employees') ability to obtain coverage and care (Families USA, 2012).

Finally, for all of the discussion of the value and potential for workplace health promotion, according to a 2004 survey fielded by the Office of Disease Prevention and Health Promotion, only 7% of U.S. employers

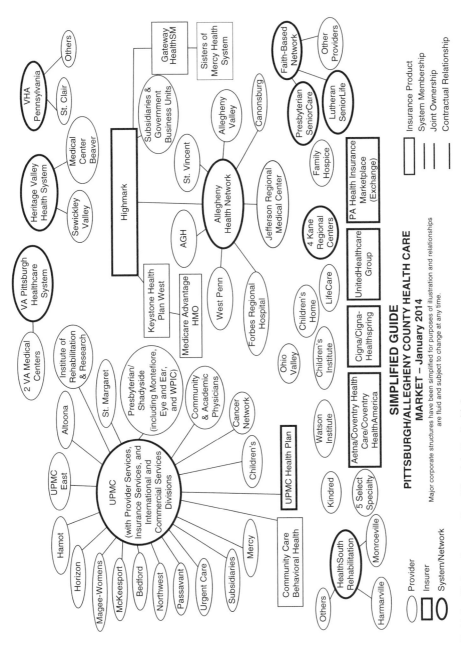

Figure 1.4 Health Care Market a Consumer Faces When Selecting Health Care

Source: B. Longest, personal note.

The following text appears within the figure:

SIMPLIFIED GUIDE
PITTSBURGH/ALLEGHENY COUNTY HEALTH CARE
MARKET – January 2014

Major corporate structures have been simplified for purposes of illustration and relationships are fluid and subject to change at any time.

Legend:
- Provider
- Insurer
- System/Network
- Insurance Product
- System Membership
- Joint Ownership
- Contractual Relationship

UPMC (with Provider Services, Insurance Services, and International and Commercial Services Divisions):
Hamot, Horizon, Magee-Womens, McKeesport, Bedford, Northwest, Passavant, Urgent Care, Subsidiaries, Mercy, Children's, Cancer Network, Community & Academic Physicians, Presbyterian/Shadyside (including Montefiore, Eye and Ear, and WPIC), St. Margaret, Altoona, UPMC East, Institute of Rehabilitation & Research

UPMC Health Plan

Community Care Behavioral Health

VA Pittsburgh Healthcare System: 2 VA Medical Centers

VHA Pennsylvania: St. Clair, Others

Heritage Valley Health System: Sewickley Valley, Medical Center Beaver

Highmark: Keystone Health Plan West, Medicare Advantage HMO, West Penn, Forbes Regional Hospital, AGH, Subsidiaries & Government Business Units, St. Vincent, Gateway HealthSM, Sisters of Mercy Health System

Allegheny Health Network: Allegheny Valley, Canonsburg, Jefferson Regional Medical Center, 4 Kane Regional Centers, LifeCare, Children's Home, Children's Institute, Ohio Valley

Faith-Based Network: Presbyterian SeniorCare, Lutheran SeniorLife, Family Hospice, Other Providers

HealthSouth Rehabilitation: Harmarville, Monroeville, Others

Kindred, Watson Institute, 5 Select Specialty

Aetna/Coventry Health Care/Coventry HealthAmerica

Cigna/Cigna-Healthspring

UnitedHealthcare Group

PA Health Insurance Marketplace (Exchange)

19

offered a comprehensive program containing five best-practice elements for achieving meaningful and sustainable outcomes: health education; links to related employee services; supportive physical and social environments for health improvement; integration of health promotion into the organization's culture; and employee screenings with adequate treatment and follow-up (Linnan et al., 2008). Significant differences in the number of comprehensive programs, as well as the number of activities offered within such programs, exist across companies of different sizes—small employers lag significantly behind larger employers. Increasing the number, quality, and types of workplace health promotion programs represents an important goal for the workplace setting in order to address health care–cost trends and remains an important public health goal.

Summary

Workplace health promotion programs are a powerful tool for improving the health and well-being of individuals and communities. The most promising programs feature a strong employer commitment and are responsive to employees' needs. The workplace is viewed as a health-promoting environment that connects employee health and the health of the organization, community, and society. Current workplace health promotion programs reflect three evolutionary phases in the quest to promote healthy individuals and healthy communities: occupational safety and health; healthy lifestyle to encourage healthier individuals' behaviors, through the provision of support and information and the development of skills; and workplace determinants of health amid the corporate and community structures that support the health of employees and their families.

The 2010 Patient Protection and Affordable Care Act for workplace health promotion programs raised a higher degree of accountability for program quality, appropriateness, and efficiency, and it identified as well the need to improve program outcomes. The expectations for accountability now hold for workplace health promotion programs, as well as all health care providers and services: to use evidence-based interventions and practices; to reduce variability in strategies, methods, and resource use that cannot be clinically justified; to increase coordination of programs through the use of information technology and team-based initiatives, all the while emphasizing prevention and disease management; and to give individuals (employees) a stronger voice in their own health and health care, and in defining what matters. Although there is great promise for workplace health promotion, controversies and pitfalls exist. Health care cost and health care systems will continue to be challenged by the need to improve health care quality, outcomes, and access to care. Much work is needed if we are to achieve the Healthy People 2020 objective, by which at least 75% of employers offer a comprehensive workplace health promotion program.

For Practice and Discussion

1. Explore the workplace health program at your school and/or place of employment. Does your organization have a coordinated and comprehensive set of health promotion and protection strategies? These should include programs, policies, benefits, environmental supports, and links to the surrounding community designed to encourage the health and safety of all employees and their families. What are examples of the organization's workplace health promotion policies, benefits, environmental supports, and links to the surrounding community?

2. Nationally, 4,609 people died from workplace injuries in 2011, which was a slight decline from 4,690 in 2010. Search the Bureau of Labor Statistics (http://www.bls.gov/home.htm) workplace injuries subject area. For your region, investigate the most dangerous occupation (workplace injuries, illnesses, and fatalities) in the past 2 years (numbers and percentages). Compare and contrast the 2 years. In each year, which occupations were the most dangerous? What is being done to protect workers in these occupations? How do these statistics compare with the national statistics? Using Figure 1.5 as a model, present your findings in a chart http://www.bls.gov/ro3/cfoipitt.htm

3. Using the Internet, search the employee benefit package offerings of the large organizations in your community (universities, school

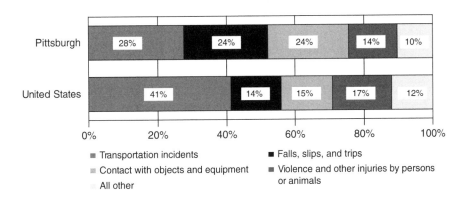

Figure 1.5   Dangerous Occupations Based on National Statistics

districts, businesses, community organizations, government). Compare and contrast their employee health benefits, including the health promotion and wellness offerings.

4.   Search and find recent articles on the implications and impact of the ACA on workplace health promotion programs at two websites: (1) Trust for America's Health (http://healthyamericans.org/), a nonprofit, nonpartisan organization dedicated to saving lives by protecting the health of every community and working to make disease prevention a national priority, and (2) the *Wall Street Journal* (http://online.wsj.com/home-page), a leading U.S. daily business newspaper. Compare and contrast the articles' topics and issues covered.

5.   Rank-order the four workplace health promotion pitfalls listed earlier, in terms of which you consider the most challenging and most urgent to address. Discuss your ranking with your classmates. What can be done to address the pitfalls?

Case Study: What Is a Workplace Health Promotion Program?—What Would You Do?

Brady Nowak, a chief people officer of a mining company, is frequently asked to explain what an employee health promotion program is in the mining industry. As she explains, "In the early years, doctors and nurses were at mines to deal with the injuries and accident victims. The work was dangerous. Conditions were unsafe. Workers died. People got hurt. I hope we are far from those times now. Today we focus on information and getting people active in their own health—fitness, nutrition, smoking cessation, and stress management are big. We are concerned with raising health costs. Keeping our workers healthy and working isn't easy. Workers' compensation, health and safety at the work sites, and workers' benefits are always part of the discussion when we talk about how to keep our workers healthy. We are constantly thinking about the work, jobs, and factories. We are looking at a corporate structure and strategic human resources that support the health of employees and their families. We talk with other business people, groups in the communities where our mines operate, insurance providers, health care organization executives, doctors, nurses, physical therapists, counselors, health educators, and government officials about health care."

The mining company president asked Ms. Nowak to create a graphic (i.e., a visual representation) to explain what an employee health promotion program is in the mining industry. The request was to make it concise, succinct, informative, and engaging, so it could be used as a poster, webpage posting, or PowerPoint slide. If you were Brady Nowak, what would you do? Create the graphic.

KEY TERMS

Workplace health promotion program

Strategic human resource management

Occupational safety and health

Healthy lifestyle

Return on investment (ROI)

Determinants of health

Patient Protection and Affordable Care Act/Affordable Care Act (ACA)

Controversies and Pitfalls

References

ADP. (2008). *After the transformation: Achieving strategic HR*. Retrieved from http://www.adp.com/tools-and-resources/case-studies-white-papers/~/media/MASWhitePapers/MASWhitePapersProtected/AchievingHR_final.ashx

Ahsmann, L. (1994). *Superior coffee and foods*. Retrieved from http://mydlc.com/illinoisshrm_wellness_site/tools/index.html

Aldrich, M. (1997). *Tenth Census of the United States. Safety first: Technology, labor, and business in the building of American work safety, 1870–1939*. Baltimore, MD: Johns Hopkins University Press.

Anthem Health Systems. (1993). *Staying alive & well at Reynolds Electrical & Engineering Company, Inc.* Indianapolis, IN: Anthem Health Systems.

Bertera, R. L. (1990). The effects of workplace health promotion on absenteeism and employment costs in a large industrial population. *American Journal of Public Health, 80*(9), 1101–1105.

Berwick, D. M., & Hackbarth, A. D. (2012). Eliminating waste in US health care. *Journal of the American Medical Association, 307*(14), 1513–1516. doi:10.1001/jama.2012.362

Carroll, A. B., Lipartito, K., Post, J., & Werhane, P. (2012). *Corporate responsibility: The American experience*. Cambridge, England: Cambridge University Press.

Centers for Disease Control and Prevention. (2013a). *Stopping the spread of germs at home, work & school*. Retrieved from http://www.cdc.gov/flu/protect/stopgerms.htm

Centers for Disease Control and Prevention. (2013b). *Workplace health promotion*. Retrieved from http://www.cdc.gov/workplacehealthpromotion/model/index.html

Centers for Disease Control and Prevention. (2015). National Institution for Occupational Safety and Health: *A–Z Index for NIOSH topics*. Retrieved from http://www.cdc.gov/niosh

Centers for Medicare & Medicaid Services. (2013). *Historical national health expenditure data.* Retrieved from http://www.cms.gov/Research-Statistics-Data-and-Systems/Statistics-Trends-and-Reports/NationalHealthExpendData/NationalHealthAccountsHistorical.html

Conova, S. (2007). Caring for Harlem's underserved workers. *In Vivo, 5*(6). http://www.cumc.columbia.edu/publications/in-vivo/january_february_2007/improving_health.html

Draper, E. (2005). *The company doctor: Risk, responsibility, and corporate professionalism.* New York, NY: Russell Sage Foundation.

Drudi, D. (2007). Railroad-related work injury fatalities. *Monthly Labor Review,* July/August.

Fabius, R., & Frazee, S. (2009). *Workplace-based health and wellness services.* Champaign, IL: ACSM.

Families USA. (2012). *Wellness programs: Evaluating the promise and pitfalls.* Retrieved from http://familiesusa.org/sites/default/files/product_documents/Wellness-Programs.pdf

Fertman, C., Allensworth, D., & Auld, E. (2010). What are health promotion programs? In C. Fertman & D. Allensworth (Eds.), Health promotion programs: From theory to practice. (pp. 3–28). San Francisco, CA: Jossey-Bass/Wiley.

Fries, J. F., Harrington, H., Edwards, R., Kent, L. A., & Richardson, N. (1994). Randomized controlled trial of cost reductions from a health education program: The California Public Employees' Retirement System (PERS) study. *American Journal of Health Promotion, 8*(3), 216–223.

Golaszewski, T., Snow, D., Lynch, W., Yen, L., & Solomita, D. (1992). A benefit-to-cost analysis of a work-site health promotion program. *Journal of Occupational Medicine, 34*(12), 1164–1172.

Jost, T. (2015, April 17). Workplace wellness programs: Federal agencies weigh in. *Health Affairs* [Blog]. Retrieved from http://healthaffairs.org/blog/2015/04/17/workplace-wellness-programs-federal-agencies-weigh-in/

Kickbusch, I., & Payne, L. (2003). Twenty-first century health promotion: the public health revolution meets the wellness revolution. *Health Promotion International, 18*(4), 275–278.

Lalonde, M. (1974). *A new perspective on the health of Canadians.* Ottawa, Ontario: Health and Welfare Canada.

Linnan, L., Bowling, M., Childress, J., Lindsay, G., Blakey, C., Pronk, S., . . . Royall, P. (2008). Results of the 2004 National Worksite Health Promotion Survey. *American Journal of Public Health, 98*(8), 1503–1509. doi:10.2105/AJPH.2006.100313

Mahan, D. (2015, February). *Medicaid expansion helps low-wage workers.* [Families USA Issue Brief]. Retrieved from http://familiesusa.org/product/medicaid-expansion-helps-low-wage-workers

McClellan, M., Kent, J., Beales, S. J., Cohen, S. I., Macdonnell, M., Thoumi, A., . . . Darzi, A. (2014). Accountable care around the world: A framework to guide reform strategies. *Health Affairs, 33*(9), 1507–1515.

McClellan, M., McKethan, A. N., Lewis, J. L., Roski, J., & Fisher, E. S. (2010). A national strategy to put accountable care into practice. *Health Affairs, 29*(5), 982–990.

Peels, D., van Stralen, M., Bolman, C., Golsteijn, R., de Vries, H., Mudde, A., & Lechner, L. (2014). The differentiated effectiveness of a printed versus a Web-based tailored physical activity intervention among adults aged over 50. *Health Education Research, 29*(5), 870–882.

Polanyi, M., Frank, J., Shannon, H., Sullivan, T., & Lavis, J. (2000). The workplace as a setting for health promotion. In B. Poland, L. W. Green & I. Rootman (Eds.), *Settings for health promotion: Linking theory and practice*. Thousand Oaks, CA: Sage.

Schoenleber, A. W. (1933). Industrial health programs: Trends which indicate that industry is beginning to acknowledge its responsibility for the medical care of employees. *Industrial Medicine, 2*, 242–249.

Schwind, H., Das, H., Wagar, T., Fassina, N., & Bulmash, J. (2013). *Canadian human resource management: A strategic approach* (10th ed.). Toronto, Ontario: McGraw-Hill Ryerson.

Soto Mas, F., Allensworth, D., & Carnara, P. J. (2010). Health promotion programs designed to eliminate health disparities. In C. I. Fertman & D. Allensworth (Eds.), *Health promotion programs: From theory to practice* (pp. 29–55). San Francisco, CA: Society for Public Health Education (SOPHE)/Jossey-Bass/Wiley.

Starr, P. (1982). *The social transformation of American medicine*. New York, NY: Basic Books.

Tze-ching Yen, L., Edington, D., & Witting, P. (1994). Steelcase: Corporate medical claim cost distributions and factors associated with high-cost status. *Journal of Occupational Medicine, 36*(5), 505–515.

U.S. Bureau of Labor Statistics. (2013, March). *Leave benefits*. Retrieved from http://www.bls.gov/opub/ted/2013/mobile/ted_20131107.htm

U.S. Department of Health and Human Services. (2000). *Healthy People 2010*. Retrieved from http://www.healthypeople.gov/2010/

U.S. Department of Health and Human Services, Office of Disease Prevention and Health Promotion. (2015a). *Education and community-based programs: Healthy People 2020*. Retrieved from https://www.healthypeople.gov/2020/topics-objectives/topic/educational-and-community-based-programs/objectives

U.S. Department of Health and Human Services, Office of Disease Prevention and Health Promotion. (2015b). *Healthy People 2020*. Retrieved from http://www.healthypeople.gov/2020/default.aspx

U. S. Department of Labor. (n.d.). *Voluntary protection programs*. Retrieved May 7, 2015, from https://www.osha.gov/dcsp/vpp/index.html

HEALTH PROMOTION APPROACHES, THEORIES, AND MODELS APPLIED TO WORKPLACE HEALTH PROMOTION

Workplace Health Promotion Approaches

When talking with employers about workplace health promotion programs, it becomes clear that organizations take different approaches to addressing the health concerns of their employees. The approaches to workplace health promotion are dynamic—ever changing to reflect individuals' and organizations' (workplaces) experiences, expectations, and dissatisfactions. As dynamic as such experiences are, individuals and organizations will nevertheless have expectations about what should happen. You will be asked and need to be able to state your approach to workplace health promotion.

Approaches to workplace health promotion help us know what might be available within any particular workplace and community. Given the changing nature of workers' health concerns and problems, all of the approaches are dynamic, fueling how we identify new and recurring needs, and creating, implementing, and evaluating new programs and services. Together the approaches form a socioecological model that spans individuals, families, workplaces, communities, health systems, and the larger environment including local, state, and federal government programs, services, and public policy.

LEARNING OBJECTIVES

- Describe approaches to workplace health promotion
- Discuss the role of health theories in workplace health promotion programs
- Identify planning models for workplace health promotion programs
- Use a set of guidelines for choosing approaches, theories, and models

Centers for Disease Control and Prevention Comprehensive Workplace Health

The Centers for Disease Control and Prevention (CDC) Comprehensive Workplace Health approach puts policies and interventions in place that address multiple risk factors and health conditions concurrently; it recognizes that the interventions and strategies chosen may influence multiple levels of the organization including individual employee behavior change, organizational culture, and the work environment. The approach champions a combination of individual- and organizational-level strategies and interventions to influence health. The strategies and interventions are grouped into four major categories (CDC, 2013).

- Health-related programs—opportunities available to employees at the workplace or through outside organizations to begin, change, or maintain health behaviors.

- Health-related policies—formal or informal written statements designed to protect or promote employee health. They affect large groups of employees simultaneously.

- Health benefits—part of an overall compensation package including health insurance coverage and other services or discounts regarding health.

- Environmental supports—the physical factors at and nearby the workplace that help protect and enhance employee health.

Recommended as part of the approach are partnerships with surrounding community organizations to offer health-related programs and services to employees when the employer does not have the capacity or expertise to do so, or to provide support for healthy lifestyles to employees when not at the workplace.

Within this approach any number of specific health risks (e.g., physical inactivity, poor nutrition, tobacco use, stress), conditions (e.g., obesity, musculoskeletal disorders, mental health), and diseases (e.g., heart disease and stroke, diabetes, cancer, arthritis) can be addressed.

NASA Integrated Employee Health Management

An integrated approach to improving the health of employees involves going beyond traditional medical or occupational health to include a variety of fitness and wellness programs as integral components to a comprehensive well-being approach. The approach spans multiple levels, adhering to a socioecological approach that provides guidelines for thinking about health decisions as being determined by multiple, including environmental and behavioral, systems.

An illustration of the integrated approach is the National Aeronautics and Space Administration (NASA)—Employee Total Health Management (Figure 2.1). In 2005 NASA found that its aging workforce was at risk for the same chronic diseases facing America's aging population as a whole, including heart disease, hypertension, obesity, diabetes, and cancer, which are frequently associated with negative lifestyle behaviors such as physical inactivity, poor eating habits, and tobacco use. In addition, the NASA work environment is highly variable, and some workers are subjected to unusually hazardous and stressful conditions. NASA was one of the first federal agencies to recognize the importance of occupational health and wellness programs for the well-being of its employees. As part of the approach, a workplace health promotion program team is formed with members from every level of the organization as well as community partner members. Frequently in large organizations a human

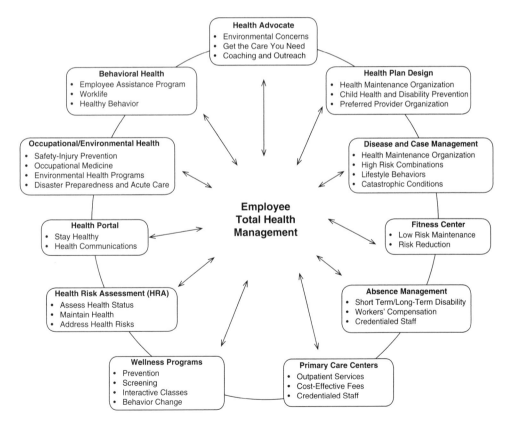

Figure 2.1   Integrated Employee Health Management—NASA Employee Total Health Management

Source: Institute of Medicine, 2005.

resource or medical staff person is assigned the responsibility for the program operation as its director. In midsized and smaller organizations, community partners and insurance providers can also fulfill this role. In the case of NASA's program, 11 program components together take in physical health and health insurance (health plan design, disease and case management, primary care centers), behavioral health, occupational and environmental health, wellness (health portal, health risk assessment, wellness program, fitness center), absence management (e.g., disability and worker's compensation), and health advocacy (e.g., coaching and outreach) (Institute of Medicine, 2005).

The integrated model shares some similarities with the coordinated health programs used in school settings and includes eight components (CDC, 2008), some of which might already exist in the workplace but have not necessarily been organized to work together (components listed below). Typically the approach is used to address specific health concerns within one or more specific components of an integrated approach. Figure 2.2 shows how the eight components might be used to address obesity in the workplace as part of the integrated model.

1. Health education: Information and instruction that addresses the physical, mental, emotional, and social dimensions of health; promotes knowledge, attitudes, and skills; is tailored to each age or developmental level; and is designed to motivate and assist individuals in maintaining and improving their health and to reduce their risk behaviors.

2. Physical education and activity: Planned, sequential instruction that promotes lifelong physical activity. Designed to develop basic move-ment skills, sports skills, and physical fitness as well as to enhance mental, social, and emotional abilities.

3. Physical health services: Designed to promote the health of individ-uals, identify and prevent physical health problems and injuries, and ensure appropriate preventive services, emergency care, referral, or management of acute or chronic health conditions.

4. Nutrition services: Integration of nutritious, affordable, ethnically and culturally diverse and appealing meals, and nutrition education in an environment that promotes healthy eating habits for all staff and employees. Diet review and counseling for disordered eating and diet-related concerns.

5. Counseling, psychological, and social services: Designed to prevent and address problems, facilitate positive work performance and healthy behavior, and enhance healthy development by providing services that focus on cognitive, emotional, behavioral, and social needs of workers (and family members).

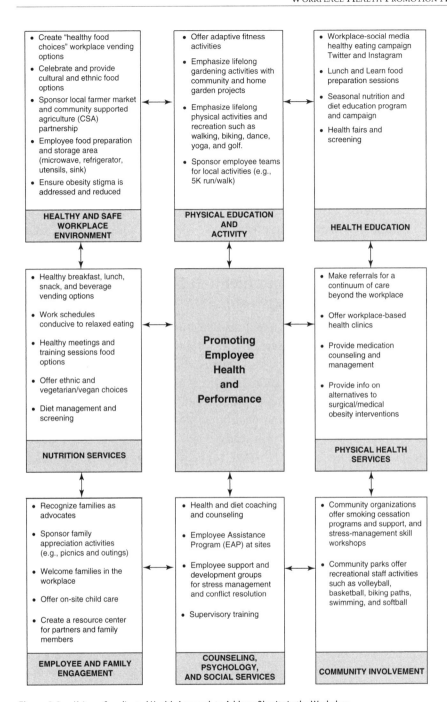

Figure 2.2 Using a Coordinated Health Approach to Address Obesity in the Workplace

6. Healthy and safe workplace environment: Designed to provide both a safe physical plant and a healthy and supportive environment that fosters high quality work performance and achievement (e.g., profits), including the physical, emotional, and social climate of the workplace.

7. Employee and family engagement: Employee health is a shared responsibility among employees, families, the workplace, and communities. Designed to actively engage employees and their families for health in meaningful and culturally respectful, culturally competent, and culturally proficient ways.

8. Community involvement: Partnerships and collaborations created and designed to maximize resources and expertise in addressing the health of employees, families, and communities.

Institute of Medicine Intervention Classifications Focused on Preventing Problems

The Institute of Medicine (IOM) classifications help us think about who at the workplace is being served and with what intervention (programs and services). According to the classifications, universal interventions are for the general population groups, without reference to those at particular risk. Selective interventions are for individuals who are at greater-than-average risk for health problems. Indicated interventions are for individuals who may already display signs of health problems. The classifications often are used to help employers make decisions about employer-offered programs and services that might be available at a workplace. Furthermore the classifications can be used to guide discussions about the shared responsibility for health among the individual (employee), family, employer, and community (including health care systems).

IOM Health Promotion and Prevention Interventions Classifications

- **Universal preventive interventions:** Focus on the whole population (all of the employees) at a workplace that have not been identified on the basis of individual risk. The intervention is desirable for everyone at work. Universal interventions have advantages when their costs per individual are low, the intervention is effective and acceptable to the population, and there is a low risk from the intervention. This is sometimes referred to as primary prevention.

     Example: Workplace programs offered to all employees, such as a walking program, health fair, and worker safety training.

- **Selective prevention interventions:** Focus on individuals or a population subgroup whose risk of developing disorders is significantly higher than average. The risk may be imminent or it may be a lifetime risk. Risk groups may be identified on the basis of biological, psychological, or social risk factors that are known to be associated with the onset of a physical or mental health disorder. Selective interventions are most appropriate if their cost is moderate and if the risk of negative effects is minimal or nonexistent. This is also referred to as secondary prevention.

  Example: Programs offered to employees with identified risk or exposure to risk factors. Nutrition programs and services for individuals with elevated blood cholesterol level and BMI, and a person impacted by the death of a close relative.

- **Indicated preventive interventions:** Focus on high-risk individuals who are identified as having minimal but detectable signs of symptoms foreshadowing a physical or mental health disorder, or biological markers indicating predisposition for such a disorder, but who do not meet diagnostic levels at the current time. Indicated interventions might be reasonable even if intervention costs are high and even if the intervention entails some risk. This is also known as tertiary prevention.

  Example: Interventions for adults with problems of aggression or elevated symptoms of depression, anxiety, and substance abuse. Employee Assistance Programs that identify, refer, and link individual to mental health treatment.

Individual Health Concerns and Problems Intervention Process Approach

The individual health concerns and problems intervention process approach is concerned with addressing the health and problems of an individual, one at a time, within the larger population (Fertman, Delgado, & Tarasevich, 2014). By definition, it is intense and time consuming to focus on attending to a person (and potentially his or her family). It is a four-step process with standard operating procedures, forms, and assigned staff members who are responsible to work with employees and families to identify and connect to health programs and services. Health coaching, crisis management, and employee assistance programs are examples of the approach. The steps may overlap, build on each other, and at times require stepping back to a previous action to gather additional information, ask a question, or address a new concern or problem. The four steps are:

1. *Initial health system connection.* Anyone (e.g., employee, supervisor, colleague, health provider) identifies that an employee may be suffering with a health concern and problem. The mechanism for the connection will vary by organization. Often it is through the health care provider or supervisor. An active health crisis (e.g., suicidal tendency, injury, violence, accident, substance use, intoxication) will also trigger the process. Organizations as part of their human resource procedures detail expected actions and documentation for such situations.

2. *Planning and recommendations.* The process includes additional information collection, clarification of needs, a consultation with the individual (and possibly with the family), goal setting, and the development of a treatment plan including recommendations.

3. *Plan implementation and interventions.* Implementation of the plan and interventions is difficult and not without challenges and struggles. It may not be a linear process but rather nonlinear, with twists and turns and at times unclear and unpredictable outcomes.

4. *Follow-up and support.* Systematic procedures are put in place for continual feedback and monitoring of participation in planned activities and progress toward stated goals. Case management is often employed to attend to the employee and his or her families. Likewise resource management, identifying the gaps and places where the process breaks down, and fixing it, is part of follow-up and support.

The individual health concerns and problems intervention process approach reflects the reality that the health concerns and problems facing many workers and their families are too numerous and too large for them to successfully confront and ameliorate without support. In addition, navigating the health care system, with its fragmentation, diverse funding streams, and eligibility requirements, adds layers of complexity that is often a barrier in itself. McKay et al. (2004) describe the approach as a 180-degree turn from clinic- and office-based practices toward high quality, consumer-driven, empirically based services in the practical setting (i.e., workplace) in which the service is ultimately to be delivered.

Total Worker Health Approach

The National Institute for Occupational Health and Safety (NIOSH) in 2004 initiated the WorkLife Initiative to improve overall worker health through better work-based programs, policies, practices, and benefits. The WorkLife Initiative supports addressing worker health and well-being by taking into account the physical and organizational work environment while at the same time addressing the personal health-related decisions and behaviors of individuals. The workplace is viewed as a site to implement programs and policies to prevent both work-related risks and chronic illnesses and injuries that are linked to employee choices. As part of the initiative, Centers of Excellence to Promote a Healthier Workforce were established to create new research in this area, effectively demonstrating the impact of improved and integrated approaches to health protection and health promotion on the improvement of worker health and safety, and defining critical elements of health-supportive workplaces.

NIOSH Centers of Excellence to Promote a Healthier Workforce

* Iowa Healthier Workforce Center for Excellence (http://www.public-health.uiowa.edu/hwce/)

* Center for Promotion of Health in the New England Workplace (University of Massachusetts, Lowell, and the University of Connecticut) (http://www.uml.edu/centers/cph-new/)

* The Harvard School of Public Health Center for Work, Health, and Well-Being (http://centerforworkhealth.sph.harvard.edu/)

* Oregon Healthy Workforce Center (http://www.ohsu.edu/xd/research /centers-institutes/croet/oregon-healthy-workforce-center/)

The NIOSH integrated approach (Table 2.1) is more expansive in its workforce coverage and health concerns. As an integrated model it focuses on occupational safety and health protection with health promotion to prevent worker injury and illness and to advance health and well-being (CDC, 2015). Furthermore it recognizes that a multitude of work- and nonwork-related factors influence employees' safety, health, ability to work, and well-being in every aspect of their lives. Employer concern about the effects of diminished employee health on productivity, absenteeism, and rising health care costs is growing. Therefore, employers are increasingly receptive to a growing body of evidence that provides the rationale for addressing health promotion in conjunction with organizational efforts to protect workers and create safe and healthful workplaces. Table 2.2 provides examples of the types of intervention proposed as part of Total Worker Health.

Table 2.1   Total Worker Health Approach http://www.cdc.gov/niosh/TWH/default.html (Total Worker Health)

Workplace	Employment	Workers
Protecting Worker Safety & Health	**Preserving Human Resources**	**Promoting Worker Health & Well-Being**
Control of Hazards & Exposures:	New Employment Patterns:	Optimal Well-Being:
• Chemicals	• Precarious Employment	• Employee Engagement
• Physical Agents	• Part-Time Employment	• Health & Well-Being Assessments
• Biological Agents	• Dual Employers	• Healthier Behaviors
• Psychosocial Factors	• Changing Demographics	• Nutrition
• Organization of Work	• Increasing Diversity	• Tobacco Use Cessation
Prevention of Injuries, Illnesses, & Fatalities	• Aging Workforce	• Physical Activity
Promoting Safe & Healthy Work:	• Multigenerational Workforce	• Work/Life Balance
• Management Commitment	• Global Workforce	• Aging Productively
• Safety Culture/Climate	Health & Productivity:	• Preparing for Healthier Retirement
• Culture of Health	• Leadership Commitment to Health-Supportive Culture	• Policy & Built Environment Supports
• Hazard Recognition Training	• Fitness-for-Duty	Workers with Higher Health Risks:
• Worker Empowerment	• Reducing Presenteeism	• Young Workers
Risk Assessment & Control:	• Reducing Absenteeism	• Low-Income Workers
• Making the Safety & Health Case	• Workplace Wellness Programs	• Migrant Workers
• Assessing All Risks	Health care & Benefits:	• Workers New to a Hazardous Job
• Controlling All Risks	• Increasing Costs	• Differently-Abled Workers
• Root Cause Analysis	• Cost Shifting to Workers	• Veterans
• Leading/Lagging Indicators	• Paid Sick Leave	Compensation & Disability:
	• Electronic Health Record	• Disability Evaluation
	• Affordable Care Act	• Reasonable Accommodations
	• HIPAA Health Information Privacy	• Return-to-Work
		• Social Security Disability Insurance

Health Theory's Role in Workplace Health Promotion Programs

A theory is a set of concepts, definitions, and propositions that presents a systematic way of understanding events or situations; it explains or predicts these events or situations by illustrating the relationships between variables. Theories must be applicable to a broad variety of situations. They are, by nature, abstract, and don't have a specified content or topic area.

The role of health theory in workplace health promotion programs is to provide a guide for studying problems, developing appropriate interventions, and evaluating their successes. Theory informs our thinking during all of these stages, offering insights that translate into stronger

Table 2.2   Interventions Consistent With Total Worker Health http://www.cdc.gov/niosh/programs
/totalworkerhealth/

- Provision of mandated respiratory protection programs that simultaneously and comprehensively address and provide supports for tobacco cessation.

- Integrated ergonomic consultations that also discuss joint health, arthritis prevention, and management strategies.

- Regularly scheduled, joint meetings of safety, occupational health, and health promotion leadership and staff to include combining the functions of safety, health, and/or sustainability committees into one entity, either intermittently or permanently.

- Development of stress management efforts that first seek to diminish workplace stressors, and only then work on building worker resiliency.

- Implementation of training and prevention programs that counter hazards and risks faced by workers both on and off the job. Topics could include falls prevention, motor vehicle safety, first aid, hearing conservation, stretching/flexibility, back safety / lifting safety, eye protection, safer work with chemicals, and weight management.

- Provision of on-site, comprehensive workplace screenings for work- and nonwork-related health risks.

- Full integration of: traditional safety programs, occupational health clinics, behavioral health, health promotion programs, coaching, employee assistance programs (EAPs), nutrition, disability and workers compensation through strategic alignment, joint reporting structures, or common funding streams.

interventions and programs. Theory can also help to explain the dynamics of health behaviors, including processes for changing them, and the influences of the many forces that affect health behaviors, including social and physical environments. We can use theory to help us identify the most suitable audiences, methods for fostering change, and outcomes for evaluation. Theory gives us tools for moving beyond intuition to design and evaluate health behavior and health promotion interventions based on understanding of behavior. Interventions grounded in theory create innovative ways to address specific circumstances. We do not depend on a "paint-by-numbers" approach, rehashing stale ideas, but use a palette of behavior theories, skillfully applying them to develop unique, tailored solutions to problems.

No single theory is dominant in workplace health promotion programs nor should it be; the problems, behaviors, populations, cultures, and contexts of health practice are broad and varied. Generally theories are viewed in one of two categories: explanatory and change. Explanatory theory describes the reasons why a problem exists. It guides the search for factors that contribute to a problem (e.g., a lack of knowledge, self-efficacy, social support, or resources), and can be changed. Change theory guides the development of health interventions. It spells out concepts that can be translated into program messages and strategies, and offers a basis for program evaluation. Change theory helps us to be explicit about our assumptions for why an intervention will work. Finally, some theories focus on individuals as the unit of change. Others examine change within families, institutions, communities, or cultures. Adequately addressing an issue may require more than one theory, and no one theory is suitable for all cases.

Effective Practice to Fit Theories to Programs

One of the greatest challenges for those designing and implementing workplace health promotion programs is learning to analyze how well a theory or model "fits" a particular organization and health issue. A working knowledge of specific theories, and familiarity with how they have been applied in the past, improves skills in this area. Table 2.3 shows the key health theories that are used in workplace health promotion programs. Theories are categorized according to the socioecological model levels of theories applied to individuals, interpersonal relationships, and workplace. Theories have a particular focus (e.g., perceptions, attitudes, environment) and set of constructs. Constructs are used to design instruments (e.g., surveys, questionnaires, tests, focus group questions) that further delineate the construct into variables that are measured, compared, and contrasted.

Table 2.3   Health Promotion Theories: Focus and Key Concepts (adapted from National Cancer Institute, 2005)

	Theory	Focus	Constructs
Individual Level	Health Belief Model	Individuals' perceptions of the threat posed by a health problem, the benefits of avoiding the threat, and factors influencing the decision to act	Perceived susceptibility Perceived severity Perceived benefits Perceived barriers Cues to action Self-efficacy
	Theory of Planned Behavior	Individuals' attitudes toward a behavior, perceptions of norms, and beliefs about the ease or difficulty of changing	Behavioral intention Attitude toward the behavior Subjective norm Perceived behavioral control
	Transtheoretical Model	Individuals' motivation and readiness to change a problem behavior over time	Stages of change Processes of change Decisional balance Self-efficacy Temptation
	Health Action Process Approach	Self-regulatory model to influence intention and behavior	Risk perceptions Outcome expectancies Self-efficacy (action, maintenance, and recovery)

Table 2.3   *(Continued)*

	Theory	Focus	Constructs
Interpersonal Level	Social Cognitive Theory	Personal factors, environmental factors, and human behavior exert influence on each other	Reciprocal determinism
			Behavioral capability expectations
			Self-efficacy
			Observational learning
			Reinforcements
	Social Networks and Social Support	Social influences on health and behavior	Emotional support
			Instrumental support
			Sharing points of view
			Informational support
Workplace Level	Communication Theory	How different types of communication affect health behavior	Media agenda setting
			Public agenda setting
			Policy agenda setting
			Problem identification, definition
			Framing
	Diffusion of Innovations	How new ideas, products, and practices spread within a society or from one society to another	Relative advantage compatibility
			Complexity
			Trialability
			Observability
	Community Mobilization	How to organize and engage people to promote health	Mobilization planning
			Awareness raising
			Building a coalition
			Taking action

They are the indicators to help explain a health behavior or guide how to change a health behavior.

Selecting an appropriate theory or combination of theories takes into account the multiple factors that influence health behaviors. The practitioner who uses theory develops a nuanced understanding of realistic program outcomes, an understanding that drives the planning process. Choosing a theory that will bring a useful perspective to the problem at hand does not begin with a theory (i.e., the most familiar theory or the theory mentioned in a recent journal article). Instead, this process starts with a thorough assessment of the situation: the units of analysis or change, the topic, and the type of behavior to be addressed. Because different theoretical frameworks are appropriate and practical for different situations, selecting a theory that "fits" should be a careful, deliberate process. Table 2.4

Table 2.4   Using Theory to Plan Multilevel Workplace Interventions (adapted from National Cancer Institute, 2005)

Change Strategies	Workplace interventions	Ecological Level	Useful Theories
Change People's Behavior	Workstation safety posters and training	Individual	Health Belief Model
			Theory of Planned Behavior
	Stress management programs		Transtheoretical Model
	Health brochures, email blasts, and social media		Health Action Process Approach
	Health coaching	Interpersonal	Social Cognitive Theory
	Group health activities		Social Networks and Social Support
	Health campaigns (e.g. good nutrition, walking)		
Change the Environment	On-site fitness center	Building (e.g. office, factory, retail store) and surrounding community	Communication Theory
	Advocating changes to company policy		Diffusion of Innovations
	Healthy and culturally aligned food options		Community Mobilization
	Community walking trails		

illustrates examples of strategies, and theories matched to a desired change, focused either on the individual or larger environment. Useful theories make assumptions about a behavior, health problem, priority population, or environment. They are consistent with everyday observations. We also consider theories used in successful programs and supported by past research in the same area or related ideas.

Workplace Health Promotion Program Planning Models

Health planning models guide the process of planning, implementing, and evaluating a workplace health program. The process is deliberate but not necessarily linear, with many twists and turns as a program develops and evolves. The workplace health promotion program planning models have their roots in the PRECEDE-PROCEED model (Green & Kreuter, 2005). The PRECEDE portion of the model focuses on program planning, while the PROCEED portion focuses on implementation and evaluation. The eight phases of the model guide planners in creating health promotion programs, beginning with more general outcomes and moving to more specific outcomes. Gradually the process leads to creation of a program, delivery of the program, and evaluation of the program (Figure 2.3).

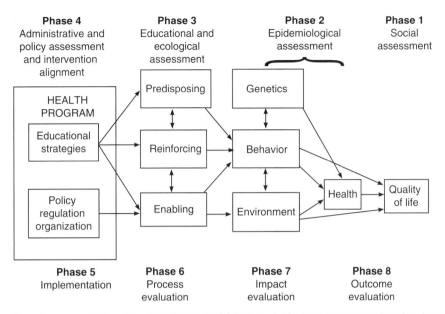

Generic representation of the PRECEDE-PROCEED model for health programming planning and evaluation that shows the main lines of causation, from program inputs and determinants of health to outcomes, by the direction of the arrows

Figure 2.3   PRECEDE-PROCEED Model
Source: Adapted from Green and Kreuter (2005).

Centers for Disease Control and Prevention Workplace Health Model

The CDC Workplace Health Model champions a planned, organized, and comprehensive set of programs, policies, benefits, and environmental supports designed to meet the health and safety needs of all employees. It is a systematic four-step process of building a workplace health promotion program (CDC, 2013).

1. An assessment to define employee health risks and concerns, and to describe current health promotion activities, capacity, and needs

2. A planning process to develop the components of a workplace health programs including goal determination, selecting priority interventions, and building an organizational infrastructure

3. Program implementation involving all the steps needed to put health promotion strategies and interventions into place and make them available to employees

4. An evaluation of efforts to systematically investigate the merit (e.g., quality), worth (e.g., effectiveness), and significance (e.g., importance) of an organized health promotion action/activity

The model seeks to put interventions in place that address multiple risk factors and health conditions concurrently, and it recognizes that the interventions and strategies chosen influence multiple levels of the organization, including the individual employee and the organization as a whole. Furthermore it considers occupational safety and health a focus in the program design and execution. As part of the planning model the CDC developed a Workplace Health Promotion website as a toolkit for employers, containing a collection of guidance, tools, and resources to assist in building or enhancing a workplace health program following the overall process shown in Figure 2.4.

The Wellness Council of America Focus on Small Business

The Wellness Council of America (WELCOA) was established in the mid-1980s through the efforts of a number of forward-thinking business and health leaders. It has influenced the face of workplace wellness in the United States. Its tenets are:

+ Health care costs are an issue of significant concern.

+ A healthy workforce is essential to America's continued growth and prosperity.

+ Much of the illness in the United States is directly preventable.

+ The workplace is an ideal setting to address health and well-being.

+ Workplace wellness programs can transform corporate culture and change lives.

WELCOA is a membership organization with its model grounded in practice and what works in organizations. For large organizations it promotes a planning model that includes leadership support, wellness team formation, data collection, action plan, intervention selection, supportive environment, and evaluation. For smaller businesses WELCOA has used its membership to develop a planning model tailored and responsive to the needs of small business that is grounded in the reality of the small business operation, which may or may not have a human resource department or office (Table 2.5). Likewise the organizational capacity and resources might not be available to offer employee wellness programs and services. Furthermore the model is not limited to business operations. The practice-oriented model can be used with any small organization and group wanting to promote the health of its employees. After gaining leadership support (e.g., from the business owner, small nonprofit director, or board of directors) and identifying and designating a wellness leader (or leaders),

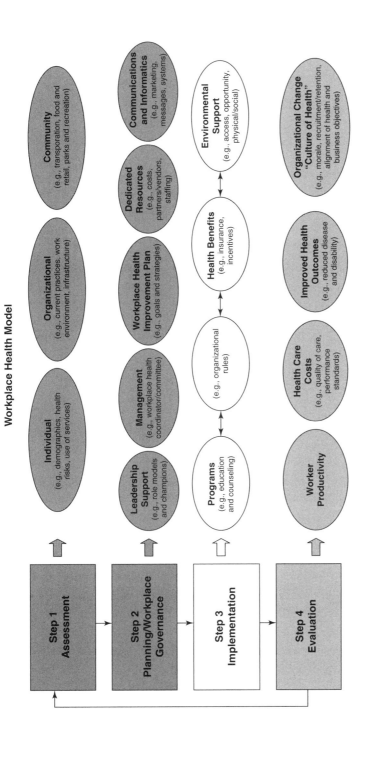

Figure 2.4 Centers for Disease Control and Prevention Workplace Health Model

Source: CDC, 2013.

Table 2.5   WELCOA Small Business Health Promotion Model

Capturing Leadership Support				Designating a Wellness Leader (or Leaders)		
Implementing Healthy Policies and Procedures	Conducting an Employee Health Interest Survey	Providing an Opportunity for Health Screening	Administering an Annual Physical Activity Campaign	Holding a Healthy Eating In-Service/Lunch and Learn	Establishing an In-House Wellness Library	Disseminating a Quarterly Health Newsletter

Partnering With and Supporting Community Health Efforts

the seven wellness activities are implemented without regard to order but rather according to the organization's needs and capacity. Underlying the organizational activities is partnering with and supporting community health efforts.

National Institute of Occupational Safety and Health: SafeWell Integrated Management System for Worker Health

The SafeWell Integrated Management System (SIMS) development was supported by Harvard School of Public Health Center for Work, Health, and Well-Being, one of the NIOSH Centers of Excellence to Promote a Healthier Workforce (Figure 2.5). The model process includes decision making, program planning, implementation, and evaluation for continual improvement toward total worker health. It engages top management and creates a culture of health by integrating workplace health programs and engaging midlevel management and employees in these efforts.

SIMS places the workplace program within the larger policy and social context. Decisions that are made within workplaces often are influenced by regulatory and legislative efforts, economic conditions, and the image the organization wants to portray in the community. While these may seem to be macro-level issues, they can impact individual health in many ways. For instance, is there access to safe, affordable recreational activities in the neighborhood? Are healthy food options available?

The main emphasis of SIMS is the integration of occupational safety and health, workplace health promotion, and the psychosocial work environment and employee benefits with three levels of engagement: the physical environment; organizational policies, programs, and practices; and individual behavior and resources. The planning, implementation, and evaluation focus on three components: (1) a systems-level coordination of programs, policies, and practices; (2) programs, policies, and practices that address the work environment/organization, and worker health and well-being;

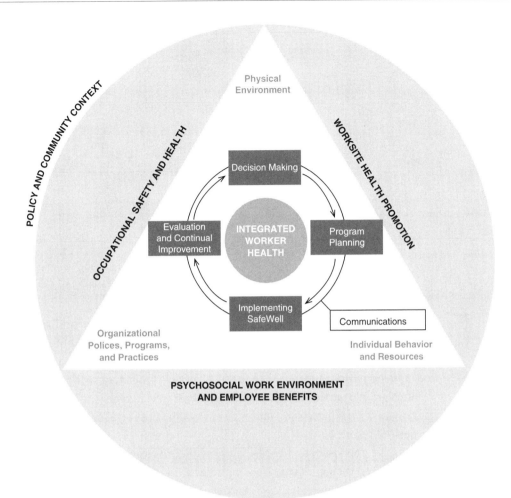

Figure 2.5   SafeWell Integrated Management System (SIMS)

and (3) coordination of occupational health and safety, workplace health promotion, and human resources. The inclusion of human resources as part of the model is consistent with the NIOSH Total Worker Health approach.

Guidelines for Choosing Approaches, Theories, and Models

Using and applying certain approaches, theories, and models is key to creating and implementing workplace health promotion programs (Figure 2.6). Knowing some of the different approaches, theories, and models that can be used to create, implement, and evaluate workplace health promotion

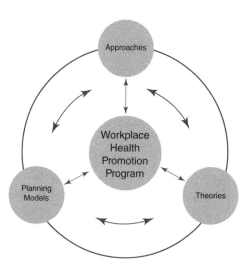

Figure 2.6   Interactive Approaches, Theories, and Models to Create Workplace Health Promotion Programs

programs is one thing—knowing which approach, theory, and model to use when is another. Unfortunately, there is no magic formula or chart to tell you which is just right for a given situation, because there is no right or wrong approach, theory, or model. One may work better than another in a particular situation—or within a certain organization, population, and workplace—to address a specific health problem or to produce a desired result.

The approaches, theories, and models are interactive (Figure 2.6). As you move through planning, implementing, and evaluating a program, certain constants help to organize and provide infrastructure for the process. With this said, the following guidelines may help you narrow down the choices (Hayden, 2014).

Guideline 1: Identify All Program Parts

Programs are complex, and like any complex machine, tool, or piece of equipment, programs have many moving parts. These parts may be called services, systems, strategies, components, activities, campaigns, guides, curriculums, modules, lunch-and-learns, health fairs, classes, initiatives, and interventions. Among and between workplace health promotion programs identical parts might be called different names. Likewise different parts with different goals often will share the same name. It can be confusing. Clarify not only the name an organization uses for each part of its health promotion program but also its purpose.

Guideline 2: Identify the Health Issue and Population Affected

As you think about the parts of your program, identify the health issue(s) you are trying to address and the population affected. Different parts of a program may use different approaches, theories, and models. For example, each problem and population may require a different health theory to be used when designing a six-week intervention, a lecture, health fair, or class curriculum. Likewise the same problem in different populations (e.g., young migrant workers, women, older workers) may require different theories.

Guideline 3: Gather Information

Next, do a literature search to learn what others have found and done about the issue. A literature search is not limited to a search of the Internet. You need to search the professional literature using an appropriate database. Ones commonly used for workplace health promotion include the following:

- CINAHL (Cumulative Index to Nursing and Allied Health Literature): available through a university or college library or a public library
- Academic Search Complete: accessed through a university or college library
- PubMed: maintained by the National Library of Medicine and National Institutes of Health, accessed directly at http://www.pubmed.gov
- NREPP (National Registry of Evidence-Based Programs and Practices): http://www.nrepp.samhsa.gov/
- RTIPs (Research-Tested Interventions): http://rtips.cancer.gov/rtips /index.do
- ERIC (Education Resource Information Center): the database for school health information, accessed directly at http://www.eric.ed.gov
- Healthy People 2020 evidence-based resources: http://www .healthypeople.gov/2020/tools-resources/Evidence-Based-Resources

Guideline 4: Identify Possible Reasons or Cause for the Problem

Take the information you found in the literature and combine it with information you know about the workplace and community. This will enable you to identify possible causes for the problem, that is, to answer the question, "Why does this problem exist?" Remember, approaches provide the big picture of how to go about addressing health problems at the workplace. Theories help explain the *why* of health behavior, that is, why people do what they do. Why is it that some people fall, use alcohol, become afflicted by head lice, go for mammograms, or do testicular self-exams, for instance, and others do not? Models provide us directions and steps to addressing employee health.

Guideline 5: Identify the Level of Interaction

Once you have determined possible causes or reasons why the health issue exists, it is time to determine under which level of interaction these reasons fall—intrapersonal, interpersonal, community, or all three. Identifying the level helps you determine which approaches, theories, and models would most likely explain the behavior and therefore would best serve as the basis for change.

Guideline 6: Identify the Approach, Theory, and Model That Match Best

Use the tables and figures in this chapter to help you identify which of the approaches, theories, and models would most likely provide a framework to address the workplace health problem, explain the behavior, enable you to plan an intervention to change the behavior, and identify a process to put the program in operation. Remember: an approach, theory, and model is most effective when all parts of it are put to use (Hochbaum, Sorenson, & Lorig, 1992). Oftentimes, however, you can effectively mix and match aspects from the different approaches, theories, and models.

When you think you have determined which approach, theory, and model would fit best, see how it applies to the following questions (National Cancer Institute [NCI], 2003):

- Is it logical given the situation you are trying to address?
- Is it similar to the approaches, theories, and models others have used successfully in similar situations found in the literature?
- Is it supported by research?

Choosing approaches, theories, and models is a lot like choosing your clothes. All of your clothes do the same thing—they cover your body—but they do so in different ways. You choose which clothes to wear depending on a host of factors, such as time of day, climate, occasion, and what your friends are wearing. For example, you wouldn't wear a bathing suit to shovel snow.

Approaches, theories, and models, just like clothes, all do the same thing. They all help address people's health concerns and problems, but they do it in different ways. You choose an approach, theory, and model depending on a host of factors such as behavioral causes of the health issue or problem, the level of interaction (intrapersonal, interpersonal, or workplace), the population, and the desired outcomes or change. Once you decide on which approach, theory, and model to use (or wear, as they are analogous to clothes), you need to apply them (or try them on) to see how they fit.

Guideline 7: Use the Approaches, Theories, and Models for All Program Parts

Once you have selected the approaches, theories, and models, use them in each aspect of your program. Use them when developing program mission statements, goals, and objectives, identifying and deciding upon the specific program parts (e.g., services, systems, strategies, components, activities, campaigns, curriculums, guides, modules, lunch-and-learns, health fairs, classes, initiatives, and interventions) as well of the timing of the different program parts. The approaches, theories, and models help in choosing the right mix of strategies and methods and can aid in communication between and among employers and employees. They provide frameworks that remain constant with each new program part, and thus facilitate talk with colleagues and peers to compare and contrast implementation and outcomes. Use the approaches to think critically about the real world challenges we all face. Conflict and struggles are expected. The approaches, theories, and models help in solving problems creatively and facing challenges. The use of approaches, theories, and models helps in replication of programs because the same frameworks can be used from one intervention and population to another. Finally, approaches, theories, and models help in designing programs that are more effective (have greater impact) and more efficient (take less time). These benefits are summarized below.

Benefits of Using Approaches, Theories and Models
1. Helps to discern program outcomes
2. Specifies programs and services for addressing concerns and problems
3. Identifies the timing for programs
4. Helps in choosing the right mix of programs
5. Enhances communication among employees and employers
6. Promotes critical thinking and creative problem solving
7. Improves replication of programs
8. Improves program efficiency and effectiveness

Summary

Effective workplace health promotion programs use approaches, health theories, and program planning models. These provide the infrastructure for the programs. Knowing some of the different approaches, theories, and models that can be used to create, implement, and evaluate workplace health promotion programs is one thing—knowing which approach, theory, and model to use when is another. Unfortunately, there is no magic formula or chart to tell you which is just right for a given situation, because there are no right or wrong approach, theory, or model. Some may work better than others in a particular situation, with a certain organization, population, and workplace to address a specific health problem or to produce a desired result.

For Practice and Discussion

1. Prepare a handout to use with a group of small business owners on the topic of approaches to workplace health promotion programs.

2. Search for peer-reviewed academic journal articles about workplace health promotion programs. How do the studies handle theory? Do the authors explicitly mention health theories? Do they present and explain theoretical constructs being examined in the study? Do they provide logical explanation of any kind, explain the theoretical foundation of the instruments used in the study, or link the variables being measured in the study to health theory? In summary what is the "status" of health theory used in workplace health promotion programs?

3. How do you reconcile the use of planning models for workplace health promotion programs with the need of organizations to also consider, as part of program planning, workers' compensation, health and safety, risk management, and employee benefits?

4. Compare and contrast the workplace health promotion program planning models mentioned in this chapter—the Centers for Disease Control and Prevention Workplace Health Model, the Wellness Council of America (WELCOA) Focus on Small Business, and the SafeWell Integrated Management System (SIMS) for Worker Health—with the PRECEDE-PROCEED model.

Case Study: Using Health Approaches, Theory, and Models—What Would You Do?

Rosa Jones, a health promotion program director, knows that workplace health promotion programs do not just "happen." No one gets up one morning saying, *Today, I am going to start a health promotion program at my job.* Workplace health promotion reflects a process of relationship building with and within an organization. Getting to know the people and what the organization does, its history, and its current direction. Programs do not happen overnight but rather over time, in little and big steps with starts, stops, bumps, twists, unforeseen events, consequences, and outcomes. Ms. Jones also knows her health promotion approaches, theories, and models and the benefits of using them. However, she knows that there is a "gap" between theory and practice. In other words, she knows that many practitioners do not know health approaches, theories, and models (it was not part of their education or professional training), and if they do know them, they do not use them in their programs. Often the attitude is, *if it is not broken, do not mess with it.* Or, if there is pressure to create and a deliver program, it precludes time to think about a program's theoretical foundation. In Ms. Jones's own words, "We have become complacent and assume that, business as usual, in our field is harmless." Wanting to address the "gap," the local area Business Group on Health (BGH) approached Ms. Jones to chair a workplace health promotion program conference focused on why workplace health promotion programs do not use health approaches, theories, and models. To get the conference planning process started BGH members asked her to develop a set of frank and hard questions that directly addressed the gap so they could begin to reflect on and set a tone for the conference.

If you were Ms. Jones, and knowing the "gap" exists, what would you do? Create a list of questions.

KEY TERMS

CDC Comprehensive Workplace Health

Integrated Employee Health Management

NASA Employee Total Health Management

Coordinated health programs

Individual health concerns and problems intervention process approach

Total Worker Health approach

NIOSH Centers of Excellence to Promote a Healthier Workforce

Explanatory and change theory

PRECEDE/PROCEED model

Centers for Disease Control and Prevention (CDC) Workplace Health Model

Wellness Council of America (WELCOA) Focus on Small Business

SafeWell Integrated Management System for Worker Health (SIMS)

References

Centers for Disease Control and Prevention. (2008). *Healthy youth! Coordinated school health program.* Retrieved from http://www.cdc.gov /healthyyouth/CSHP/

Centers for Disease Control and Prevention. (2013). *Workplace health promotion.* Retrieved from http://www.cdc.gov/workplacehealthpromotion/model /index.html

Centers for Disease Control and Prevention. (2015). *Total worker health.* Retrieved from http://www.cdc.gov/niosh/TWH/default.html

Fertman, C., Delgado, M., & Tarasevich, S. (2014). *Promoting child and adolescent mental health.* Burlington, MA: Jones & Bartlett Learning.

Green, L., & Kreuter, M. (2005). *Health program planning: An educational and ecological approach* (4th ed.). New York, NY: McGraw-Hill.

Hayden, J. (2014). *Introduction to health behavior theory.* Burlington, MA: Jones & Bartlett Learning.

Hochbaum, G. M., Sorenson, J. R., & Lorig, K. (1992). Theory in health education practice. *Health Education Quarterly, 19*(3), 295–313.

Institute of Medicine. (2005). *Integrating employee health: A model program for NASA.* Washington, DC: National Academies Press.

McKay, M. M., Hibbert, R., Hoagwood, K., Rodriguez, J., Murray, L., Legerski, J., & Fernandez, D. (2004). Integrating evidence-based engagement interventions into "real world" child mental health settings. *Brief Treatment and Crisis Intervention, 4*(2), 177.

National Cancer Institute. (2005). *Theory at a glance: A guide for health promotion practice* (2nd ed.). Washington, DC: U.S. Department of Health and Human Services. (NIH Publication No. 05-3896).

CHAPTER 3

HUMAN RESOURCE MANAGEMENT MAKES HEALTH A PRIORITY

Human Resources, the Workplace Health Promotion Program's Gatekeeper

Workplace health promotion programs are an integral part of an organization's human resource management. The traditional human resource management and decision-making process is top down. Senior management makes policy and procedures that are administered by middle management and implemented by lower-level management (e.g., shop-floor supervisors) to employees. It is a hierarchical, linear process that limits interaction between levels as well as feedback and input from the employees impacted by the decisions. The process in part gave rise to the formation of unions as a means for workers to have a voice in workplace conditions. And while large organizations now have diverse approaches to human resource decision making, the traditional approach still largely exists in small and even midsized organizations, which may be dependent on an individual owner, founders, or partners to perform many if not all of the organization's management functions (e.g., marketing, sales, production, personnel, billing, payroll).

In larger organizations, human resource management increasingly is known as strategic human resource management and defined as an administrative entity that systematically links the needs of an organization and aims to provide it with an effective workforce while meeting the needs of its members and other constituents in the society. Individuals with job titles such as Chief

LEARNING OBJECTIVES

- Discuss human resource management as the workplace health promotion program gatekeeper

- Explain how human resource management is organized and functions

- Explain health insurance benefits and providers

- Identify four human resource management actions for quality workplace health promotion programs

People Officer and Senior Director of Total Rewards, as well as individuals with more traditional titles such as Vice President for Human Resources, now exercise exhaustive and ongoing evaluations of an organization's internal and external environments. Internally considerations include the organizational mission and goals, organizational strengths and culture, and organizational strategies. Externally considerations include the economic, technological, social, political, cultural, legal, and demographic challenges. Within the context of this internal and external evaluation, human resource programs are planned, implemented, and evaluated, and are part of every decision made by an organization's leadership, whether it be about marketing, production, services, expansion, or accounting. Companies (i.e., human resource departments) are in a competition for employees. Workplace health promotion programs are one of the elements used to compete, recruit, and retain individuals in an organization (Schwind, Das, Wagar, Fassina, & Bulmash, 2013).

Human Resource Management and Human Resource Departments

Although human resource management is central to all organizations, not all organizations will have a dedicated human resource department. The field of human resource management thus focuses on what managers—especially human resource specialists—do and what they should do as it relates to human resource systems. These systems, in turn, create value by facilitating and enabling employees to achieve their goals. Human resource management activities are geared to:

- Assist the organization to attract the right quality and number of employees
- Orient new employees to the organization and place them in their job positions
- Develop, disseminate, and use job descriptions, performance standards, and evaluation criteria
- Help establish adequate compensation systems and administer them in an efficient and timely manner
- Foster a safe, healthy, and productive work environment
- Ensure compliance with all legal requirements insofar as they relate to management of the workforce
- Help maintain a harmonious working relationship with employees and unions where present

- Foster a work environment that facilitates high employee performance

- Establish disciplinary and counseling procedures

A human resource department is a specialized group with a primary focus of ensuring the most effective use of human resource systems by individual managers and the organization overall. Human resource departments are more typical in midsized to large organizations.

Human resource departments are service and support departments. They exist to assist employees, managers, and the organization. Their managers do not have the authority to order other managers in other departments to accept their ideas. Instead the department staff has staff authority, which is the authority to advise but not direct managers in other departments.

Line authority, possessed by managers of operating departments, allows these managers to make decisions about production, performance, and people. Operating managers are the ones normally responsible for promotions, job assignments, and other people-related decisions. Human resource specialists advise line managers, who alone are ultimately responsible for employee performance. While human resource departments show considerable variation across organizations, they must continuously focus on six groups of interactive activities (Figure 3.1).

1. Planning human resources: An organization must determine its demand and supply of various types of human resources by planning. Key to this process is collecting information through analyses of the various jobs, including required job behaviors and performance standards. The results of job analysis and human resource plans shape the overall human resource strategies in the short run and facilitate employment and training planning.

2. Attracting human resources: Recruitment is the process of finding and attracting capable job applicants who will form a pool of high-quality candidates. Recruitment is shaped and guided by a series of legal requirements (e.g., equal employment opportunity laws, affirmative action policies). Furthermore the selection process is a series of specific steps used to decide which recruits should be hired, and it aims to match job requirements with an applicant's capabilities.

3. Placing, developing, and evaluating human resources: New employees need to be oriented to the organization's policies and procedures and placed in their new job positions. Likewise, existing employees need to be kept updated on new and revised policies and procedures. All employees must also be developed to prepare them for future responsibilities through systematic career planning.

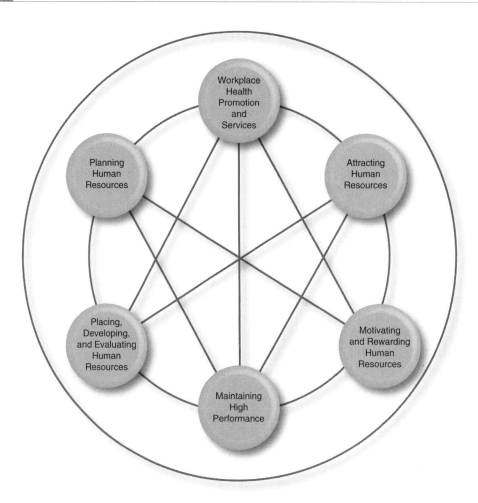

Figure 3.1   Human Resource Activities
Source: Adapted from Schwind et al., 2013.

Performance appraisals give employees feedback on their performance and can help the human resource department identify future training needs. This activity also indicates how well human resource activities have been carried out, since poor performance might often mean that selection or training activities need to be redesigned.

4.   Engaging and motivating employees: Organizations are successful when employees are able to meet the organizational goals as well as their own personal goals within their job. Compensation (salary) and benefits (e.g., vacation days, insurance, retirement) are part of engaging and motivating employees. Furthermore employee engagement and motivation are also partially determined by internal work procedures, climate, and schedules, so these conditions must be continually modified to maximize performance.

5.   Maintaining high performance: Most effective organizations have well-established employee-relations practices including good communication between managers and employees, standardized disciplinary procedures, and counseling systems. Internal work procedures and organizational policies are continuously monitored to ensure that they meet the needs of a diverse workforce and ensure safety to every individual.

6.   Promoting health and safety: Rising health care costs for employers and employees now require the strategic and systematic integration of distinct environmental, health, and safety policies and programs into a continuum of activities that both enhance the overall health and well-being of employees and prevent work-related injuries and illness. Key components are human resource best practices that link employee, employer, family, community, and health care.

The Society for Human Resource Management (www.shrm.org), the world's largest human resource management association, promotes the development of six human resource professional competencies. Figure 3.2 shows the competencies as a three-tier pyramid with the Credible Activist competency the most important for high performance as an HR professional and effective HR leader. Demonstrating these competencies can help professionals ensure managers that they are capable of helping the human resource function create value, contribute to the business strategy, and shape the company culture.

Although great emphasis is placed on the strategic role of human resources, effective execution of the necessary administration services, such as filing open jobs, paying employees, benefits enrollment, keeping employee records, and completing legally required paperwork (such as W-2 forms and EEO reports) is still important. Furthermore technological advances have made human resource management and information systems more efficient and effective, which in turn has benefited the administration of services and freed up time for human resource departments to focus on strategic issues. Successful human resource professionals must be able to share information, build relationships, and influence persons both inside and outside the company, including managers, employees, community members, government workers, customers, vendors, and suppliers.

Human Resource Professions With Responsibilities for Workplace Health Promotion

Responsibilities for workplace health promotion programs are typically spread across a number of human resource professionals within an organization. Therefore the company's management team can expect to

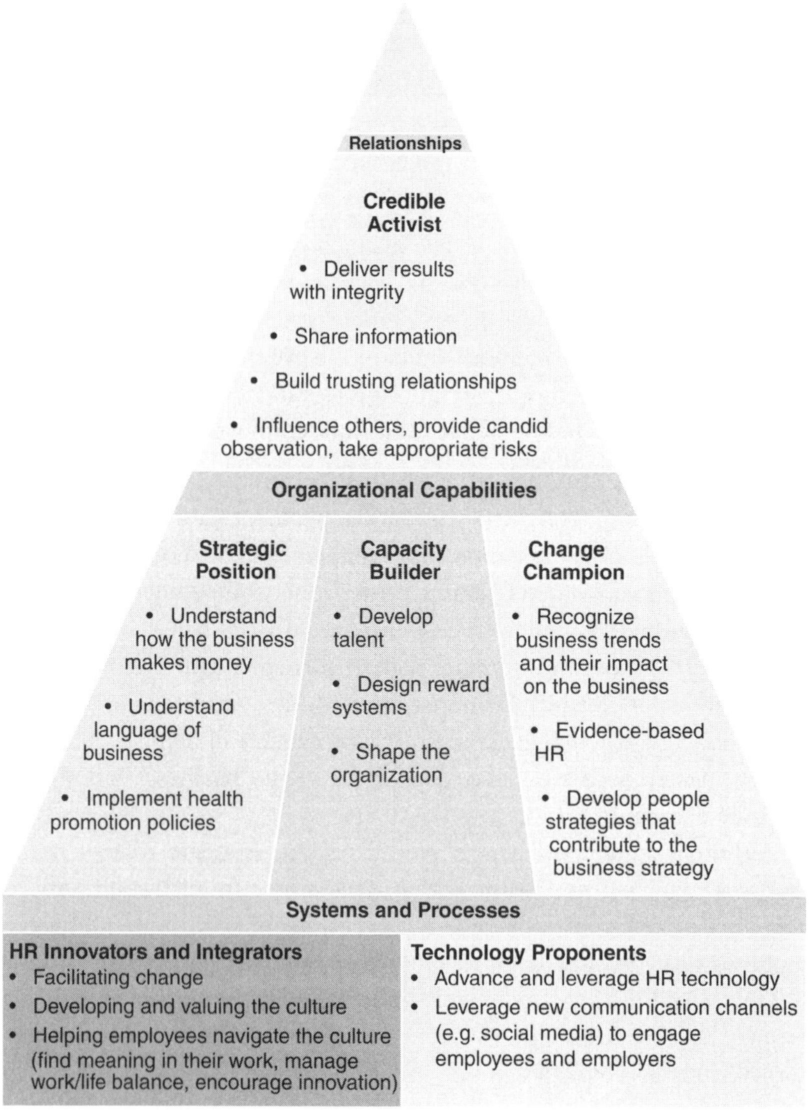

Relationships

Credible Activist

- Deliver results with integrity

- Share information

- Build trusting relationships

- Influence others, provide candid observation, take appropriate risks

Organizational Capabilities

Strategic Position	**Capacity Builder**	**Change Champion**
• Understand how the business makes money	• Develop talent	• Recognize business trends and their impact on the business
• Understand language of business	• Design reward systems	• Evidence-based HR
• Implement health promotion policies	• Shape the organization	• Develop people strategies that contribute to the business strategy

Systems and Processes

HR Innovators and Integrators
- Facilitating change
- Developing and valuing the culture
- Helping employees navigate the culture (find meaning in their work, manage work/life balance, encourage innovation)

Technology Proponents
- Advance and leverage HR technology
- Leverage new communication channels (e.g. social media) to engage employees and employers

Figure 3.2   Human Resource Professional Credible Activist Competency Pyramid With the Six Competencies
Source: RBL Group and Michigan Ross School of Business, 2012.

work with professionals who provide human resource services (health and fitness programs and equipment) and others who provide products (e.g., health and disability insurance). Line supervisors and managers are involved with programs, but the organization's human resource professionals are the gatekeepers and individuals with whom an organization will consult to at least make the initial program decisions.

The human resource professionals with responsibilities for health promotion typically have position titles such as medical director, health

Table 3.1   Human Resource Professions With Responsibilities for Workplace Health Promotion

Job Title	Brief Job Description
Medical director (M.D.)	Oversees health care, safety, and wellness needs of the employees. Serves as a medical policy advisor to the company. Is accountable for and provides professional leadership and direction to the utilization/cost management and clinical quality management functions. Works collaboratively with executive leadership who interface with medical management such as provider relations, member services, benefits, and claims management.
Health and wellness program manager	Oversees the strategy, management, and execution of employee health and wellness services. Directs the development and implementation of new or modifications to existing programs (e.g., integrated health management, quality improvement initiatives, preventive health programs, clinical consulting, and employer worksite wellness offerings).
Benefits and compensation specialist	Manages benefits plans (medical, dental, FSA, HSA, disability, life insurance) and well-being programs. Analyzes compensation data within an organization and evaluates job positions to determine classification and salary. Administers employee insurance, pension and savings plans, and works with insurance brokers and plan carriers.
Workers' compensation manager	Responsible for analyzing injury reports and workers' compensation claims, thus monitoring, assisting, evaluating, and reporting on claims. Determines compensability and benefits due on long-term indemnity claims; monitors reserve accuracy and files necessary documentation with state agency.
Health and safety director (Certified Safety Professional [CSP] certification preferred)	Reviews, evaluates, and analyzes work environments and design programs and procedures to control, eliminate, and prevent disease or injury caused by chemical, physical, and biological agents or ergonomic factors. Responsible for implementation and improvement of the corporation's safety, environmental, and health and wellness programs including regulatory and system compliance for, but not limited to: OSHA, EPA, DNR, and DOT. Conducts safety training and education programs, and demonstrates the use of safety equipment.

and wellness director, benefits and compensation specialist, workers' compensation coordinator, and health and safety director (Table 3.1). A medical director operates as part of the corporate executive leadership managing all aspects of the organizational health and safety policy, procedures, and programs. The medical director is the corporate expert on national health care policies and regulations. A health and wellness director would be most involved with program delivery and implementation and long-term outcomes related to employee health status and job performance. Specialists in the area of benefits and compensation deal with job analysis, salary, and benefit packages (e.g., health insurance) that may structure and determine the health promotion program parameters for the employees. Workers' compensation involves analyzing injury reports and monitoring, evaluating, and reporting on workers' compensation claims. They develop action plans to resolution, coordinate return-to-work efforts, and approve claim payments and may negotiate settlements. The health and safety director is concerned with workplace environment design to control, eliminate, and prevent disease and injury caused by chemical, physical, and biological agents or ergonomic factors.

A second set of human resource professionals involved with health promotion program delivery at the workplace can be internal or external to the organization (Table 3.2). These professionals provide health promotion programs, services, and equipment. Fitness center directors and staff operate facilities such as on-site gyms, pools, and recreational activities providing for an additional fee the staffing, insurance, and facility maintenance. Screening service providers administer health screening including blood screening and reporting at worksites. Specialty health professionals—such as health coaches, nurses, nutritionists, personal trainers, physical therapists, and employee-assistance professional counselors—offer personalized services tailored to individual employee needs. Case managers work with individuals on disease management (e.g., diabetes and cardiac problem prevention), and with workers' compensation claimants as well as employees on short- and long-term disability.

Often an organization contracts through another company the hiring of professionals to provide services for and supervise its workplace wellness programs. Likewise insurance companies employ many of these professionals to staff their health promotion programs and services. The insurance companies employ the individuals as part of their efforts to manage health cost for both the employees (e.g., by lowering employee monthly insurance premium cost deducted from salary) and employers (e.g., by lowering the cost of employer contribution per employee).

A third set of human resource professionals serving the workplace health promotion arena incudes those working in the health insurance industry (Table 3.3). These positions are in addition to the ones held by professionals listed in Table 3.2. Health insurance companies employ insurance agents and brokers, on-site coordinators, and health informatics and information management directors. Increasing numbers of insurance companies design and deliver workplace health promotion programs, frequently called "products," which are part of an organization's health insurance plan.

Table 3.2   Workplace Health Promotion Programs, Services, and Equipment Providers

Job Title (with preferred credentials and training)	Brief Job Description
Fitness center staff	Supports the facilitation of fitness assessments (including health history, height, weight, circumference measurements, body composition, heart rate, blood pressure, submax VO2 bicycle testing, flexibility testing through the use of a sit and reach test, and muscular strength and endurance tests utilizing push-up and sit-up protocols). Conducts equipment orientations including both cardiovascular equipment and resistance equipment. Assists with health promotion activities and programs.
Biometric screening manager	Manages the development and delivery of biometric screenings to employees. Responsibilities include pre-event coordination; event setup and management, as well as setup and management of the screening software program and other equipment; supervision of on-call and vendor staff; communication and coordination with client representatives; and post-event activities.
Specialty health professionals	Health coaches, nurses, nutritionists, personal trainers, and physical therapists provide services to identified populations of individuals within the employee population. Often services are structured as part of employee incentives to lower health care premiums, oversee disease management (diabetes, cardiovascular, stress, smoking), and physical activity.
Workers' compensation case manager	Provides case management services, focusing on quality and cost effectiveness, to various injured workers, facilitating communications, and coordinating benefits at the onset of injury/illness. Ensures that employees receive adequate and timely support regarding: the quality of diagnoses and treatment plans; conformance with treatment plans; satisfactory rate of recovery; and, when applicable, return to work on undefined or accommodated duty as therapeutically indicated.

Likewise, health insurance offered in the health exchanges as part of the Affordable Care Act also provides workplace health promotion programs. Navigators provide these services. To become an insurance broker or agent, one must be licensed through the state for each position and oftentimes for separate types of insurance. Brokers typically are required to have more education or experience than an agent. Insurance agents can be either captive or independent. A captive agent is an agent who works for only one company. A captive agent will sell policies only for that insurer. An independent agent is one who works as an agent for a variety of different insurers. An independent agent can provide policies from several insurers and give comparisons across providers. Each state has individual requirements regarding

Table 3.3   Health Insurance Workplace Health Promotion Professionals

Job Title	Brief Job Description
Insurance brokers	Offer a whole host of insurance products. Brokers have the duty to analyze a business and secure correct and adequate coverage for the business. This is a higher duty than the pure administrative duty of insurance agents.
Insurance agents	Serve as intermediaries between the insurance company and the insured. Agents are responsible for the timely and accurate processing of forms, premiums, and paperwork. Agents have no duty to conduct a thorough examination of a business or to make sure it has appropriate coverage.
On-site health promotion program coordinators	Corporate on-site health promotion planning, design, implementation, delivery, and evaluation (including but not limited to: health screenings, awareness events, health communications, health challenges, lifestyle interventions, health education, company-wide incentives, and program analysis). Integrate online wellness portal platform with on-site activities. Help develop reports on participation and activities. Leverage health plan, wellness, and community resources. Act as company and community liaison.
Navigators	An individual or organization trained and able to help consumers, small businesses, and their employees as they look for health coverage options through the Marketplace, including completing eligibility and enrollment forms. These individuals and organizations are required to be unbiased. Their services are free to consumers. Navigator positions were created as part of the Affordable Care Act.
Actuaries	Design and price insurance policies, such that they remain competitive and maintain profits. Extensively use analytics, economics, and mathematics skills and tools to evaluate risks. Set guidelines for each risk class and category.
Underwriters	Use the data of the individual (organization) customers to decide in which risk class and category the particular customer falls in. Evaluate each client's risk and decide how much coverage the client can be given, and at what premium cost.
Health informatics and information management directors	Oversee the collection, storage, retrieval, analysis, and interpretation of corporate health care data and information. Directs the preparation and analysis of data for an organization's decisions related to employee health, safety, health care, medical and legal issues, reimbursement, research, planning, and evaluation.

the broker and agent license exam and licensure process requirements, so check your state for more detailed information. Generally one can expect to be required to fulfill prelicensure education and a background check before taking the exam. After passing the exam and receiving a license, regular renewal and continuing education is usually necessary.

Table 3.4   Health Promotion Program Vendor Staff

Job Title	Brief Job Description
Pharmacy benefits management (PBM) staff	Oversees prescription drug claims processing and payment. May also be responsible for developing and maintaining formulary, contracting with pharmacies, and negotiating discounts and rebates with drug manufacturers.
Employee assistance program professionals	Counselors, social workers, psychologist, and health educators who address social and emotional concerns. Information, outreach, and short-term counseling typically offered, as well as treatment referrals.
Clinical services medical staff	Physicians, nurses, and physician assistants who offer pre-employment and job standard examinations, vaccinations, return to work evaluations, vision and hearing testing, and risk exposure assessment.

A fourth set of human resource professionals working in the health promotion arena includes those individuals associated with vendor services particularly related to health care services (Table 3.4). The staff is employed by organizations external to the workplace organization, and which offer expertise in a particular health concern or service. The vendor organizations typically work with many workplaces offering contracted, competitive services that are tailored to a workplace level of need and financial commitment.

Health Insurance Benefits and Providers

Large national health insurance companies are involved in workplace health promotion programs. Table 3.5 compares the top five health insurance companies in the United States by the number of members and revenues. In 2015 the top five companies (UnitedHealthcare, Anthem, Aetna, Cigna, and Humana) together served 169 million people and collected over $270 billion in revenue while the entire United States' health insurance industry grossed almost $670 billion. Including these top five, a total of 125 health insurance companies each control at least 0.10% of the market share of the entire health insurance industry in the United States. Health insurance company mergers are anticipated as a result of the ACA. The National Committee for Quality Assurance (NCQA) ranks the performance of health insurance companies by variables such as consumer satisfaction, prevention and treatment.

Insurance company products or services are called health insurance plans or packages (Table 3.6). Different types of health insurance packages (plans) can determine much of what, how, and to what extent a workplace health promotion program can be implemented for employees.

Table 3.5   Top Five Health Insurance Companies in the United States

	Companies				
	UnitedHealthcare	**Anthem**	**Aetna**	**Cigna**	**Humana**
Number of Members	>85 million	36 million	22 million	14 million	12 million
Revenue	$110.6 billion	$61.7 billion	$35.54 billion	$29.1 billion	$39.13 billion

Table 3.6   Health Insurance Package Types and Characteristics

Characteristics	Package Types								
	Indemnity	HSA (health savings account)	PPO (preferred provider organization)		POS (point of service)			HMO (health maintenance organization)	
Network	No Network	Variable	PPO Physician Network		HMO Network, PPO Network, and Out of Network			HMO (primary care) Network	
Coverage	"Covered" Medical expenses from any provider	"Covered" Medical expenses from any provider	Within Network	Out of Network	HMO Network	PPO Network	Out of Network	Within Network	Out of Network
		Other expenses paid from by HSA	Covered with fixed fee (copayment)	Covered with fixed percent (coinsurance)	Covered	Covered	Covered	Covered w/ referral	Not Covered
Pros	No network restrictions	Lower premium Can use account to pay for not covered medical expenses	Ability to make self-referrals		Many options available			Usually the most affordable	
Cons	Higher premium	High deductible required	Higher out-of-network fees		Higher out-of-network fees			Must stay within network	

Health Insurance Plan Types

The five most commonly used types of health insurance plan are indemnity, health savings account (HSA), preferred provider organization (PPO), point of service (POS), and health maintenance organization (HMO). Traditional indemnity plans are at one end of the spectrum, and HMOs are at the other. Indemnity plans allow the participant to visit any doctor of their choosing and receive reimbursement from their insurance company. An HMO participant must choose a primary care physician who must then refer them to any further care within a specific network of providers. PPO and POS plans combine features of both indemnity plans and HMOs. Traditionally a PPO plan will differ from an HMO plan in the fact that both in-network and out-of-network providers are insured. However, the two have different fixed fees associated with them. Generally, it is cheaper to go to a provider within the network, but participants have the option to visit outside the network if they choose to. Furthermore POS plans traditionally offer participants two or three provider network options, each with a different set of benefits. These choices generally include a PPO network, a HMO network, and out-of-network benefits each with a different associated set of fees. A new option, created by Congress in 2003, is an HSA. It combines a high-deductible health plan (HMO, PPO, or indemnity) with a tax-advantaged savings account that can be used to pay various medical expenses, such as deductibles and coinsurance.

Each package offered includes many varying components that are important when implementing a workplace health promotion program for employees. The four basic components of any health insurance package are the premium, deductible, copayment, and coinsurance percentage. The premium is the amount the policyholder or sponsor (e.g., an employer) pays to the health plan to purchase health coverage. A deductible is the amount of expenses that must be paid out of pocket before an insurer will pay any expenses. Generally speaking, the higher the premium, the lower the deductible, and vice versa. A copayment is the amount that the insured person must pay out of pocket before the health insurer pays for a particular visit or service. Coinsurance is a percentage of the total cost that the insured person may also be required to pay, usually after the deductible is met. These components have set values that vary between every package depending on the amount of coverage being offered and specifics of the plan.

For example, a person may have an insurance package with a $500 monthly premium, a $20 copayment for primary care visits, a $500 deductible, and 20% coinsurance. This person will pay the $500 premium every month. If that person goes to the doctor, he or she would have to pay a copayment of $20 for that visit. If that person then needs to have a $10,000 surgery, he or she will have to pay the $500 deductible, while 80% of the remaining $9,500 will be paid by the insurance company, and the remaining 20% (coinsurance) will be paid by the insured person. Individuals must choose a package that finds a personal balance between all of these components based on how much coverage they want, what kind of care network they want, and how much they want to spend out of pocket each month and per visit.

Authority and Responsibility for Package Design, Selection, and Implementation

Getting insurance (commonly called enrolling) occurs in one of four ways. First, a person may purchase employer-offered health insurance. Most employers will offer health insurance benefits to their full-time employees. Each company will vary as to the options they make available to their employees. These plans usually receive a group discount from the provider and the company will often pay a significant part of the monthly premium for their employees. For this reason, employer-offered health insurance is usually the most financially reasonable and popular option. In the case of persons who are unemployed or self-employed, or if their employer does not offer health insurance coverage, they can purchase individual or private insurance from a private provider. This allows them to individualize the plan to their specific needs. For this same reason, they must be careful to shop around before purchasing individual packages, because coverage and prices vary greatly between companies. In addition to these options, they may purchase health insurance from the Health Insurance Marketplace (Exchanges) thanks to the ACA. This gives qualified individuals the chance to compare and purchase insurance packages from competing providers in their specific area, which lowers costs for buyers. Also, the insurance packages offered through the Marketplace are often subsidized based on several factors, which could bring costs down even more. Finally, individuals may also qualify for health insurance coverage through one of the federal or state government safety net programs such as Medicare, Medicaid, or High Risk Pools. These programs are available to specific populations such as older adults and low-income individuals, usually at a free or greatly reduced price to the individual.

Four Human Resource Management Actions for Quality Workplace Health Promotion Programs

Workplace health promotion programs are part of an organization's human resource management, which can be defined as: the leadership and management of people within an organization using systems, methods, processes, and procedures that enable employees to achieve their own goals that in turn enhance the employees' positive contribution to the organization and its goals. Human resource management is not an end in itself; it is a means to help an organization to achieve its primary organizational objectives. Anyone within an organization can be an initial contact person to talk with about a workplace health promotion program. However, almost universally the organization's human resource professional(s) or department members are the ones responsible for the organization's health promotion program. They provide access to the organization, its employees, and leadership as well as to the systems and resources to create, implement, and evaluate a workplace health promotion program. Four human resource management actions in particular engage, support, and sustain an organization's health commitment.

The first action—knowing how employees perceive an organization's response to their health concerns and problems—helps human resource management to tailor and fit programs and services to employees. Such awareness contributes to a workplace that is supportive to all individuals. It values and recognizes employees as members of the workplace.

What Employees Have to Say About Health Programs and Services

1. Confidentially is important when addressing the health of employees and their families. Individuals do understand, however, that there are times when employers may have to share their information with others (e.g., if the worker is at risk for harm, accident, job injury).

2. Employees are most likely to talk with individuals they know and trust, regardless of their training (e.g., medical personnel, human resource staff, community organizational staff).

3. Ongoing employee supervisor interaction is critical to gaining the trust of employees and making them feel supported around health.

4. Health promotion programs and services provide many positive benefits for employees.

5. Employers (e.g., supervisors, front line management) need to be open to and learn more about employees' backgrounds and cultures, although employees recognize that it is unrealistic for employers to know every distinct culture that may be represented with a workplace.

6. Workplaces play an important role in reducing barriers to accessing health services.

7. Human resource personnel, supervisors, and front line staff need to be trained on health issues and policies. Employees feel that, in contrast to how human resource personnel, supervisors, and front line staff respond to employee's physical health problems, they are much less informed about how to respond to employees' mental health issues.

8. A positive workplace environment is critical to the health of all employees.

9. Employees with health issues may require special attention and may have individual needs. Employees with health problems, however, don't want to be treated differently because of their health status.

10. Employees want a voice in their workplace health promotion programs. They recognize that they have a unique perspective on the workplace and its culture and climate.

The second action is to ensure that human resource management is ethical. Health is a personal issue. In the past decade, increased public awareness of professional behavior, coupled with the passage of federal and state legislation controlling the helping professions, has underscored the importance of ethical concerns in workplace health promotion programs. Professionals have responded to the dilemmas of service provision by developing codes of ethics or statements of ethical standards of behavior for the members of their profession. These codes and standards reflect professional concerns and define the guiding principles of professional activities. As an aid to ethical decision making in dilemmas arising in service delivery, such standards or codes help clarify the professional's responsibilities to clients, the agency, and society. Typically, a code of ethics includes items that state the goals or aims of the profession, that protect the client, that provide guidance to professional behavior, and that contribute to a professional identity for the helper. A complete understanding of a code of ethics or ethical standards requires knowledge of the code's strengths and purposes as well as its limitations.

Workplace health promotion professionals are expected to have and adhere to certain codes of behavior. A code of ethics is binding only to the members of the group or organization that adopts it (see Table 3.7). Most codes of ethics stipulate that the worker's first responsibility is to enhance and protect the individual's (i.e., employee's) welfare. Codes also give guidance about the helper's responsibilities to employers, to colleagues in the profession and other fields, and to society in general. The primary functions of a code of ethics or ethical standards are to establish guidelines for professional behavior and to assist members of the profession in establishing a professional identity (Sargent, Corey, Cory, & Callanan, 1998; Welfel, 1998). Other purposes include providing criteria for evaluating the ethics of a professional's practice and serving as a benchmark in the enforcement of ethical standards (Kenyon, 1999).

Ethical codes do have limitations; they cannot cover every situation. They do, however, present a framework for ethical behavior, although their

Table 3.7   Workplace Health Promotion Professional Codes of Ethics

Society for Human Resource Management
http://www.shrm.org/hrdisciplines/ethics/Pages/default.aspx

American College of Sport Medicine
www.acsm.org/join-acsm/membership-resources/code-of-ethics

National Association of Nutrition Professionals
http://nanp.org/code-of-ethics

American Psychological Association
http://www.apa.org/ethics/code/index.aspx

American College of Occupational and Environmental Medicine
http://www.acoem.org/codeofconduct.aspx

Certified Health Educators Specialist
http://www.nchec.org/credentialing/ethics

exact interpretation will depend on the situation to which they are being applied. As a result of this vagueness, codes may have a limited range, and some codes of ethics will likely conflict with others regarding some standards of behavior. Such conflicts pose problems for professionals who are members of more than one professional organization.

The third action for workplace health promotion programs is to be culturally competent: to facilitate employees' access to and engagement with the goal of eliminating health disparities and promoting health equity. Actions and activities are required that honor the workers' autonomy, including their right to retain their own cultural orientation in regard to their health. At the same time, each organization has its values and ways of doing things, its own culture. These assumptions of organizations and staff sometimes create challenges for a program that aims to be culturally competent. Examples of program ideas and actions that may get in the way include the following:

- People who ask for help must be on time.

- Eye contact from the person seeking help is desirable.

- Technology is useful and not to be feared.

- Paperwork is essential.

- Staff should be distant and uninvolved with service recipients or applicants.

- All programs are suitable for all employees.

- Everyone should be treated exactly the same.

* Employees seeking help should follow our rules.

* The causes of problems are logical and rational.

* Experts know what is best for persons who ask for help.

* Drop-in care is impossible.

* Formal settings such as the workplace, hospitals, and clinics are the best places in which to provide care.

* Visiting hours in institutions should be limited.

* Medication is good.

* Mental health problems can be dealt with by strangers.

* People should be responsible for paying for their health care.

Culturally competent workplace health promotion programs are not designed with the notion that "one size fits all"; rather, such programs offer a variety of alternatives and options to fit a variety of people. Workers have access to as much choice as possible in a culturally competent organization. In addition, culturally competent programs realize and acknowledge that society has not always been fair to everyone and that oppression and discrimination are real. Culturally competent programs have as an underlying philosophy that each and every person deserves dignity and has value. An organization that wants to establish a culturally competent workplace health promotion program should consider three critical points: (1) Long before an individual becomes part of a workplace, his or her health (physical and mental) has an established history; (2) workplaces, neighborhoods, and homes shouldn't be hazardous to a person's health; (3) employees need to have the opportunity to make the choices that allow them to live a long, healthy life, regardless of their income, education, or ethnic background (Robert Wood Johnson Foundation, 2009).

The following list includes six questions for organizations that want to assess their workplace health promotion programs and reflect upon the quality of their culturally competent practices.

Questions an Organization Should Ask When Assessing and Reflecting Upon Attempts to Be Culturally Competent

1. How do staff, volunteers, and leadership represent the diverse population served by the organization?

2. Do youth and families genuinely have a voice in program and service planning and implementation?

3. Is there outreach to populations who may be underserved or may not feel welcome or safe in approaching the organization?

4. Are programs and services offered in neighborhoods and communities that are underserved or most greatly affected, and if that is not possible, are connections made and networks built with local religious communities or businesses?

5. Is the organization linguistically culturally competent?

6. Does the organization aggressively advocate for the rights of all youth and families who are affected by the social problems (i.e., social determinants) of concern within the school community?

Finally, workplace health promotion programs need to be aligned with the vision of the human resource department and the wider organization. The fourth human resource management action required is twofold: to keep health as part of all organizational leadership decisions; and to remain visible, dedicated, and alert to the promotion of health at the workplace while being cognizant of individual, organizational, and environmental influences.

In keeping health promotion as part of the organizational vision, each workplace health promotion program reflects a unique mix of health priorities spread across six priority health domains specified by the Healthy People 2020 initiative: physical health, mental and behavioral health, physical activity, nutrition, physically and psychologically safe and healthy environment, and health education in an eHealth environment with practices supported by electronic processes and communications (U.S. Department of Health and Human Services, 2015). The health priorities identified as part of the program planning process (and used as well to build the program) are key to health being aligned and visible within the organizational goals.

Workplace Health Promotion Program Priority Health Domains (U.S. Department of Health and Human Services, 2015)

*   Physical health

*   Mental and behavioral health

*   Physical activity

*   Nutrition

*   Physically and psychologically safe and healthy environment

*   Health education in an eHealth environment

Summary

Human resource management is the gatekeeper for workplace health promotion. Human resource management is increasingly becoming known as strategic human resource management, which systematically links the needs of an organization and aims to provide it with an effective workforce while meeting the needs of its members and other constituents in the society. Many of the human resource management professions with their distinct career pathways, positions, and professional organizations are involved with addressing employees' health needs. Health insurance offered through the employer organization or Health Exchanges (Marketplace) will impact how an organization addresses employee health. Four human resource management actions are key to quality health promotion programs: knowing employee program perceptions, establishing and following codes of ethics, achieving cultural competency, and keeping the workplace health promotion program priorities aligned (visible) with the overall organization's goals and strategic human resource management.

For Practice and Discussion

1. Explore the management approach section of the Johnson & Johnson Corporation website (http://www.jnj.com/about-jnj/management-approach). How does the corporation's approach to its workforce impact the employees' health and the workplace environment?

2. Many different types of human resource positions work in the area of employee health and safety (including benefits, workers' compensation, disability, retirement). How do you determine what positions might be most important for employee health promotion in any given organization?

3. Investigate the workplace health promotion program options as part of the health insurance coverage offered through the Health Exchange/Marketplace website (https://www.healthcare.gov/). Compare and contrast the options. What are implications of the options for midsized and small organizations that want to promote the health of their employees and employee family members?

4. Imagine you're a member of a local fitness club that has contracts with several employers in your area to provide health screening and physical activity programs. The fitness club director has offered you a free one-year club membership if you help the fitness club to secure a contract with the software company where you are employed as director of the human resource department. The fitness director is

willing to identify health risks of individual employees to help you tailor and fit programs to specific employees, which will help you lower health care costs for your organization. What are potential ethical issues with such an incentive? What are your options?

5. Culturally competent workplace health promotion programs are not designed with the notion that one size fits all; rather, such programs offer a variety of alternatives and options to fit a variety of people. Culturally competent workplace health promotion programs have as an underlying philosophy that each and every person deserves dignity and has value. What are ways that a workplace health promotion program can be culturally sensitive and respectful?

Case Study: Strategic Human Resource Management—What Would You Do?

Jon Graham, Vice President for Strategic Human Resources, talks fondly about the 1980s when he worked in the personnel office. He shares, "I did it all: hiring, suspending, and firing employees; processing and distributing paychecks; keeping track of sick days and vacation days. I enrolled the employees in benefit plans. What I did was merely administrative and nothing more." Today Graham is responsible for his company's strategic human resource department. His charge is to transform the department to become more than what is called *transactional*; his job is to make the HR department play a bigger role in the strategic direction of the organization. For example, his team put in place a global health resources information system and a workplace health promotion program. Not only did the successful implementation of both change the role and responsibilities of the human resource organization, but it also added value to the company. It helped transform the organization from one with slow-moving functional silos into a high-performance company. The human resource decisions were a key element in this transformation. It is clear that the members of the strategic human resource department were a driver of this change. They did not simply implement someone else's plan. They created the plan. They were the plan leaders.

If you were Jon Graham, knowing the global health resources information system and workplace health promotion program changed the role of human resources within the organization, what would you do to sustain and build on this change?

KEY TERMS

Human resource management	HMO
Strategic human resource management	Deductible
Human resource department	Coinsurance
Human resource activities	Premium
Human resource professionals	Copayment
Society for Human Resource Management	Employer-offered health insurance
Human Resource Competency Study	Health Insurance Marketplace (Exchanges)
Insurance companies (Providers)	Individual/private insurance
Agent	Employee voice
Broker	Codes of ethics
Indemnity	Cultural competence
HAS	Workplace health priorities
PPO	Workplace health priority alignment
POS	

References

Kenyon, P. (1999). *What would you do? An ethical case workbook for human service professionals.* Pacific Grove, CA: Brooks/Cole.

National Committee for Quality Assurance. (2014). *NCQA health insurance plan ratings methodology: April 2014.* Retrieved from http://www.ncqa.org /Portals/0/Report%20Cards/Rankings/HPR_Rankings_MethodologyOverview _Final.pdf

RBL Group & Michigan Ross School of Business. (2012). Human Resource Competency Study. Retrieved from http://hrcs.rbl.net/hrcs/index/history

Robert Wood Johnson Foundation (2009, April). *Beyond health care: New directions to a healthier America.* Retrieved from http://www.rwjf.org/content /dam/farm/reports/reports/2009/rwjf40483

Sargent, J.-A., Corey, G., Cory, M., & Callanan, P. (1998). Issues and ethics in the helping professions. *Canadian Journal of Counselling and Psychotherapy/Revue (canadienne de counseling et de psychothérapie, 32*(4).

Schwind, H., Das, H., Wagar, T., Fassina, N., & Bulmash, J. (2013). Canadian human resource management: A strategic approach. Ontario, Canada: McGraw-Hill Ryerson.

U.S. Department of Health and Human Services, Office of Disease Prevention and Health Promotion. (2015). *Healthy People 2020.* Retrieved from http://www.healthypeople.gov/2020/default.aspx

Welfel, E. R. (1998). *Ethics in counseling and psychotherapy: Standards, research, and emerging issues.* Pacific Grove, CA: Brooks/Cole.

PART TWO

PLANNING

CHAPTER 4

PROGRAM PLANNING AND INITIAL ACTIONS

Workplace Health Promotion Program Planning Elements and Management

Workplace health promotion program planning is a series of decisions, from general and strategic decisions to specific operational details, based on the gathering and analysis of a wide range of information. The decisions made as part of planning determine the program implementation and evaluation. Planning creates the program foundation and structure.

In planning a workplace health promotion program we manage a number of elements, including:

- Meaningful participation of key stakeholders
- Time
- Money and other resources
- Data gathering and interpretation
- Consideration of the role of health promotion approaches, theories, and models
- Decision making
- Planning tools

When these elements are managed well, program outcomes may be greater than expected. If not managed well, problems are likely to occur. Participation by stakeholder groups (i.e., employers and employees) is critical to achieving the best results—a lack of participation may lead to decisions being overruled, delayed, challenged, or questioned by either internal or external stakeholders. Mismanagement of time and missed deadlines can result in lost opportunities, decreased impact of the program,

LEARNING OBJECTIVES

- Describe the planning process and management of workplace health promotion programs
- Explain decision making involved in workplace health promotion program planning
- Define *needs assessment* and explain its relevance to workplace health promotion programs
- Discuss workplace health readiness
- Discuss workplace capacity for health

and greater stresses. Poor management of budgets and other resources may lead to unanticipated costs and even an inability to implement the program. Ill-informed decisions result from misleading, weak, or incomplete information and data. Health approaches, theories, and models ground the programs; without them we do not know why our programs succeed and fail. Good decisions take time, creativity, and a supportive climate. Planning tools provide us with the concrete details that need to be known to implement and evaluate the program.

Participation

Much has been written about the importance of meaningful participation in health promotion programs. From the outset identify the key stakeholders (these can include the employer, employees, families, health insurance carriers, and health care providers). Consider their roles (who will be informed, make decisions, provide information, or provide hands-on support). Develop a process for participation. For example, when decisions will be made, by whom, and by what process (e.g., Is consensus required? How will priorities be set?).

In planning, the process is important. Focus on the process of developing a workplace health promotion program, not only on its end result. This includes:

1. Working *with* people, rather than for them
2. Involving employees and employers in the program design
3. Ensuring the employees and employers understand the program implementation
4. Using evaluation tools and strategies that are clear to employees and employers

Time

The time required to plan a workplace program depends on a number of circumstances and variables. In the workplace, because participation is so important, time for program planning is often longer than for other kinds of planning. There are many trade-offs, and the ideal level of desired participation can sometimes be in tension with political and organizational considerations, cost, and other deadlines. What you come up with as a timeline will be a compromise—try to allow for as much time as possible to involve employees and employers appropriately.

Money and Other Resources

It is wise to create an inventory of available resources. This includes allocated budgets: both "above-the-line" cost items for which program-specific funds must be found, and also use of staff time, equipment, and space (already budgeted and therefore "below-the-line" costs). Other resources to be considered include expertise, contributions in kind from partnerships, and collaborations. Forgoing other opportunities with the organization, partners, and the community at large (e.g., collaborations) also creates costs. It is essential to know what these costs and resources are from the outset, and keep reviewing this inventory. Managing time itself means calendar time, a one-way movement through key dates and times. When discussing money and resources, remember that time is also money—every hour spent in the process costs additional resources and money already allocated, as well as the opportunity to make progress on other projects! However, time spent involving people can pay off over the long term with greater support for the program and commitment of resources to complete it.

Data Gathering (Needs Assessment)

Think about where to obtain the information (data) needed to guide planning efforts. Keep in mind that an approach to data gathering (needs assessment) can depend on:

- Seeing health as more than the absence of disease
- Being clear about the role of approaches, theories, and models and examining all determinants of health when assessing needs and designing a program
- Seeing positive directions and capacities of employees, employers (workplaces), and communities, rather than focusing only on problems and deficits
- Looking for ways to collect positive data throughout the planning process

Data is gathered from the employer and employees to make decisions. It is important to always ask why a piece of data is being collected, what question it will be used to answer, and how it will be used to make a decision. Likewise, federal legislation and regulations will guide and influence what data is collected so as to protect individuals' rights and privacy.

Considering the Role of Health Promotion Approaches, Theories, and Models

The health promotion approaches, theories, and models used to collect and interpret data make a difference in planning.

Health promotion approaches, theories, and models all do the same thing. They help address people's health concerns and problems, but they do it in different ways. Choosing an approach, theory, and model depends on a host of factors such as behavioral causes of the health issue or problem, the level of interaction (intrapersonal, interpersonal, or workplace), the priority population, and the desired outcomes or change. Once you decide on which of the approaches, theories, and models to use, you need to apply them to see how they fit.

Each approach, theory, and model makes you look for a different kind of information about your population of interest and suggests a range of different kinds of strategies. Each adds its contribution to the other, so that most health promotion programming is a mixture of approaches, theories, and models.

Decision Making

Decisions have to be made throughout the planning process. It is important to be aware of who has to be involved in decisions, and to know who needs to be consulted and who needs to be kept informed. Fundamentally, as part of the planning process, try to decide how best to proceed and realistically what to expect from the workplace to implement and support any proposed program. The following list includes questions to ask as part of the planning process. Based upon the answers, you can make decisions about how to shape and tailor a program to the workplace.

Planning Process Questions That Shape and Tailor Health Promotion Program Decision Making

1. What is the current status of health promotion effort (i.e., what do they have now)?

2. What are the workplace health-related benefits (e.g., insurance, disability, leave)?

3. What is the motivation for action (i.e., why do they feel the need to do something)?

4. What is the organization's track record in regard to addressing employee issues (e.g., health)?

5. What is the consensus on the program priorities?

6. Who are health program champions and advocates? What is the support of the program?

7. What are the program mission (vision) statement, goals, and objectives?

8. What is the action plan? What do they want to do? What program do they want to create and build?

Planning Tools

Planning tools can provide the concrete details you will need to know to implement and evaluate the program. They will help you to reach consensus (i.e., agreement among the stakeholders) on what the program will be, and help as well to get the program design on paper. In building the program, determine priorities that consider program importance and feasibility (Price, Dake, & Ward, 2010). Create program mission statements, goals, and objectives using techniques such as SMART goals. Make decisions about program components that focus on organizational efforts related to disease management. Select program vendors and service providers for employee wellness (Chen, Sheu, & Chen, 2010). As part of the planning, generate reports that detail program implementation. The reports include logic models and Gantt charts as well as budgets. From these documents an action plan can be prepared to tell the shareholders the program inputs (e.g., staffing, materials, equipment), activities, interventions, goals, timelines, and resources (e.g., funding). Using all of the planning tools, create program snapshots (a program vision) and a step-by-step guide to implement the program (Breny Bontempi, Fagen, & Roe, 2010).

Major Report Headings and Elements for a Program Planning Report to Detail Program Design and Implementation (adapted from Egger, Spark & Donovan, 2004)

Scope

*   Program description
*   Priority populations
*   Key activities and outcomes (disease management, wellness)
*   Interventions (evidence-based)
*   Logic model
*   Rationale (business case)

Key stakeholder (employer and employee)/partners interest and support

*   Partnerships and collaborations
*   Vendors and service providers

Program resources

- Permanent staff
- Consumables
- Budget
- Level of confidence in cost estimates
- Cost implications (return on investment)

Recommendations and decisions

- Action plan
- Policies, procedures, and legal requirements
- Gantt chart

Data Gathering Equals Needs Assessments

Understanding how the health of a group of individuals at a workplace might be improved requires information on both their current health status and their ideal health status. Collection of that information is called a needs assessment. A needs assessment is a formalized approach to collecting data in order to identify the needs of a group of individuals. Workplace health promotion health needs assessments have their roots in public health community needs assessments that focus on individuals living in a specific geographic area such as a city, county, state, or nation. Community needs assessments are developed to understand the etiology of public health problems and to address them through primary, secondary, and tertiary prevention programs (Centers for Disease Control and Prevention [CDC], 1995). Needs assessments reflect the three levels of influence in the ecological health perspective: intrapersonal, interpersonal, and population (McLeroy, Bibeau, Steckler, & Glanz, 1988; Rimer & Glanz, 2005).

Similar to a community health needs assessment, a workplace health program needs assessment consists of four basic steps: (1) determining the scope of the assessment, (2) gathering data, (3) analyzing the data, and (4) reporting the findings. Before you do anything, it is best to think about each one of the steps and map out to the best of your ability what will happen in each step. This is important so that you can explain to employers and employees what they can expect from the process as well as how long it will take to complete the needs assessment.

1. Determine scope. Work with the employers and employees to determine the purpose and scope of the needs assessment. Ask who will be involved and what are the decisions that will be made based on

the needs assessment. Think carefully and critically about what information is needed to make the decisions. Who ultimately will use the results to make decisions about the health programs? Take an ecological approach to the needs assessment.

2. Gather the data. Gather only the needed data. Consider culturally appropriate data gathering approaches tailored to the population and setting. Gather multiple types of data—both quantitative (e.g., health risk assessments) and qualitative (e.g., interviews and focus groups). In the workplace as well as in the community, all data collection and reporting is required to adhere to federal requirements of the Health Insurance Portability and Accountability Act of 1996 (HIPAA) Privacy, Security and Breach Notification Rules and the Patient Safety and Quality Improvement Act of 2005 (PSQIA) Patient Safety Rule (http://www.hhs.gov/ocr/privacy/)

3. Analyze the data. Use clear methods that people can understand.

4. Report and share the findings. Identify your options to share the needs assessment findings. Think about how best to communicate the findings. In sharing the information, identify factors linked to health problems. Validate the need before continuing with the planning process. Tailor all communications to the stakeholders.

Needs assessments use primary and secondary data. Primary data is collected directly from the individual using a range of methods and tools both quantitative (e.g., medical examinations, questionnaires, surveys) and qualitative (e.g., interviews, focus groups, observation). From secondary data, which has been collected by someone for another purpose, you can get the "big" picture of a health problem. Working with secondary data you can view a variety of approaches to defining and analyzing a problem. Secondary data sources of information may be divided into two categories: internal and external. Internal data is collected in the course of an organization's everyday operations. Absenteeism, presenteeism, worker productivity, health care utilization, and workers' compensation claims are some of the data that might be available. The main sources of external secondary health data are government (federal, state, and local), voluntary health associations, private foundations, national and international institutions, professional associations, and universities. These organizations collect the data to monitor and report health concerns and problems, and to develop and refine health policy and programs. Some of the many sources of publicly available health data can be found in Table 4.1.

Workplace health needs assessments start with defined priority populations: employer (organization) and employees. As part of workplace health

Table 4.1   Publicly Available Secondary Health Data Sources

Secondary Data Source	Web Address
Behavioral Risk Factor Surveillance System	http://www.cdc.gov/brfss/technical_infodata/surveydata.htm
Health Care Cost and Utilization Data	http://www.ahrq.gov/data/hcup/
Joint Canada/ United States Survey of Health	http://www.cdc.gov/nchs/about/major/nhis/jcush_mainpage.htm
Longitudinal Studies of Aging	http://www.cdc.gov/nchs/lsoa.htm
Medical Expenditures Panel Survey	http://www.meps.ahrq.gov/mepsweb/data_stats/download_data_files.jsp
National Health and Nutrition Examination Survey	http://www.cdc.gov/nchs/about/major/nhanes/datalink.htm
National Health Interview Survey Occupational Health Supplement	http://www.cdc.gov/niosh/topics/nhis/
National Hospital Discharge Survey	http://www.cdc.gov/nchs/about/major/hdasd/nhds.htm
National Survey of Family Growth	http://www.cdc.gov/nchs/NSFG.htm
Surveillance Epidemiology and End Results Program	http://seer.cancer.gov/data/access.html

promotion program planning, data is collected from both the employer and employee (Figure 4.1). The first information collected is gathered about and from the employer (organization), seen at the top of Figure 4.1. This information in turn sets the parameters for the information gathered about the employees. The initial organizational information focuses on workplace health readiness and capacity for health. Next we focus on the organization's champions and advocates for workplace health, the climate and culture to promote employee health, the legal issues in health policies and procedures, and the workplace health promotion teams, partnerships, and collaborations. Employee data sources shown at the bottom of Figure 4.1 may include but not be limited to demographic profiles, health status (health records), health risk assessment (HRA), biometric screening, workers' compensation and disability claims and costs, medical care claims (service utilization) and costs, pharmacy claims and costs, absenteeism, and employee assistance participation. Evaluation results (process, impact, outcome) from current workplace health priority program practices, interventions, and services can be considered. As part of planning, the information is integrated and analyzed to create the program action plan, which is shown at the center of Figure 4.1. Included in the plan are the program health priorities, mission statement, goals, objectives, logic model, Gantt chart, and budget.

In large and midsized organizations the health insurance provider data is a primary data source for workplace health promotion programs. The data is collected directly from the employee using HRAs, health records,

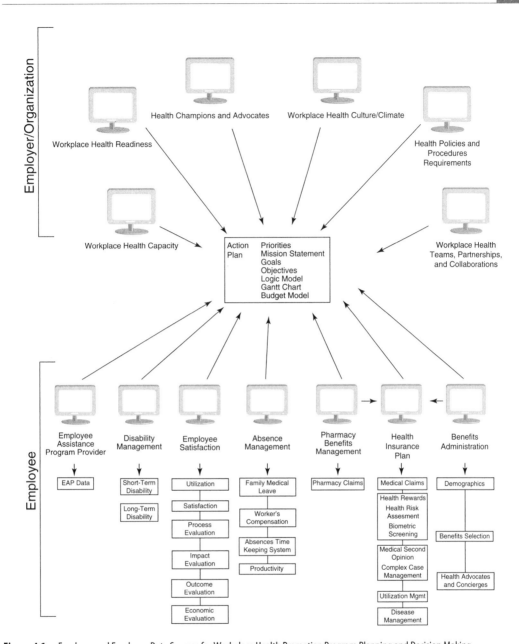

Figure 4.1   Employer and Employee Data Sources for Workplace Health Promotion Program Planning and Decision Making

biometric screenings, medical claims, and service utilization. Likewise the health insurance providers and program vendors are the secondary data sources. The secondary data consists of the everyday information collection that occurs as part of health care service delivery (e.g., health care utilization, prescriptions). Both primary and secondary data are collected for the individual employee (and family members, depending on coverage) but reported in the aggregate with no personally identifiable information. Other sources of workplace health data incorporated into needs assessment may include employee disability (short and long term) and OSHA data legally required and reported.

Workplace needs assessment data does not need to be (and is not) limited to only health insurance–driven data sources. Community-wide data sources are also considered, especially the secondary data sources. Furthermore for small organizations data sources may be limited to only the community assessments. For example, migrants and low-wage employees often rely upon community-based health services offered at federally qualified health centers, public health agencies, and local human service organizations (e.g., health clinics, community-based agencies, and community health services and programs). For this population these local organizations may use their data to identify and assess health needs for a population that can be addressed at the workplace.

Workplace Health Readiness

The first data collected as part of planning is the state of the organization's workplace health readiness. In talking with leaders and executives of businesses, large organizations, schools, universities, government offices, and health care institutions (and including small and midsized businesses and organizations), it becomes clear that they are concerned about the impact that employee illness, chronic poor health, low job satisfaction, and turnover have on productivity and contribution to lost company earnings. Likewise it becomes clear that what workplaces are willing, able, and ready to do to address employee health varies. In other words, differences are found in workplace health readiness: a workplace's expertise and experience necessary to successfully impact employee health (Change Agent Work Group, 2009).

Size of a workplace matters when assessing readiness as far as potential resources and level of program sophistication, but it is not a foregone conclusion that size determines program effectiveness to address employee health needs. For example, the health promotion program outcomes of small workplaces can be equal to those found in large organizations when small workplaces form community partnerships and are part of collaborations (Partnership for Prevention, 2011).

Workplace health readiness is a continuum, meaning a line from one end to the other (see the following list). The early phases relate to the awareness and the necessity to address employee health needs. The later phase involves being more appropriate and responsive to employee health needs. For some organizations employee health is not a priority. This is not to say that the organization is unaware of the need to address employee health but rather that organizational resources and supports for employee health are placed in other areas. This is most common in new, small, and entrepreneurial workplaces focused on survivability and sustainability.

Workplace Health Readiness Continuum

1. Not a priority: The workplace resources and supports are placed or utilized in areas other than employee health.

2. Awareness: The workplace has a basic understanding of the need to change its approach to employee health.

3. Transition: The workplace is in a transition, beginning to facilitate and engage in activities that impact employee health.

4. Integrated: The workplace has a fully integrated employer health promotion program strategy.

Table 4.2 defines five elements that can be used to assess a workplace's health readiness at each continuum point. It is expected that the particular phase of readiness will vary over time as a workplace progresses to address employee health.

Each of the elements can be further delineated at each point in the continuum. For example, Table 4.3 shows greater detail as to what might be expected in relation to diagnostics, informatics, and health metrics at each phase.

Another aspect of organizational health readiness is employee benefit availability, including health insurance coverage options, disability, and leave, all of which play a role in shaping workplace health promotion programs. If health insurance is available, it is important to know if a workplace is fully or self-insured. The general underwriting rule is that it becomes an advantage to self-fund if an employer has 1,000 employees or more. Under self-insured plans, employers also eliminate costs associated with broker fees and state insurance premiums and commission taxes. They might avoid compliance with state-mandated benefits regulations and federal Employee Retirement Income Security Act (ERISA) regulations. Often, too, employers gain more control and freedom over plan design. Fully insured plans offer predictability and safety—albeit at a cost—and as the size of an organization increases the benefits of self-insured plans are attractive (Sammer, 2011). Even though self-insured plans state that they

Table 4.2   Workplace Health Readiness Elements (adapted from Change Agent Work Group, 2009)

Elements	Not a Priority	Awareness	Transition	Integrated
1. Vision for health	Resources and supports for employee health are not available	Focuses on reducing short-term health care costs	Transitions to health management with limited goals	Focuses on employer health asset management and business outcomes with explicit goals
2. Management participation and commitment	Focus on other priorities	Limited to human resources and benefits managers	Some involvement beyond human resources with accountability defined by specific initiatives	Senior leadership responsible for ensuring the workforce is healthy
3. Workplace policies and the work environment	Minimal health and safety compliance	No wellness goals	Initial, "easy" changes to policy and work environment	Policies and work environment fully support wellness goals
4. Diagnostics, informatics, and health metrics	None	A few basic metrics reported annually	Demographics and disease burden analyzed; analysis drives programs on a limited basis	Health policies and initiatives fully linked to demographics and disease burden; periodic, regular review of metrics; all metrics have goals
5. Health goals and program elements	Individual employee responsibility	A few programs with little or no integration	More sophisticated program elements and some integration	Full suite of integrated programs using state-of-the-art techniques

cover all risks, an employer typically does not assume 100% of the risk for catastrophic claims. Rather, the employer buys a form of insurance known as stop-loss or excess-loss insurance to reimburse the employer for claims that exceed a predetermined level. This coverage can be purchased to cover catastrophic claims on one covered person (specific coverage) or to cover claims that significantly exceed the expected level for the group of covered persons (aggregate coverage).

Employers that offer health insurance benefits finance those benefits in one of two ways: either they purchase health insurance from an insurance company (fully insured plans), or they provide health benefits directly to employees (self-insured plans).

Typically, these plans differ by the factors shown in the following list.

Table 4.3   Workplace Health Readiness Element Transition Related to Diagnostics, Informatics, and Health Metrics (adapted from Change Agent Work Group, 2009)

Not a Priority	Awareness	Transition	Integrated
Resources and supports for employee health metrics collection are not available.	Organization administers HRAs, but not subject to schedule. A few basic metrics around major diagnostic categories, cost, and participation are reported periodically. Demographics and disease burden have not been analyzed.	HRAs are administered every two to three years to all employees; family members may be included, too. Demographics and disease burden are understood and drive programmatic initiatives on a limited basis. Some additional metrics that are leading indicators of cost and changes in population health status are reported, a few with goals.	HRAs are completed annually on employees and family members. The organization offers strong incentives for biometric testing and communicates its value to employees. Health policies and initiatives are fully linked to demographics, risk factors, and disease burden. Comprehensive metrics, including those tracking the total value of health, are reported periodically, all with goals.
		Organization has only limited measurements of the value added by investments in health. Selected health elements are included in strategic business activities.	Organization insists on credible measurement of the value added by investments in health, including specific improvements in biometric results, shifts in health risks, and utilization gaps according to evidence-based medicine. All health elements are included in major strategic business activities.
		Organization monitors participation and outcomes metrics to track changes in the population health status.	In addition to monitoring participation and change metrics, organization has metrics for risk and cost tracking of the total value of health.
		Modeling tools are used to estimate impact of health-related lost time on productivity and to identify medical conditions affecting the workforce. This information is used to create a health and productivity business case.	Comprehensive self-report surveys are conducted to identify the impact of lost time on productivity and to identify which medical conditions would benefit from interventions.

Fully Insured and Self-Insured Workplace Comparisons—Who Assumes the Insurance Risk, and What the Plan Characteristics, Employer Size, and Market Share Are (Employee Benefit Research Institute, 2009)

Fully Insured Plans

Risk: In a fully insured plan, the employer pays a per-employee premium to an insurance company, and the insurance company assumes the risk of providing health coverage for insured events.

Plan characteristics: In fully insured arrangements, premiums vary across employers based on employer size, employee population characteristics, and health care use. Premiums can also change over time within the same employer because of changes in the demographics of the employed group. However, employers are charged the same premium for each employee.

Employer size: Small employers that offer health benefits are typically fully insured. In 2008, 88% of workers in firms with 3–199 employees were in fully insured plans. Smaller firms are typically located in one office or region (if they are on the large side of small).

Market share: Overall, 45% of workers with health insurance were covered by a fully insured plan in 2008.

Self-Insured Plans

Risk: In a self-insured plan, instead of purchasing health insurance from an insurance company and paying the insurer a per-employee premium, the employer acts as its own insurer. In the simplest form, the employer uses the money that it would have paid the insurance company and instead directly pays health care claims to providers. Self-insured plans often contract with an insurance company or other third party to administer the plan, but the employer bears the risk associated with offering health benefits.

Plan characteristics: Large employers often offer multiple self-insured health plans to different classes of workers. Benefits may vary for management and labor, and benefits may vary by occupation or even hours of work. Even when an employer offers a uniform benefits program across all locations and geographic regions, the cost of providing the program—commonly known as the premium equivalent—will vary because the cost of health care services is not uniform across the United States.

Employer size: In 2008, 89% of workers employed in firms with 5,000 or more employees were in self-insured plans.

Market share: Overall, 55% of workers with health insurance were covered by a self-insured plan in 2008.

Understanding workplace readiness influences the program plan and implementation. It provides a context for a workplace's effort to address employees' health. It is the starting point from which to build the program. Readiness evolves and progresses. An organization travels along the health readiness continuum in a journey of incremental steps that will yield incremental successes.

Workplace Capacity for Health

Once you know the health readiness of a workplace, focus next on the workplace capacity for health to determine what resources are available in the workplace to address identified health concerns and problems—for example, health promotion materials, technology (computers, software packages, Internet access, websites, and so on), staff, programs, funding, and services—as well as the gaps and needs in these areas (Gilmore & Campbell, 2005). A key element of a workplace capacity for health assessment is the engagement of potential program participants (employees), employers, and stakeholders (e.g., shareholders, community members, family members) to mobilize forces to address and solve the health problems or concerns identified in the needs assessment.

The areas covered by the assessments can be quite broad. For example, they might include policies; procedures; health services and health promotion resources (e.g., staff, space, materials, technology, and funding); service gaps and linkages; networks; health insurance and benefits; legal requirements and compliance; and accreditations. Furthermore the assessments might cover an organization's experience and lessons learned from its own growth and development incorporating change and trying new initiatives such as a health promotion program (Senge, 1990). Assessing the capacity of a workplace to operate and support a health promotion program provides early insight into the culture and climate of a setting (Moos, 1979). Finally, other often-assessed areas include relationships that support health; opportunities to promote personal health for everyone at the site; and support systems for and barriers to implementation of the program.

The following are a sample of the growing number of available health capacity assessment tools from varied sources that are widely used.

CDC Worksite Health ScoreCard (http://www.cdc.gov/dhdsp/pubs /docs/HSC_Manual.pdf)

The CDC Worksite Health ScoreCard (HSC) is a tool designed to help employers assess whether they have implemented evidence-based health promotion interventions or strategies in their workplace to prevent heart disease, stroke, and related conditions such as hypertension, diabetes, and obesity (CDC, 2014). The tool contains 125 questions that assess how evidence-based health promotion strategies are implemented at worksites. The scorecard surveys employers in 16 areas including organizational supports (18 questions), tobacco control (10 questions), nutrition (13 questions), lactation support (6 questions), physical activity (9 questions), weight management (5 questions), stress management (6 questions), and depression (7 questions). Figure 4.2 shows questions from the organization support area. Employers use this tool to assess how a comprehensive health promotion and disease prevention program is offered to their employees, to help identify program gaps, and to decide the health program priority areas.

School Health Index

School Health Index: A Self-Assessment and Planning Guide was developed by the National Center for Chronic Disease Prevention and Health Promotion (CDC, 2012) in partnership with school administrators and staff, school health experts, parents, and national nongovernmental health and education agencies for the purposes of:

• Enabling schools to identify strengths and weaknesses of health and safety policies and programs

• Enabling schools to develop an action plan for improving student health, which can be incorporated into the school improvement plan

• Engaging teachers, parents, students, and the community in promoting health-enhancing behaviors and better health

The School Health Index has two activities that are completed by teams from a school: the eight self-assessment modules and a planning for improvement process. The self-assessment process involves members of the school community coming together to discuss what the school is already doing to promote good health

The CDC Worksite Health ScoreCard:

An Assessment Tool to Prevent Heart Disease, Stroke, and Related Conditions Worksheet

Organizational Supports

Organizational Supports During the past 12 months, did your worksite:	Yes	No	Score
1. Conduct an employee needs and interests assessment for planning health promotion activities? *Answer "yes" if, for example, your organization administers focus groups or employee satisfaction surveys to assess your employee health promotion program(s). Answer "no" if your organization administers general surveys that do not assess your employee health promotion program(s).*	☐ (1 pt.)	☐ (0 pts.)	
2. Conduct employee health risk appraisals/assessments through vendors, on-site staff, or health plans and provide individual feedback plus health education? *Answer "yes" if, for example, your organization provides individual feedback through written reports, letters, or one-on-one counseling.*	☐ (3 pts.)	☐ (0 pts.)	
3. Demonstrate organizational commitment and support of worksite health promotion at all levels of management? *Answer "yes" if, for example, all levels of management participate in activities, communications are sent to employees from senior leaders, the worksite supports performance objectives related to healthy workforce, or program ownership is shared with all staff levels.*	☐ (2 pts.)	☐ (0 pts.)	
4. Use and combine incentives with other strategies to increase participation in health promotion programs? *Answer "yes" if, for example, your organization offers incentives such as gift certificates, cash, paid time off, product or service discounts, reduced health insurance premiums, employee recognition, or prizes.*	☐ (2 pts.)	☐ (0 pts.)	
5. Use competitions when combined with additional interventions to support employees making behavior changes? *Answer "yes" if, for example, your organization offers walking or weight loss competitions.*	☐ (2 pts.)	☐ (0 pts.)	

Figure 4.2   CDC Worksite Health ScoreCard Organizational Support Question Sample
Source: Centers for Disease Control and Prevention, 2014.

and to identify strengths and weaknesses. The School Health Index assesses the extent to which a school implements the types of policies and practices recommended by the CDC in their research-based guidelines for school health and safety policies and programs.

Heart Check (http://www.health.ny.gov/diseases/cardiovascular/heart _disease/docs/heartcheck.pdf)

The Heart Check Scoring Sheet survey provided by the New York State Department of Health's Healthy Heart Program assesses how well a workplace environment supports a variety of health behaviors (New York State Department of Health, 2013). The Healthy Heart Program (HHP) works to reduce cardiovascular disease, illness, and death by making it easier for people to engage in healthy behaviors. The 250-question Heart Check survey looks at the ways in which a workplace environment supports employee wellness and healthy living. It asks questions and gathers information about workplace smoking policies, nutritional support, and physical activity opportunities available through the employer, and considers the organization's administrative ability—or "readiness"—to support workplace-based wellness programs. Stress reduction and health screening testing are also part of the survey.

Checklist of Health Promotion Environments at Worksites

The Checklist of Health Promotion Environments at Worksites (CHEW) was designed as a direct observation instrument to assess characteristics of worksite environments that are known to influence health-related behaviors (Oldenburg, Sallis, Harris, & Owen, 2002). The CHEW is a 112-item checklist of workplace environmental features hypothesized to be associated, either positively or negatively, with physical activity, healthy eating, alcohol consumption, and smoking. The three environmental domains assessed are (1) physical characteristics of the worksite, (2) features of the information environment, and (3) characteristics of the immediate neighborhood around the workplace.

Designing Healthier Environments at Work Assessment Tool
(http://mihealthtools.org/work/)

This online assessment developed by the Michigan Department of Community Health's Cardiovascular Health, Nutrition and Physical Activity Section helps organizations determine ways to create a healthier work environment—one that supports employees in moving more, eating better, and leading a tobacco-free lifestyle (State of Michigan, 2014). At the site are five different tools that can be used together or separately depending on the workplace. The five are:

1. An assessment tool to identify changes your worksite can make to support health

2. A feedback report with suggestions for improvement

3. An action planning tool that allows you to choose the improvements you want to make and to document progress and completion

4. Survey tools to capture employee interests and feedback; and

5. A success story tool to document and share your worksite's achievements

Safety and Health Management Systems eTool

The Safety and Health Management eTool (Occupational Safety & Health Administration, n.d.-a) is used as part of a four-component approach for small and midsized employers to assess their capacity for health and safety. The four components are management commitment and employee involvement, workplace analysis, hazard prevention and control, and training for employees, supervisors and managers. Figure 4.3 shows the action areas for each component.

HERO EHM Best Practice Scorecard (http://www.the-hero.org /index.html)

HERO was established to create and disseminate Employee Health Management (EHM) research, policy, leadership, and infrastructure to advance the principles, science, and practice of EHM. The HERO Employee Health Management (EHM) Best Practices Scorecard is designed to help employers, providers, and other stakeholders learn about and determine EHM best practices (Mercer, 2014). Earlier versions of the Scorecard were available in 2006, with Version 4 launched in 2014. The online Scorecard questionnaire is divided into six sections representing the foundational components that support exemplary employee health management programs. While no inventory of best practices will include all innovative approaches to EHM, the HERO Scorecard includes those most commonly recognized by industry thought leaders and in published literature.

Employers answer detailed questions about their EHM program design, administration and experience. Results are analyzed and reported by section. The report also includes the average score for all respondents nationally and for three employer "sizes" so that employers may compare themselves to a peer group. The Scorecard also includes a separate section on program outcomes. Responses in this section do not contribute to an organization's best practice score, but are used for benchmarking and to study relationships between specific best practices and outcomes.

Management Commitment and Employee Involvement

☐ Develop and communicate a safety and health policy to all employees.

☐ Demonstrate management commitment by instilling accountability for safety and health, obeying safety rules and reviewing accident reports.

☐ Conduct regular safety and health meetings involving employees, managers and supervisors.

☐ Assign responsible person(s) to coordinate safety and health activities.

☐ Integrate safety and health into business practices (e.g., purchases, contracts, design, and development).

☐ Involve employees in safety and health-related activities (e.g., self-inspections, accident investigations, and developing safe practices).

☐ Recognize employees for safe and healthful work practices.

Worksite Analysis

☐ Evaluate all workplace activities and processes for hazards.

☐ Reevaluate workplace activities when there are changes in:

☐ Processes ☐ Materials ☐ Machinery

☐ Conduct on-site inspections, identify hazards, and take corrective actions.

☐ Provide a hazard reporting system for employees to report unsafe and unhealthful conditions.

☐ Investigate all accidents and near misses to determine their root causes.

Hazard Prevention and Control

☐ Eliminate and control workplace hazards (e.g., engineering controls, workstation design, and work practices).

☐ Establish a preventive maintenance program.

☐ Keep employees informed of safety and health activities and conditions.

☐ Plan for emergencies (e.g., create an evacuation plan, train employees, and conduct fire drills).

☐ Record and analyze occupational injuries and illnesses.

Training for Employees, Supervisors and Managers

☐ Provide training on specific safe work practices before an employee begins work.

☐ Provide additional training for new work processes and when accidents and near misses occur.

☐ Provide refresher training on a routine basis.

Figure 4.3 Safety and Health Management eTool Action Areas for Each Component

Source: Occupational Safety & Health Administration (n.d.-a).

National Committee for Quality Assurance Wellness & Health Promotion Accreditation (http://www.ncqa.org/Programs/Accreditation/WHPAccreditation.aspx)

The National Committee for Quality Assurance (NCQA) is a private, 501(c)(3) not-for-profit organization dedicated to improving health care quality. Since its founding in 1990, NCQA has been a central figure in driving improvement throughout the health care system, helping to elevate the issue of health care quality to the top of the national agenda. NCQA Wellness & Health

Promotion (WHP) Accreditation is a comprehensive assessment of full-service wellness providers (NCQA, n.d.). WHP accreditation helps employers get their money's worth when selecting wellness providers by identifying vendors that are most likely to deliver on employers' priorities, such as improving workforce health and reducing absenteeism. WHP evaluations assess: (1) wellness program implementation; (2) services to empower participants to boost their health; and (3) private health information protection. The accreditation program aligns with the Affordable Care Act.

Summary

Workplace health promotion program planning is a series of decisions, from general and strategic decisions to setting forth specific operational details, based on the gathering and analysis of a wide range of information. The decisions made as part of planning determine the program implementation and evaluation. Planning creates the program foundation and structure. It is the process for designing and building the program. Planning a workplace health promotion program requires the managing of a number of elements, including meaningful participation of key stakeholders, time, money and other resources, data gathering and interpretation, considering the role of health promotion approaches, theories, and models, and decision making. The information (data) comes from the organization (employer) and employees. The first information collected is gathered about and from the organization. This information in turn sets the parameters for the information gathered about the employees. The initial information (data) collected as part of the planning process focuses on workplace health readiness and workplace capacity for health.

For Practice and Discussion

1. As you enter into planning a workplace health promotion program, how do you best manage the planning elements in the planning process?

2. Figure 4.1 illustrates data sources for information you can use to make decisions about a workplace health promotion program. List the data sources and propose potential decisions that might be made using them. Compare and contrast the data sources, information, and potential questions.

3. Using the health readiness continuum propose an algorithm (formula) to determine organizational health readiness. How might workplace

variables such as size, employee population, product, and location impact the algorithm?

4. With employer self-insured health plans, a company can design efficient and effective benefit programs that fit its budget and its employee needs. Self-insured plans offer a high level of flexibility and customization, allowing businesses to select from an array of benefit plan configurations and administration options. Typically the plans include health providers based on where employees live and availability of primary care providers and specialists; catastrophic intervention programs to manage chronic and severe cases requiring aggressive treatment programs; pharmacy benefit options including formulary prescriptions and mail order options; and stop-loss plans based on risk tolerance. Considering a large business (2,000-plus employees) with locations in six different states discuss why each of these features are recommended and how they might be modified to best fit the employees.

5. Compare and contrast two workplace health capacity tools. How might their implementation vary in small, midsized, and large organizations?

Case Study: Program Planning Needs Assessment Challenges—What Would You Do?

Ashley Largo, the health promotion program coordinator, B.I.G. Manufacturing, needs to figure out what is honestly happening in regard to the employees' health, both from her employer and employee points of view. She says "I try not to waste people's time and energy. Nor do I want to waste the organization's resources and money. There is too little of it to go around." She is aware that she needs to balance input from the employer and employees. Ms. Largo faces three challenges in doing the needs assessment for the workplace health promotion program.

First, the general perception is that the company sets the rules and determines the management, administration, and reporting logistics associated with a needs assessment. The feeling is that because the business is paying for it, the business gets to determine what it covers, what questions are answered, what, how, and when data is collected, and how any reports generated by the needs assessment will be shared as well as used (if at all) to make decisions about the workplace health promotion programs. Second, the employer's tolerance for risk is low. Ms. Largo presented the assessment as a process that is respectful, well thought out, and safe (i.e., it will not cause problems or interfere with business operations). The cost of the needs assessment was not an issue, but rather the business leadership was most concerned about a poorly implemented and executed needs assessment that might create negative outcomes, such as bad publicity, which could hurt business and potentially lose customers and clients, hurt feelings, cause employees to be scared, confidentially broken or trust lost. They were anxious that the needs assessment might hurt production and that a lot of work (lots of staff time and salary) would be required to rebuild trust.

Third, before ever getting to collect data from employees, a lot of work, time, and energy would be required. The employees feel distant from the decisions being made on their behalf in relation to their (employee) health. The reality is that the business leadership makes the decisions about what health plans to offer (e.g., health coverage, leave, disability). The leadership wants employee program participation to lower costs and increase productivity. But the employees believe that they are last to have programmatic input, which is causing resistance and reluctance to participate. This sentiment was well captured by an employee who, when told about the needs assessment, said, "If it helps the company, I am not interested; if it helps me, I am interested."

All of these factors cause Ms. Largo to hesitate to use her business leadership skills to do more related to employee health. The situation has caused an innovative, progressive, and creative organization to be conservative in nature and cautious to take risks with employees' personal lives (i.e., health issues). If you are Ms. Largo, responsible for the workplace health promotion program planning and decision making, and know the importance of shared responsibility among all stakeholders (i.e., employers and employers) to ensure program participation and support, what do you do? How do you proceed with the planning process?

KEY TERMS

Planning

Planning elements

Workplace health readiness

Workplace health readiness continuum

Fully insured

Self-insured

Stop-loss or excess-loss insurance

Workplace capacity for health

Health Ontario Comprehensive Workplace Health Promotion Initiative

CDC Worksite Health ScoreCard

School Health Index

Heart Check

Checklist of Health Promotion Environments at Worksites (CHEW)

Designing Healthier Environments at Work Assessment Tool

Safety and Health Management eTool

HERO EHM Best Practice Scorecard

National Committee for Quality Assurance (NCQA) Wellness & Health Promotion Accreditation

References

Breny Bontempi, J. M., Fagen, M. C., & Roe, K. M. (2010). Implementation tools, program staff and budget. In C. Fertman & D. Allensworth (Eds.), *Health promotion programs: From theory to practice* (pp. 153–175). San Francisco, CA: Jossey-Bass/Wiley.

Centers for Disease Control and Prevention. (1995). *Planned approach to community health: Guide for the local coordinator*. Atlanta, GA: U.S. Department of Health and Human Services, Centers for Disease Control and Prevention, National Center for Chronic Disease Prevention and Health Promotion.

Centers for Disease Control and Prevention. (2012). *School Health Index: A self-assessment and planning guide*. Retrieved from http://www.cdc.gov /healthyyouth/shi/

Centers for Disease Control and Prevention. (2014). *Health ScoreCard Manual*. Retrieved from http://www.cdc.gov/dhdsp/pubs/docs/HSC_Manual.pdf

Change Agent Work Group. (2009). *Employer health asset management*. Retrieved from http://www.aon.com/attachments/improving_health.pdf

Chen, W. W., Sheu, J.-J., & Chen, H.-S. (2010). Making decisions to create and support a program. In C. Fertman & D. Allensworth (Eds.), *Health promotion programs: From theory to practice* (pp. 121–150). San Francisco, CA: Jossey-Bass/Wiley.

Egger, G., Spark, R., & Donovan, R. (2004). *Health promotion strategies and methods*. North Ryde, Australia: McGraw-Hill Ryerson.

Employee Benefit Research Institute. (2009, February 11). *Health plan differences: Fully-insured vs. self-insured*. Retrieved from http://www.ebri.org /pdf/ffe114.11feb09.final.pdf

Gilmore, G., & Campbell, M. (2005). *Needs and capacity assessment strategies for health education and health promotion* (3rd ed.). Burlington, MA: Jones & Bartlett.

McLeroy, K. R., Bibeau, D., Steckler, A., & Glanz, K. (1988). An ecological perspective on health promotion programs. *Health Education Quarterly, 15*(4), 351–377.

Mercer. (2014). *The HERO Employee Health Management Best Practices Scorecard in collaboration with Mercer*. Retrieved from http://www.mercer.com /content/dam/mercer/attachments/global/Health/13600-HB_HERO_ Scorecard_Form_NA_FIN1%2010_03_2014.pdf

Moos, R. H. (1979). *Evaluating educational environments: Procedures, measures, findings, and policy implications*. San Francisco, CA: Jossey-Bass.

National Committee for Quality Assurance. (n.d.). *Wellness and health promotion accreditation*. Retrieved May 6, 2015 from http://www.ncqa.org /Programs/Accreditation/WellnessHealthPromotionAccreditation.aspx

New York State Department of Health. (2013). *Heart check: Assessing worksite support for a heart healthy lifestyle*. Retrieved from http://www.health.ny .gov/diseases/cardiovascular/heart_disease/docs/heartcheck.pdf

Occupational Health & Safety Administration. (n.d.-a). *Effective workplace safety and health management systems.* OSHA Fact Sheet. Retrieved May 6, 2015 from https://www.osha.gov/Publications/safety-health-management-systems.pdf

Occupational Health & Safety Health Administration. (n.d.-b). *Safety & health management systems etool.* Retrieved from https://www.osha .gov/SLTC/etools/safetyhealth/index.html

Oldenburg, B., Sallis, J. F., Harris, D., & Owen, N. (2002). Checklist of Health Promotion Environments at Worksites (CHEW): Development and measurement characteristics. *American Journal of Health Promotion, 16*(5), 288–299.

Partnership for Prevention. (2011). *Leading by example.* Retrieved from http://www.prevent.org/data/files/initiatives/lbe_smse_2011_final.pdf

Price, J. H., Dake, J. A., & Ward, B. (2010). Assessing the needs of program participants. In C. I. Fertman & D. D. Allensworth (Eds.), *Health promotion programs: From theory to practice.* San Francisco, CA: Jossey-Bass/Wiley.

Rimer, B., & Glanz, K. (2005). *Theory at a glance. A guide for health promotion practice.* Retrieved from http://www.cancer.gov/cancertopics /cancerlibrary/theory.pdf

Sammer, J. (2011). Is self-insurance for you? *HR Magazine, 56*(5). Retrieved from http://www.shrm.org/publications/hrmagazine/editorialcontent/2011/0511 /pages/0511sammer.aspx

Senge, P. (1990). *The fifth discipline: The art and practice of the learning organization.* New York, NY: Random House.

State of Michigan. (2014). *Designing healthy environments at work.* Retrieved from http://mihealthtools.org/work/

ASSESSING THE STRENGTH OF WORKPLACE HEALTH PROMOTION CHAMPIONS, ADVOCATES, CULTURE, AND CLIMATE

Champions and Advocates for Workplace Health Promotion

As part of the program planning, it is important to identify the organization's champion and advocate for employee health at every level of the organization, from the senior management to the factory floor. Champions know the workplace, health concerns, and problems faced by the employees, employers, and their families. As programs are planned, implemented, and evaluated, champions provide insight into how the many organizations, groups, and individuals (also called stakeholders) involved with promoting health at the workplace interact and work together. They support and help address potential challenges to implementing a program. They know the history of the concerns and problems and what has worked before in solving them, as well as what has not worked. Frequently, champions are called key informants because they know important or key information about an organization.

Advocates fight for resources, time, funding, and space for the program's operations. They build trusting and honest relationships that form the foundation for the work of planning, implementing, and evaluating an effective workplace health promotion program. They know the system—all of the people who have a stake in getting the programs up and running, and those involved in sustaining and expanding existing programs as well as creating and

LEARNING OBJECTIVES

- Identify champions and advocates for workplace health promotion

- Describe a workplace climate and culture to promote employee health

- Explain the importance of health-promoting policies and procedures

- Summarize legal issues in health policies and procedures

adding new ones. They fight for policies that are supportive within the organization and beyond. Talking at department meetings, community meetings, and serving on boards of community organizations are all part of being an advocate. Advocates work to change public legislation at the local and state (maybe even national) levels to protect and promote the health of employees, employers, and their families.

There is no set formula or procedure to locate and identify health champions and advocates. You may already know them, as they are often the individuals involved with past and current workplace efforts. Visiting a company is a good way to observe functioning programs and speak with employees. In the process, you can get a sense of who might be influential in the program implementation and employees' participation. These opinion leaders are key to eventual program diffusion (Locock, Dopson, Chambers, & Gabbay, 2001).

Part of the reason for assessing champions and advocates is to understand who they are working with and their support systems. It is all too easy for one person's commitment and enthusiasm to flag over time, particularly because health concerns and problems are not likely to be considered the workplace's number-one priority. The synergy that results when people work together helps to sustain enthusiasm and support for the effort, even through difficult times. Getting a sense of the breadth and depth of support can provide you a preview of what to expect in terms of realistic organizational actions as well as being a source for ongoing frank discussion and feedback as a program is planned, implemented, and evaluated.

Health Promoting Workplace Culture and Climate

Workplace culture refers to a workplace's persona, which is made up of the attitudes of those within the workplace, as well as how people relate to each other and how they feel about and treat one another (see Box 5.1). Workplace culture reflects the norms of the workplace, what happens within the workplace, and what the people within the workplace care about and pay attention to. Exhibit 5.1 shows a Workplace Culture Survey that employers complete to help them better understand their workplace's culture. Figure 5.1 shows a workplace safety culture survey completed by employees to address the physical safety aspects of workplace health and well-being. Both provide examples of what to consider and expect as you walk through the doors of an organization the first time to talk about a workplace health promotion program (Carroll & Harrison, 1998; O'Reilly & Chatman, 1996; Schein, 1985).

BOX 5.1   FEDEX CULTURE MAKES THE DIFFERENCE (FEDEX, 2015)

There is no magic formula for making employees want to stay, but one common thing companies do is foster a sense that their employees are part of a whole working toward a greater mission. Employers with distinctly different businesses with very different missions are consistent when assessing why people stay. For example in the case of FedEx it is not by accident that the company's people are happy. FedEx Ground has built recognition into the corporate culture with weekly "Bravo Zulu" awards, which derive the name from the naval term for "well done."

The award is an "attaboy" from anyone in the company who feels the recipient has done something noteworthy. It's not the only award given—there are some with money and trips attached—but it is a way of being gracious about work that is, in a term, well done.

And it is no accident that people come first in the company's overriding philosophy of "people, service, profit" because, as a vice president of human resources said, "If you treat your people right, they will give great service, which will generate more business and higher profits that you can reinvest into your people."

The focus on FedEx's people includes training employees for leadership roles and promoting from within. There is also the opportunity for lateral movement so people can expand their skills sets instead of remaining in the same job for their entire careers.

"When people see that FedEx sign or see one of those airplanes, they feel a little bit like 'I'm part of the FedEx family, I'm here making a difference,'"

One FedEx employee, when commenting on why the company is a great place to work, said, "I have freedom to perform and I am allowed to suggest, communicate, and implement change. Of the people I work with day to day, there is opportunity for ongoing education, development, and career growth."

Another stated, "I work for a company that attracts the best people. In turn, this makes my job easier because there are competent people to work with in getting tasks [and] goals accomplished. The job is always challenging because FedEx Ground and its people will always strive to be better [and make] continuous improvement. I've worked for several major transportation companies, and FedEx Ground is the best by far."

A director of human resources said, "The culture behind our business is important: getting behind our people and letting them know that we value what they do."

Knowing the culture of a workplace is the way to discover what is important and valued. You probably cannot find a workplace in which employee health is not a value held by everyone. However, it is one of many values (primarily producing a service, good, or product) that compete for people's time and energy to uphold and champion. Workplace health promotion champions and advocates need to know and respect the other

EXHIBIT 5.1   Workplace Culture Survey (adapted from Association of California School Administrators, 2008)

Directions: Rate each norm/value on the following scale: 1 = Almost always characteristic of our workplace; 2 = Generally characteristic of our workplace; 3 = Seldom characteristic of our workplace; 4 = Not characteristic. For each norm/value, please provide a recent illustrative example of how that norm is demonstrated through individual or organizational behavior.

Norm/Value	Rating	Recent Illustrative Examples
Moral Purpose: The workplace is driven by a commitment to make a positive difference in the lives of employees and their community.		
Professional Community: Commitment to examining practices with a focus on improving employee performance.		
Experimentation: Ongoing professional development with an interest in trying new practices and evaluating the results.		
High Expectations: A pervasive push for high standards-based performance for employees and all staff, using multiple data sources to inform assessments and personnel processes.		
Public Service: Staff understands that their role is to serve the community. Staff respects and honors community values, culture, and contributions.		
Trust and Confidence: A pervasive feeling that people will do what's right between and across groups. No "us vs. them."		
Support for Personal and Professional Growth: Individual coaching and mentoring are pervasive.		
Tangible Support: Financial and material assistance aligned to the goals determined within a cycle of continuous improvement. People have what they need to do their work.		
Reaching Out to the Knowledge Base: Use of research, reading of professional journals, attending workshops.		
Appreciation and Recognition: Acknowledgment of quality employee work and effort.		
Caring, Celebration, Humor: A sense of community with shared purpose and joy. Personal balance and health are values.		

EXHIBIT 5.1   *(Continued)*

Norm/Value	Rating	Recent Illustrative Examples
Appreciation of Leadership: Specifically, leadership provided by supervisors, directors, owners, managers, and other staff.		
Clarity of Goals and Outcomes: There is a coherent vision and action plan tied to measurable goals that employees and employer could articulate and relate to their own work.		
Protection of What's Important: Workplace goals, priorities, and core cultural values.		
Involvement of Stakeholders in Decision Making: Those who will be affected by decisions are involved in making them; diverse points of view are included and honored.		
Traditions: Rituals and events that celebrate and support core workplace and community values.		

values and norms within the workplace, and to show and demonstrate how diverse, distinct norms and values are complementary and synergistic, championing and reflecting a broad, diverse range of values.

Workplace climate describes the quality of everyday life at the workplace and the way people feel inside the workplace, and how these factors affect performance and health. It is what people experience within the workplace. It refers to the sense employees, customers, consumers, and families have of feeling included and appreciated. Workplace climate also refers to the physical and emotional safety of a workplace and how the environment around the workplace affects the workplace itself (Neal, Griffin, & Hart, 2000).

How employees perceive a workplace's climate is measured using surveys that ask people about their experiences in the workplace. For example, employees are asked to indicate how much they agree with the following statements:

"Managers encourage employees to think independently" and "Employees in this workplace respect each other's differences." Surveys for workplace personnel include questions on workplace leadership and professional relationships. Common are questions on issues such as bullying, race, and interpersonal relationships. Likewise the surveys can be used to find out what a workplace's strengths and needs are, and can be used both for needs assessment and to evaluate changes over time. Exhibit 5.2 is an example of an employee climate survey which asks employees about

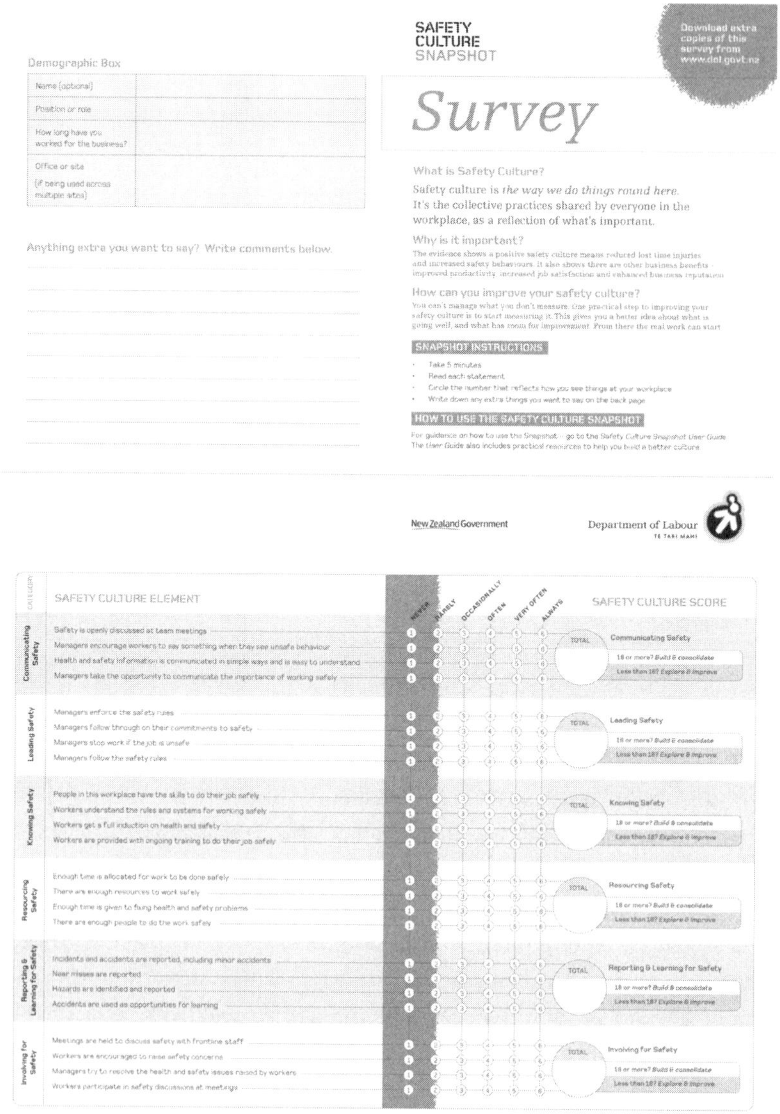

Figure 5.1   New Zealand Safety Culture Snapshot
Source: http://www.osh.govt.nz/index.asp

a number of areas in order to get a sense of the employee's workplace building climate.

Entering a workplace knowing the culture and climate provides a framework for establishing a workplace health promotion program. Being aware of a workplace culture and climate, even before starting to talk about the specifics of the work, provides a sense of how the workplace operates and how its workers might perceive advocates for program implementation.

EXHIBIT 5.2   Workplace Climate Survey

Dear Employee,

We are interested in finding out what you think about health and well-being, that is, your feelings, thoughts, relationships, and behavior. We greatly appreciate your time and effort in completing this survey.

	Strongly Agree	Agree	Disagree	Strongly Disagree	Do Not Know
1. I like coming to my workplace.					
2. I feel safe at my workplace.					
3. I have someone to talk to at my workplace if I need help or advice.					
4. I think the workplace rules are fair.					
5. Our workplace deals fairly and quickly with bullying and harassment problems.					
6. I get information about health and well-being issues.					
7. I learn about different health issues, including health and well-being.					
8. I feel like I belong.					
9. I get to do work that I enjoy and find interesting.					
10. I have friends at my workplace.					
11. I know who to go to if I need help with health and well-being issues.					
13. There are staff members who understand my issues.					
14. My employer shows that the health and well-being of employees is important.					

On the basis of information gathered, judge how hard staff can be challenged to create programs and services, engage employees, families, community members, customers, consumers and employers, as well as to advocate and champion for policies and procedures to promote and protect health and well-being. The following list presents what you might encounter as the consequence of a strong push to promoting health in a workplace culture and climate.

Health-Promoting Workplace Culture and Climate (adapted from Australian Government Department of Health, n.d.)

1. A workplace that promotes health and well-being.

    *   Workplace staff understands the importance of health and well-being, its impact on job performance, and the significant contributions the workplace makes to the improvement of employee health.

2. Respectful relationships, belonging, and inclusion.

    *   Workplace staff expects and model respectful and responsive relationships within the workplace.

    *   Belonging and inclusion for all workplace members is specifically addressed in workplace strategic planning, policies, and practices.

    *   The workplace environment and communication reflects the diversity of the workplace.

    *   Leadership and staff create opportunities for employees, staff, families, and the wider workplace to be involved in a range of activities and contribute to workplace planning.

3. Collaborative working relationships with employer and employees.

    *   Workplace planning, policies, and practices support collaborative working relationships.

    *   Workplace staff implements strategies to proactively develop collaborative working relationships to promote employees' health, well-being, and work performance.

4. Support for employee families.

    *   Workplace staff has knowledge and skills to communicate effectively with family members related health and well-being.

    *   Policies and practices support employees to identify and, where appropriate, facilitate access for family to supportive health resources and services.

5. Understanding health difficulties and improving ways to seek health.

    *   Workplace staff has an understanding of health difficulties, including common signs and symptoms, health problems' impact on employees and families, and factors that put employees at risk.

    *   Workplace staff understands that getting help and support early is important for employees and families experiencing difficulties.

    *   The workplace provides an inclusive and accepting environment for community members who may be experiencing difficulties with their health.

- The workplace has policies and practices that support employees and families to seek help for health difficulties.

6. Responding to employees experiencing health difficulties.

    - Workplace staff has a shared understanding of its role, and its boundaries, in addressing the needs of employees experiencing health difficulties.

    - The workplace has protocols and processes for recognizing and responding to employees experiencing health difficulties, including helping employees to remain engaged in their education.

    - Staff has knowledge and skills for recognizing and supporting employees experiencing health difficulties, including how to access and connect to support.

    - The workplace has effective working relationships and clear pathways with services, and supports families to access these services.

    - The workplace facilitates working together with families and professionals who are involved in caring for their employees' health and learning.

Importance of Workplace Health Policy and Procedures

Part of understanding a workplace health promoting culture and climates is reviewing policies and procedures that impact and influence worker health, safety, and well-being. Workplace policy reflects the goals and ethos of the workplace. It is part of the workplace's overall strategy to promote employee health and welfare, which is closely linked to the management of employee behavior. The policies and procedures set the boundaries for how workplaces, families, and communities operate and interact. They help everyone be clear about who is responsible and accountable for making sure workplaces, families, and communities are working together to address employees' health concerns and problems.

Reviewing policies and procedures provides a window into the level of organizational operation and support for employee health. The strongest organizations have policies and procedures that are consistent with what is presented and described as part of an organization's literature and program operations.

Policies are written and there are many reasons to put workplace policy in writing. A written policy may be required by a law or by the organization's insurance carriers. It makes legal review possible. It provides a record of the organization's efforts and a reference if the policy is challenged. It may protect the employer from certain kinds of claims by employees. A written policy is easier to explain to employees, supervisors, and others. Putting the policy in writing also helps employers and employees concentrate on important policy information.

As you review policies and procedures, keep in mind that effective policies are developed using a broad and thorough consultation process. Effective policy is based on laws. Policies and procedures:

1. Ensure compliance with current laws and regulations. Provide the authority for the policies and procedures developed, as well as standardizing and documenting the workplace's agreed position on, and accepted procedure for, dealing with health-related incidents, concerns, and problems.

2. Demonstrate the responsiveness of the workplace to issues of workplace and community concern.

3. Provide a planned and coordinated response to health concerns and problems (e.g., suicide, threats, harassment, crisis response, tobacco use, and substance abuse). This ensures the efficient use of workplace resources and promotes a better outcome for all parties involved. It should define confidentiality and provide for access to counseling and referral services where necessary.

4. Create and support a health-promoting workplace and building climate with set guidelines for employees and employers about acceptable and unacceptable behaviors on workplace premises.

5. Provide a step-by-step outline of actions to take when an incident occurs, and incorporate appropriate and consistent disciplinary measures, if necessary.

6. Clarify roles, rights, and responsibilities of all workplace members in relation to health concerns and problems (e.g., suicide, threats, harassment, crisis response, tobacco use, and substance abuse).

7. Ensure that workplace staff members are not placed at risk by their actions through a clear statement of the workplace's legal and procedural responsibilities.

8. Clarify roles, rights, and responsibilities of all workplace staff in relation to health concerns and problems (e.g., threats, harassment, crisis response, tobacco use, and substance abuse).

In reviewing workplace health promotion policy and procedures, consider all of the above. Likewise, look for policy to clearly state that all workers are responsible for being ready to work when they arrive at the workplace and for avoiding behaviors that could threaten their own safety and health or that of their coworkers. The policy makes clear that all employees will be educated about the policy, will be expected to understand it, and will know what they can do—given their particular work roles—to help make the policy succeed. The policy clarifies options for addressing coworkers' problem behaviors, as well as the meaning of (a) taking responsibility for one's own behavior, (b) showing compassion by helping others, (c) and being honest about problems that threaten health and safety in the workplace. The policy states that the organization will train supervisors to ensure that they (a) understand all applicable laws and regulations, (b) know how to communicate effectively with their subordinates, and (c) are consistent and fair when carrying out and enforcing the policy.

Finally, the policy names the major consequences of violating the workplace policy and of failing to obtain and benefit from organization-provided assistance. Possible consequences could range from a note in the record to suspension from work; transfer to a less safety-sensitive or security-sensitive position; demotion; or firing. The policy states that the organization prefers to avoid severe penalties—by preventing problems in the first place and by responding comprehensively as soon as a problem is identified—and will apply those penalties only when other actions have failed.

The most important task for every organization is to ensure that the policy meets the needs of its employees and workplace. Whether or not laws and regulations apply, an effective policy comprises a number of generally agreed upon elements. Organizations can write (or adapt) and organize content on the key topics using whatever language and structure will best communicate the information to their workers. Organizations do not need to start from scratch. They can borrow and adapt information from policies put together by other organizations in their industry. For example, since the Drug-Free Workplace Act (discussed later in this chapter) was passed, many national, regional, and local programs have been set up to help employers create effective policies. The programs provide free or low-cost information, technical assistance, or model policies that organizations can customize to meet their particular needs.

Basic Elements of an Effective Policy

Statement of Purpose

1. Background

   How was the policy developed? (For example, was it developed in meetings with union representatives or employees representing different segments of the workforce, after consultation with other businesses in the same industry, or in collaboration with the organization's legal counsel?)

2. Goals

What are the workplace laws and regulations (federal, state, or local) with which the organization must comply (if applicable)?

What other goals does the organization expect to achieve? (For example, does it hope to reduce or eliminate drug-related workplace accidents, illnesses, and absenteeism?)

Does the organization want to address a specific health concern (e.g., alcohol, tobacco, violence) in the context of accomplishing a broader goal of promoting worker health, safety, and productivity? Many successful policies have taken this approach.

3. Definitions, Expectations, and Prohibitions

How does the organization define health concern and problem?

What employee behaviors are expected?

Exactly what behaviors are prohibited?

Who is covered by the policy?

When will the policy apply? (For example, will it apply during work hours only, or also during organization-sponsored events after hours?)

Where will the policy apply? (For example, will it apply in the workplace, outside the workplace while workers are on duty, in organization-owned vehicles while workers are off duty?)

Who is responsible for carrying out and enforcing the policy?

Will the policy include any form of screening or testing?

Are any employees covered by the terms of a collective bargaining agreement, and, if so, how do the terms affect the way the policy will be carried out and enforced for those employees?

Implementation Approaches

1. Benefits and Assurances

How will the organization help employees comply with the policy?

How will the organization protect employees' confidentiality?

How will the organization help employees who seek help for health-related problems?

How will the organization help employees who are in treatment or recovery?

How will the organization ensure that all aspects of the policy are implemented fairly and consistently for all employees?

2. Consequences and Appeals

What are the consequences of violating the policy?

What are the procedures for determining whether an employee has violated the policy?

What are the procedures for appealing a determination that an employee may have violated the policy?

3. Dissemination Strategies

How will the organization educate employees about the policy? (For example, the organization can train supervisors, discuss the policy during orientation sessions for new employees, and inform all employees about the policy using a variety of formats—such as a section in the employee handbook, posters in gathering places at work sites, or information on the organization intranet.)

Legal Issues in Health Policies and Procedures

Workplace compliance and adhesion to protect and safeguard the legal rights of employees and their families is another aspect of understanding a workplace health promoting culture and climate. Programs need to comply with the laws to avoid legal liability. Workplace health promotion programs take into consideration a number of legal requirements and federal legislation to protect the rights and safety of individuals at the workplace. Assessing the workplace health promoting culture and climate includes understanding how the legal requirements have and will shape a workplace health promotion program.

Health Insurance Portability and Accountability Act (HIPAA) regulates health providers sharing information with each other and with workplaces—for example, when confidential information is housed in health programs and services at a workplace. Protection of an employee's right to privacy (confidentiality safeguards) is a key element of any workplace health promotion program. Employers must respect and protect the specific wishes of their employees about how much information to share with their supervisor and coworkers.

Confidentiality is an agreement not to disclose any information obtained when there is an expectation that the information will be kept private. Privacy is the control over the extent, timing, and circumstances of sharing oneself with others. Confidentiality is essential to establishing and maintaining a strong health provider–employee relationship. Some assurance of privacy is needed, or individuals may avoid seeking the help that they need. Soler and Peters (1993) outline several reasons to protect the privacy of individuals and families. Potentially embarrassing information about a family or employee, such as HIV status or health history, can create discrimination or judgment by workplace staff or other employees rendering the individual vulnerable to mistreatment.

Limits to confidentiality do exist. In working with employees in their workplace, health providers must talk about the exceptions to the promise of privacy because there are times when keeping information confidential can block helping an employee or cause harm. Harm to self (or others) breaks all confidentiality deals. The American Psychological Association (1981) notes that confidentiality must be broken when a "clear danger to the person or to others" exists (p. 626). Usually employees present one of three circumstances requiring the health providers to break the confidentiality agreement:

1. A threat to harm self

2. A threat to harm another requires warning this person of the threat, if it's credible

3. Disclosure of any form of physical or sexual abuse and/or neglect requires reporting to civil authorities

Occupational Safety and Health Act is the primary federal law that governs occupational health and safety in the private sector and federal government in the United States. Congress enacted the legislation in 1970. Its main goal is to ensure that employers provide employees with an environment free from recognized hazards, such as exposure to toxic chemicals, excessive noise levels, mechanical dangers, heat or cold stress, or unsanitary conditions. Furthermore it may also protect coworkers, family members, employers, customers, and many others who might be affected by the workplace environment.

The Act created the Occupational Safety and Health Administration (OSHA), an agency of the Department of Labor. OSHA was given the authority both to set and enforce workplace health and safety standards. The Act also established the National Institute of Occupational Safety and Health (NIOSH), an independent research institute in the then-Centers for Disease Control. NIOSH has three overarching goals:

+ Conduct research to reduce work-related illnesses and injuries

+ Promote safe and healthy workplaces through interventions, recommendations, and capacity building

+ Enhance global workplace safety and health through international collaborations

Workers' compensation insurance (commonly known as workers' comp) provides coverage for an employee who has suffered an injury or illness resulting from job-related duties. Coverage includes medical and rehabilitation costs and lost wages for employees injured on the job. In 1917, the U.S. Supreme Court upheld the constitutionality of compulsory insurance requirements, opening the doors for every state to require employers to purchase workers' compensation coverage. Then, as now, each state instituted different requirements. The laws place responsibility of workplace injuries and diseases on the industry in which it occurred rather than with the general public. Different from other laws and legal requirements, workers' compensation was never contemplated as a separate issue considered for national legislation. It was always bundled with other issues such as the Social Security Act, disability insurance, and new occupational health and safety regulations (Howard, 2002).

Each state workers' compensation laws define who is considered an employee (e.g., anyone working under contract for hire, expressed or implied; executive officers of corporations; state, county, or city employees; volunteer firefighters). The laws define employers who are exempt from having to provide workers' compensation to their employees (e.g., agriculture employers/employees, domestic worker in private homes, federal employees). The types and duration of the benefits are defined (e.g., temporary total disability, temporary partial disability, permanent partial disability, permanent total disability). Likewise, the laws define due process and adjudication systems.

Drug-Free Workplace Act of 1998 mandated that companies seeking contracts with the government must maintain a drug-free workplace. Additionally, the Department of Transportation requires companies operating any commercial vehicle in interstate commerce to have a drug-free workplace policy. This Act requires any organization that receives a federal contract worth at least $100,000 to establish drug-free workplace policies, procedures, and programs. It requires that all organizations receiving federal grants of any size establish and maintain drug-free workplace policies, procedures, and programs.

Drug-Free Workplace Act of 1998, Minimum Organizational Requirements

1. *Prepare and distribute a formal drug-free workplace policy statement.* This statement should clearly prohibit the manufacture, use, and distribution of controlled substances in the workplace and spell out the specific consequences of violating this policy.

2. *Establish a drug-free awareness program.* The program should inform employees of the dangers of workplace substance abuse; review the requirements of the organization's drug-free workplace policy; and offer information about any counseling, rehabilitation, or employee assistance programs that may be available.

3. *Ensure that all employees working on the federal contract understand their personal reporting obligations.* Under the terms of the Act, an employee must notify the employer within 5 calendar days if he or she is convicted of a criminal drug violation in the workplace.

4. *Notify the federal contracting agency of any covered violation.* Under the terms of the Act, the employer has 10 days to report that a covered employee has been convicted of a criminal drug violation in the workplace.

5. *Take direct action against an employee convicted of a workplace drug violation.* This action may involve imposing a penalty of some kind or requiring that the employee participate in an appropriate rehabilitation or counseling program.

6. Maintain an ongoing good faith effort to meet all the requirements of the Act throughout the life of the contract.

Omnibus Transportation Employee Testing Act of 1991 requires mandatory drug and alcohol testing for certain employees holding commercial driver's licenses who operate commercial motor vehicles. This includes pre-employment (for drugs only), post-accident, reasonable suspicion, return to duty, and follow-up testing. Commercial motor vehicle is defined as a motor vehicle used in commerce to transport passengers or property (e.g., gross vehicle weight rating of at least 26,001 pounds, vehicle transport at least 16 passengers including the driver, hazardous vehicle transport). According to the Act, all employers in the transportation industry are required to test safety-sensitive employees at certain key points in their professional careers. These key points include pre-employment (before the employee is hired), whenever there is reasonable suspicion that the employee has been involved in drug use, immediately after the employee is involved in an accident, and before allowing the employee to return to duty following suspension for drug abuse. Any employee who is found to have a substance abuse problem must be referred by the employer to a trained substance abuse professional. This person will be responsible for evaluating the employee's treatment needs and assessing the employee's ability to return to work.

Clean Air Act (http://www.epa.gov/air/caa/): In 1990, Congress dramatically revised and expanded the Clean Air Act, providing the Environmental Protection Agency (EPA) even broader authority to implement and enforce regulations reducing air pollutant emissions. The 1990 amendments also placed an increased emphasis on more cost-effective approaches to reduce air pollution. States implement most environmental statutes on behalf of the federal government. To help with this, the federal government provides assistance to states for administration of the programs and for infrastructure.

Good indoor air quality (IAQ) in the workplace is a critical component of a healthy and comfortable work environment. IAQ affects individuals' health, productivity, performance, and comfort. One workplace that has received a lot of attention is schools. The EPA developed the IAQ Tools for Schools—Framework for Effective School IAQ Management (Figure 5.2) and Action Kit to offer comprehensive guidance for districts just beginning to address IAQ or those already working on IAQ management (U.S. EPA, 2013). However, the IAQ tools are not limited to use in school buildings but are also widely used at workplaces to improve staff productivity by managing the environmental quality of a plant or facility.

Family and Medical Leave Act of 1993 (FMLA): The FMLA, administered by the U.S. Department of Labor, applies to most employers of more than 50 employees. A covered employer must grant an eligible employee up to a total of 12 work weeks of unpaid leave (for covered conditions) during any 12-month period. Among the reasons eligible employees are entitled to leave are the instances in which an employee is unable to work because of a serious health condition. "Serious health condition" is defined as an illness, injury, impairment, or physical or mental condition. For details of the FMLA, frequently asked questions, employer coverage and employee eligibility criteria, and other provisions of the law, go to www.dol.gov/whd/FMLA.

Americans with Disabilities Act (ADA) (www.eeoc.gov): Title 1 of the Americans with Disabilities Act of 1990, which took effect July 26,

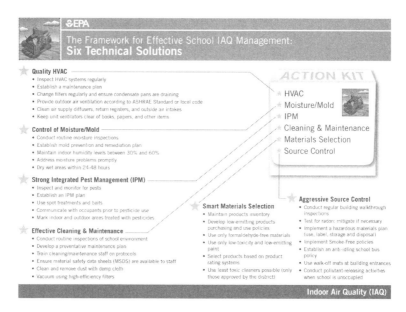

Figure 5.2   EPA Indoor Air Quality Management Framework

1992, prohibits private employers, state and local government, employment agencies, and labor unions from discriminating against qualified individuals with disabilities in job application procedures, hiring, firing, advancement, compensation, job training, and other terms, conditions, and privileges of employment, An individual with a disability is a person who:

•   Has a physical or mental impairment that substantially limits one or more of his/her major life activities

•   Has a record of such an impairment

•   Is regarded as having such impairment

To receive the protections of the Americans with Disabilities Act as "reasonable accommodations," the employee must be willing to disclose to the employer that he or she has a disability. The congruence between the formal statements of the business and the informal climate of the workplace with regard to its health friendliness plays a significant role in an employee's willingness to self-disclose to request a "reasonable accommodation." Interviews with employees who have self-disclosed reinforce the importance of flexible workplace practices, and supervisor and coworker support. The employer is not required to provide accommodations that would pose an "undue hardship" on the operation of the business (Table 5.1). Similarly, workers cannot be forced to accept accommodations that are neither requested nor needed.

Table 5.1   Some Examples of Reasonable Accommodations for Persons as Required by the Americans with Disabilities Act

Schedule modification	Changes in policy
• Allowing workers to shift schedules earlier or later	• Extending additional paid or unpaid leave during a hospitalization
• Allowing workers to use paid or unpaid leave for appointments related to their mental disability	• Allowing an employee to make phone calls during the day to personal or professional supports
• Allowing an employee to work part-time temporarily (e.g., when first returning from an absence)	• Providing a private space in which to make such phone calls
	• Allowing workers to consume fluids at their work stations throughout the work day (e.g., if needed due to medication side effects)
Modifications to the physical environment	**Job modification**
• Providing an enclosed office	• Arranging for job sharing
• Providing partitions, room dividers, or otherwise enhancing soundproofing and visual barriers between workspaces	• Reassigning tasks among workers
	• Reassigning the employee to a vacant position
Provision of human assistance	**Provisions of assistive technology**
• Allowing a job coach to come to the worksite	• Providing a portable computer to enable an employee to work at home or at unusual hours
• Participating in meetings with the worker and his/her job coach or other employment service provider	• Providing software that allows the worker to structure time and receive prompts throughout the work day
Supervisory techniques	
• Offering additional supervisory sessions	
• Offering additional training or instruction on new procedures or information	

Accessibility means that people of all ages and abilities have reasonable access to programs and materials, and have the opportunity to participate. Physical accessibility focuses on the way information is delivered through signage, materials, technology, and interpersonal exchanges. Programs and opportunities include and address the needs of a diverse group of employees, including those with physical disabilities, varied levels of literacy, those working night and evening shifts, and individuals working in varied locations (Table 5.2). It is important that individuals with different types of disabilities and/or those with special skills assist in helping ensure disability access and inclusivity.

Finally, the ADA generally prohibits employers from obtaining medical information from employees through disability-related inquiries or

Table 5.2   Health Promotion Programs Inclusive of, and Accessible to, Diverse Groups of Employees

Night and Evening Workers

Employees working evening and night shifts are frequently unable to attend lunch and learn programs, webinars, audio and video conferences, or other education opportunities that are presented to day staff. CDs, DVDs, and other recorded methods of providing content to off-tour staff are only partial substitutes; staff members need to be given the time to take advantage of different materials. Whenever possible, programs should be offered in an equitable manner.

Remote and Community-Based Clinic Employees

Because of distance, remote or community-based outpatient clinic workers are often not able to attend classes and other wellness opportunities provided to employees at larger medical centers. Video conferencing can provide a link if staffing permits. However, as with night and evening employees, programs should be offered in an equitable manner.

Physical Accessibility

Physical barriers and distance present potential challenges to an employee's ability to access programs and services. Required are accessible gyms, health and wellness fairs, clinics, and walking paths.

Communication

Communication barriers limit an employee's access to information and services. This may include health screening surveys, health information pamphlets, direct services (e.g., coaching), and training programs. Important issues to consider include accessibility for those with low vision or blindness, hard of hearing or deaf, low literacy, non-English speaking, and cognitive limitations. Each of these groups may benefit from materials available in formats other than standard print.

medical examinations. It does, however, allow employers to conduct voluntary medical examinations as part of an employee health program, including a workplace health promotion program. With the passage of the Affordable Care Act the question then becomes, when do the incentives offered or penalties imposed under a health promotion program render participation involuntary? To address this concern the U.S. Equal Employment Opportunity Commission (EEOC) clarified when disability-related inquiries and medical examinations conducted under workplace health promotion programs are voluntary. First, an employee health program, including any disability-related inquiries and medical examinations, must be reasonably designed to promote health or prevent disease. It must have a reasonable chance of improving health of or preventing disease in participating employees and must not be overly burdensome, a subterfuge for violating the ADA or other employment discrimination laws, or use a highly suspect method to promote health or prevent disease (Jost, 2015).

Collecting biometric information from employees, for example, without providing employees with follow-up information or advice or without using aggregate information to design programs to treat specific conditions, would not reasonably promote health. A program is not reasonably designed to promote health if it imposes, as a condition to obtaining a reward, an overly burdensome amount of time for participation, requires unreasonably intrusive procedures, or places significant costs on employees. Programs should not simply shift costs from employers to targeted employees based on their health.

For a workplace health promotion program to be deemed voluntary, an employer may not require an employee to participate in a program, deny coverage under its group health plans or particular group health plan benefits, or take any adverse action against an employee who refuses to participate in a health promotion program or achieve certain outcomes under such a program. An employer may not retaliate against, interfere with, coerce, intimidate, or threaten an employee who does not participate in a wellness program.

For an employee's participation in a program to be considered voluntary, an employer must provide a notice clearly explaining what medical information will be obtained, how the medical information will be used, who will receive the medical information, how its disclosure will be restricted, and how the employer will prevent improper disclosure of the medical information.

If the health promotion program is administered as part of a group health plan, it is also subject to HIPAA privacy and security, which means that information provided to an employer must generally be deidentified and information that an employer might have access to under general EEOC confidentiality rules might only be accessible with employee authorization.

Summary

As part of the program planning, it is important to identify champions and advocates who are key informants about past and current efforts to promote employee health, safety, and well-being in an organization. They support and guide the development of a health-promoting workplace culture and climate. Gathering information about a workplace health-promoting culture and climate results in knowing how staff can be challenged to create programs and services and to engage employees, families, community members, customers, consumers, and employers, as well as to advocate and champion for policies and procedures to promote and protect health and well-being. Key to the process is understanding organizational policies and procedures that support and promote health. Finally, workplace compliance and adhesion to protect and safeguard the legal rights of employees and their families is examined as part of understanding a workplace health promoting culture and climate.

For Practice and Discussion

1. Where in your life have you been a program champion and advocate? What did you do? What challenges did you face? Who supported your efforts and what role did the support of others play in the efforts?

2. Think about an organization where you have worked. What was the health promotion culture and climate at the workplace? Identify three consequences of the workplace health promotion culture and climate. If you could change one aspect of the health culture and climate, what would you change, and why?

3. As part of some new job orientations for individuals starting a new position, the organization's company policies and procedures will be reviewed. Think about an organization where you have worked. What was your experience learning about company policies and procedures? What were you told and what were you left to learn on your own? What was a consequence of knowing or not knowing a policy or procedure?

4. Small and midsized businesses often experience a gap or discrepancy between their employee health promotion programs and company policies and procedures. Frequently stated policies and procedures will differ with what happens with an employee depending on the role of the individual in a business. Likewise supervisors often are uncomfortable dealing with employee health concerns, so they are left to fester and go unattended, which potentially increases company liability. Research and recommend strategies for businesses to develop health-promoting policies and procedures they can implement and support.

5. You are a lunchtime speaker for a meeting of the New Haven Manufacturer's Association (http://www.newhavenmanufacturers.com/). The association promotes and advocates causes important to the manufacturing community in both the greater New Haven, Connecticut, region and beyond, educates members on business, and provides a forum for the exchange of ideas and issues. Prepare a 15-minute presentation on legal considerations when thinking about your workplace health promotion program. As part of your presentation, the association director requested that you provide a user-friendly approach for members to assess their compliance with current federal, state, and local legal requirements.

Case Study: Finding Champions and Advocates—What Would You Do?

Maria Ruiz is health promotion director at a large state higher education university system. She is charged with creating smoke-free campuses across the university's multiple campuses. The system's Board of Directors approved and support policies that allow campuses to be smoke-free or tobacco-free. In 2014, one of the larger University campuses became tobacco-free. The use of any tobacco products was prohibited in university buildings and on university grounds. The tobacco-free campus policy is part of the university's commitment to creating a healthy and sustainable environment for all members of the campus community, and is designed to be positive and health directed.

Building on the success of the first tobacco-free campus, Ms. Ruiz is directed to work with other campuses to be tobacco-free. If you were Ms. Ruiz, what would you do?

KEY TERMS

Champions	Occupational Safety and Health Act
Advocate	Drug-Free Workplace Act of 1998
Opinion leader	Workers' Compensation Insurance
Workplace culture	Omnibus Transportation Employee Testing Act of 1991
Workplace climate	
Policy	Clean Air Act
Procedure	Indoor air quality (IAQ)
Effective policy elements	Family and Medical Leave Act of 1993 (FMLA)
Health Insurance Portability and Account-ability Act (HIPAA)	Americans with Disabilities Act (ADA)

References

American Psychological Association. (1981). *Ethical principles of psychologists.* Washington, DC: Author.

Association of California School Administrators. (2008). *School culture survey.* Retrieved from http://www.acsa.org/FunctionalMenuCategories/Media /EdCalNewspaper/2008/Dec15/Climatesurvey.aspx

Carroll, G. R., & Harrison, J. R. (1998). Organizational demography and culture: Insights from a formal model and simulation. *Administrative Science Quarterly*, *43*(3), 637–667. doi:10.2307/2393678

FedEx (2015). *Recognition programs and awards.* Retrieved from http://www.fedex.com/gb/about/our-people/recognition.html

Howard, C. (2002). *Workers' compensation, federalism, and the heavy hand of history: Studies in American political development.* Retrieved from http://www.hks.harvard.edu/inequality/Seminar/Papers/Howard.PDF

Jost, T. (2015, April 17). Workplace wellness programs: Federal agencies weigh in. *Health Affairs* [Blog]. Retrieved from http://healthaffairs.org/blog/2015/04/17/workplace-wellness-programs-federal-agencies-weigh-in/

KidsMatter Australian Primary Schools Mental Health Initiative. (2012). *KidsMatter primary framework.* Retrieved from https://kidsmatter.edu.au/primary/about-kidsmatter-primary/framework

Locock, L., Dopson, S., Chambers, D., & Gabbay, J. (2001). Understanding the role of opinion leaders in improving clinical effectiveness. *Social Science and Medicine, 53*(6), 745–757.

Neal, A., Griffin, M. A., & Hart, P. M. (2000). The impact of organizational climate on safety climate and individual behavior. *Safety Science, 34*(1–3), 99-109. doi:10.1016/S0925-7535(00)00008-4

O'Reilly, C. A., & Chatman, J. A. (1996). Culture as social control: Corporations, cults, and commitment. *Research in Organizational Behavior, 18*(7), 157–200.

Schein, E. H. (1985). *Organizational culture and leadership.* San Francisco, CA: Jossey-Bass.

Soler, M. I., & Peters, C. M. (1993). *Who should know what? Confidentiality and information sharing in service integration.* Des Moines, IA: National Center for Service Integration.

U.S. Environmental Protection Agency. (2013). *Indoor air quality tools for schools*, 3. http://www.epa.gov/iaq/schools/pdfs/framework.pdf

CHAPTER 6

ASSESSING WORKPLACE HEALTH PROMOTION TEAMS, PARTNERSHIPS, AND COLLABORATIONS

Teams, Partnerships, and Collaborations: A Socioecological Approach to Promote Employee and Employer Health

Workplace health promotion programs depend on teams, partnerships, and collaborations. One of your first tasks in planning a program is to determine the already established as well as the potential health teams, partnerships, and collaborations in the workplace, and to investigate aspects of how they work—for instance: the competition for membership, their available resources, and their support and effectiveness. Look for teams, partnerships, and collaborations to take a socioecological model approach to promote employee and employer health (Figure 6.1). The socioecological approach considers all levels when addressing the health needs of employees and employers. While working at each level (e.g., family, employee, workplace, community), you can assess how to help the teams, partnerships, and collaborations best fit programs to local needs and strengths. In this approach, the teams, partnerships, and collaborations are the links that unite the different levels to address health concerns and problems, and to promote health.

Teams occur mostly at the workplace (e.g., factory floor, office) level with participation of employees (and families) and employers from the site. At the workplace local health care providers, education, and human service agencies and programs might be part of the teams.

LEARNING OBJECTIVES

- Discuss the socioecological model to assess teams, partnerships, and collaborations for workplace health promotion

- Summarize how workplace teams promote health at the workplace

- Explain workplace health promotion partnerships

- Identify effective workplace health promotion collaborations

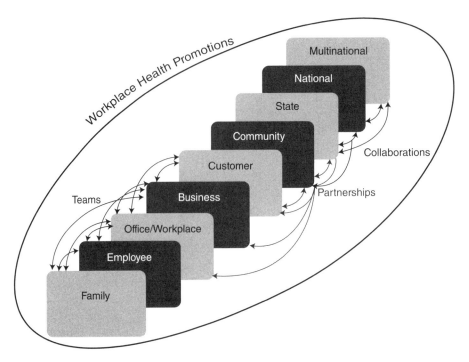

Figure 6.1   Teams, Partnerships, and Collaborations Linking the Levels of Promoting Employee and Employer Health

Partnerships typically are formed at the organization and company level including all of the different organization and company locations that join with a broader range of health care provider services and programs. Health insurance providers (e.g., brokers, agents, insurance companies), state government programs, and other businesses often are partnership members. Collaborations reach even higher, to the state, national, and multinational level, to address broad public policies. Collaborating partners will seek and accept input from many of the levels (e.g., employee, workplace, health care, community), but the collaboration leadership tends to reside at the state, national, and multinational level. All three together contribute to the health of employees, employers, and families.

Workplace Teams

A team is a group of interdependent individuals who share responsibility for specific outcomes for their organization (e.g., workplace). The minimum defining features are shared responsibility and interdependence. Team members are interdependent if each depends on the others to carry out his or her role, to accomplish goals, or create a product. For example, a team at a workplace addressing employee and employer health and safety might be composed of staff who are supervisors, union representatives, employees, human resource department personnel, managers, safety inspectors, health insurance brokers and agents, and medical staff. Each member brings expertise from his or her professional role and experience at the workplace, shares the goal of helping and supporting employees and employers, and works with other team members to create a plan of action, and to identify resources and supports to address the health needs of the employees and employer. Teams are site specific. Therefore in large and midsized organizations such as businesses with multiple sites (e.g., manufacturing and mining sites), large school districts with many buildings, and health care systems with multiple facilities and clinics, each site might have its own team.

The value of teams for organizations can be seen in the actions of most large corporations to form teams to address the most difficult challenges. For example, Hewlett-Packard (Box 6.1) uses a small global team of full-time employees that enlists volunteers throughout the company to serve on its larger virtual team to address how HP can contribute to environmental sustainability in its marketplaces and workplaces. Teams can embrace the

---

BOX 6.1   SUSTAINABILITY AND SOCIAL INNOVATION TEAM (HEWLETT-PACKARD, 2015)

At Hewlett-Packard (HP), a board-level discussion in 2009 set the wheels in motion to transform the company's social impact strategy. In 2011, environmental sustainability was integrated into that strategic mission. HP's current Sustainability and Social Innovation (SSI) group is a small global team of full-time employees that enlists volunteers throughout the company to serve on its larger virtual team. By design, SSI partners with a range of public and private organizations in the areas of health, education, and the environment. Among its innovative partnerships, SSI works closely with Mothers2Mothers, an NGO devoted to improving the health of mothers living with HIV and eliminating pediatric AIDS.

The director of partner and program development in the SSI group uses what she calls the "MacGyver" approach—a way of being extremely innovative but also pragmatic and resourceful when developing solutions. She concedes that the need for speed and results is tempered by the importance of developing sustainable solutions that can be scaled up. There are rarely any "quick fixes," she says, and the collaboration necessary for long-term success requires careful management. In the partnership with Mothers2Mothers, HP has tapped into a range of internal talent and resources to improve the NGO's systems and processes. And what gets busy people at HP fired up to work with Mothers2Mothers? Not surprisingly, it is the opportunity to have a positive impact on the world and the satisfaction of tackling challenging problems in innovative and collaborative ways.

characteristics of entrepreneurs but work within organizations to address complexity by serving as internal change agents. Teams can develop the strategies, products, services, processes, and business models to help companies solve short- and long-term issues. This work and progress is not done through one or two charismatic individuals. Instead, progress results from the people working together in teams.

Workplace Health Promotion Teams Among Many Workplace Teams

Workplace health promotion programs are like all other business and workplace initiatives. They are operated by a team: a workplace health promotion team. The team is often just one of many employee-related human resource teams that are found in organizations. Listed below are some human resource teams that many organizations form and support. As part of the planning process you need to understand how the health promotion team operates within the workplace environment and among all of the other teams operating in the workplace.

Human Resource Teams Operating in Workplaces

- Environmental Health and Safety Team: Promotes safety practices, procedures and processes to ensure compliance with internal and external guidelines. Teams design, implement, and evaluate comprehensive health and safety programs that will maintain and enhance health, improve safety, and increase productivity. Occupational health and safety professionals include occupational and environmental health nurses, occupational medicine physicians, industrial hygienists, safety professionals, and occupational health psychologists.

- Crisis Response Team: Guides an organization's response to an ongoing crisis as the situation evolves and evaluates the need for specific response services on an ongoing basis. These might include debriefing and assistance with grief and bereavement (e.g., facilitate a grief/bereavement employee services for employees affected by the loss).

- Equal Employment Opportunity Committee: Reviews the job descriptions to ensure that the requirements do not cause exclusion of candidates from protected classes. The EEO Committee uses documentation provided by the human resource office to review procedures followed by the office and to ensure that all EEO guidelines and procedures have been met, such as monitoring the search and selection procedures to ensure equal opportunity.

- Employee Relations Committee: Oversees union relations and ensures fair and equal employment without reference to an individual's race; color; sex; sexual orientation; age (over 40); marital status; ancestry; national origin; religious creed; having a GED rather than a high school diploma; handicap or disability, or the use of a guide or support animal for disability, or relationship to a person with a disability.

- Benefits and Compensation: Reviews and recommends for approval to the Board of Directors compensation guidelines, benefits whose costs are budgeted, and related matters including philosophy, policies, programs and long-term planning, and financial considerations for employees.

- Staff Training and Development: Identifies needs and develops programs for personal and professional development of employees in order to improve performance, aid in career advancement, and increase job satisfaction. Examples of responsibilities are oversight of the new-employee programs to welcome and orient new staff; such oversight provides up-to-date and useful company information and resources as well as an evaluation of the company staff development seminars or supervisory workshops (individual, group, online) for personal and professional development for staff.

- Risk Management: Develops and oversees an organization's risk management program. Responsibilities can include identifying the organization's risk exposure, developing a risk control program, and establishing a risk-financing strategy. Working with the professional risk manager, the committee will coordinate such risk management activities as loss control efforts, claims reporting, insurance purchasing, and safety program implementation. Potential team members include risk managers, claims/security officers, and insurance brokers.

The team membership (e.g., number of people, selection criteria, compensation), as well as the tasks, responsibilities, and activities are directly related to the size of the organization. Workplace health promotion teams for multinational, Fortune 500 companies, federal and state government, Veterans Administration, large university systems, and national health care organizations have dedicated directors and staff, compensated and assigned to direct, implement, and evaluate their corporate health promotion programs. Common are multilevel teams (executive to factory level) addressing how to promote employee health. Midsized organizations (e.g., school districts, local hospital systems, large retailers, regional food suppliers and supermarkets, regional and local human services and arts organizations) also operate workplace health promotion teams. Each of these teams might stand alone, or be blended with the functions of another team. In large corporations and organizations the committees might report to the corporation board of directors with legally mandated responsibilities and reporting requirements. In small organizations with fewer than 50 employees (local business, community organizations, recreational associations) as well as in single-owner proprietorships, committee structures differ. Frequently the small organizations partner with other like organizations and health insurance providers (e.g., brokers, agents, insurance companies, marketplaces/exchanges), in state government programs to address employer and employee health. The need to promote employee health is no different for small, midsized, and large employers, in fact it may be greater for the small employer, given the dependence of small businesses and organizations on their employees to produce a product or deliver a service. But most small business owners will tell you that they simply do not have the time to involve employees in the decision making of the organization's human resource department when it relates to health policy, procedures, and programs.

Workplace Health Promotion Teams Link to the Factory Floor

Primary in the planning process is to determine how the workplace health promotion teams link to the factory floor. That connection with employees is the center and source of the teams' greatest impact. Teams need direct contact with employees wherever they work, be it a factory, hospital, school, farm, mine, nursing home, bodega, big box retailer, dry cleaner, or community center. Each workplace reflects the employers' and employees' values, belief systems, norms, ideologies, rituals, and traditions, and these are further shaped by the surrounding community's political, social, cultural, and economic forces (e.g., home, neighborhood, city, state, country). At the heart of the workplace are the workers and supervisors. Workplaces reflect this relationship. They reflect the individual supervisors' style, organization, attitudes, morale, practices, and expectations. They reflect the employers' lives and families. The workers producing the product and providing the service are the recipients of the workplace wellness program. The workplace health promotion team members work for their employer but always need to keep the workers and factory floor in mind as the program is developed and implemented in the workplace.

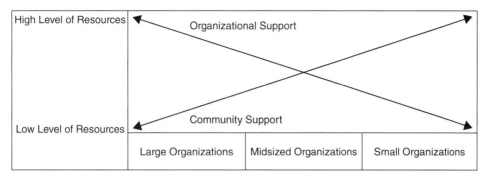

Figure 6.2 Organizational Size Health Promotion Teams' Support and Resource Balance

Assessing a Workplace Health Promotion Team: Organization Size Matters

Organization size matters when assessing a workplace health promotion team. At large corporations expect mainly organizational support and resources. Small businesses, however, rely on community support and resources (Figure 6.2). In large and midsized organizations, workplace health promotion team decisions are structured and reviewed through formal policies and procedures often requiring multiple layers of review and approvals. Chief executive officers, chief operating officers, chief people officers, chief financial officers, presidents, chancellors, and human resource vice presidents, as well as board presidents and board members, might expect to be the ultimate health promotion program decision makers based on an overall organizational strategic business plan and its objectives. Small business owners and executives typically make the decisions in consultation with a health promotion team but are the ultimate decision makers largely based on the organizations' fiscal condition and government regulation (i.e, Affordable Care Act). For indigent, migrant, and underserved populations of workers, community human services that outreach into the community and workplace may be the only opportunity a worker has to receive any health care services, including dental care for themselves and their families.

Assessing a Workplace Health Promotion Team: Key Questions

Answers to a few key questions help to assess the role of teams in an organization's workplace health promotion efforts. A first question to answer about a health promotion team is whether or not the team has established a program vision to drive their efforts. Do members know where the team is going; can they articulate and picture its desired outcome? Teams add stability, credibility, and importance to a workplace health promotion program. Consensus and consistency among team members provide the foundation for the team's efforts. Furthermore the team members give a human face to the program—literally, in organizational photographs, newsletters, and events. Team members frequently are seen handing out items, such as informational brochures on health topics, or coordinating health activities and events. In addition, they can conduct surveys and solicit ideas from fellow employees. Team members want to be clear about what and why they do what they do.

Look for a workplace health promotion team to have members from all parts of the organization (see the following list) who can envision how health (or the lack of it) affects different aspects of the organization. On a team you need people who can think strategically, make realistic plans, and anticipate pitfalls—people who know where to look for support and where to anticipate resistance. You also want a diverse group in terms of health. A smoker can give you realistic feedback on your smoking cessation program. Someone who is overweight and doesn't exercise can "tell it like it is" and help your team understand why some well-meaning plans may not work. And if that person supports your programs, it may inspire others.

Potential Wellness Team Members

- Senior and mid-level managers
- Front-line employees
- Benefits managers
- Union representatives
- Human resources personnel
- Marketing and communications directors
- Safety coordinators
- Information systems representatives
- Health care representatives
- Community health programs and services

If the organization is unionized, union support is critical. In most organizations it is best to have union representation on the workplace wellness team. Unions represent the employees who will benefit from the wellness program. Their buy-in is key. You will want to know the union's involvement with the employee health promotion efforts. Ask if the case for union involvement has been made. Compelling arguments might focus on occupational health and safety or on moderating increases in health insurance premiums. It is possible you may need to locate the union president. You do that by contacting the district's business office or human resource department or the union's state affiliate. Affiliates can be found on the union's website. If the union president cannot find the time to represent the union on the team, she or he might know a union member who would be willing to champion the issue on the union's behalf (Noe, Hollenbeck, Gerhart, &Wright, 2013).

Effective Workplace Health Promotion Teams

Effective workplace health promotion teams encourage employers and employees to perceive health promotion as an organizational priority with a broad range of talents and views. To assess a health promotion team's effectiveness, look to see if the organization keeps the team's involvement fresh and fun (Hunnicutt, 2007). See the list of the Wellness Council of America (WELCOA)'s tips for a successful team. Effective teams communicate to the employer and employees that the team pulls in health-related data and puts out helpful, human responses. They don't just meet—the team members gather ideas, brainstorm, plan, implement, and analyze results on behalf of the organization and for the health of everyone associated with the workplace.

WELCOA Successful Health Promotion Team Tips (Hunnicutt, 2007)

- Have "worksite health promotion team member" written into the job descriptions of team members. This will ensure health promotion is a defined duty in their workload.

- Promote the health promotion team throughout the organization. Doing so helps employees see workplace health promotion is a priority and reminds them that the team is there to help with their health promotion goals. It also inspires participation and team involvement. Make it official by creating a team name, motto, and logo.

- Develop a team with strong leadership. Your team will need vision, energy, altruism, a spirit of inclusiveness, and a genuine desire to help others. Your team leader should be someone who can create agendas, handle conflict, set priorities, motivate others, meet goals and deadlines, and communicate throughout the organization.

- Add diversity to your team. Try to include representation from all different functional areas, experience levels, ages, and fitness levels. A larger organization could have a team of 14–20 people. A small organization may do well with four to seven people.

- Meet regularly. Face-to-face meetings once or twice a month are best.

- Distribute agendas *before* the meeting to keep members informed and meetings on task.

- Assign someone to take minutes and distribute them.

- Communicate often. Educating the organization on your priorities and letting others know how to get involved helps employees embrace the health promotion program.

- Participate in continuing education about health and health promotion.

Effective teams remember that the business of business is business (all organizations operate to create, produce, and provide a product or service). Teams won't get anywhere pushing ideas that cut into productivity. Teams and management have to be on the same side, or teams will lose the support they need to get more health promotion into the organizational culture. Be realistic—not too many organizations will sponsor 30-minute naps, but a 10-minute stretch break may float. Health promotion teams aim to enhance work life, not replace it with healthy activities.

Partnerships: What to Look For

A partnership is a group of interdependent local organizations represented by individuals who share responsibility for specific outcomes across organizations at the local level. Similar to teams, the minimum defining features are shared responsibility and interdependence. Partnership members use their organization's role and its experience working with employees and employers, combined with their shared goal of helping and supporting them to create resources and supports within and across a community, to address employee and employer health needs. For example, local small business partnerships with business owners, local hospitals, mental health agencies, drug and alcohol programs, health insurance brokers and agents, and faith-based organizations develop and sustain a range of health programs and services with multiple entry points and funding. The goal is to create an accessible, consumer-driven continuum of health programs and services. Partnerships also occur across large organizations with multiple sites, perhaps spanning states, regions, and nations.

During the planning process it is important to look for a diverse range and type of existing and potential partnerships to support the workplace health promotion programs. Workplace partnerships create resources and supports within and across a community and region to address employee and employer health needs. Partnerships reflect the commitment and investment of people and resources to address employee health needs. Partnerships require specifically defined roles and responsibilities, and usually the commitment of resources (fiscal and other), for the implementation of specific interventions usually delineated in a formal document. They develop and sustain a range of health programs and services with multiple entry points and funding. They are "an undertaking to do something together. . . a relationship that consists of shared and/or compatible objectives and an acknowledged distribution of specific roles and responsibilities among the participants which can be formal, contractual, or voluntary, between two or more parties" (Skage, 1996).

Expect to find a number of different partnerships as part of workplace health promotion programs. Partnerships vary based on their goals (Table 6.1). In the spirit of creating healthy towns, neighborhoods, and schools local businesses and organizations make donations of money and perhaps in-kind donation of materials and supplies for an activity or event. Community events such as 5K runs are the model for these local health oriented (partnership) donations with their annual T-shirts printed on the back with the names of the organizations that donated to the activity. In addition to the public recognition, organizations may receive tax credits.

Many large corporations align themselves with national health organizations, forming national and local sponsorships (partnerships) to be the sponsor of marathons, golf tournaments, youth recreation and sports programs, family-friendly hikes and walks, biking programs, and summer fresh food farmers' markets. As part of a sponsorship an organization gives financial support for a set period of time or cycle that can last for years. Typically sponsors receive public recognition. It is not unusual that an activity will use the names of the sponsors in its publicity and advertisements (e.g., Bank of America Chicago Marathon). These sponsorships (partnerships) support the community and can potentially address major health concerns. For example, the Komen Million Dollar Council Elite is a special group of sponsors and partners who have committed to invest a financial contribution of $1 million annually in the fight to end breast cancer. Each of these organizations commits to find new and innovative ways to raise awareness about breast cancer and encourage people from all walks of life to get involved in finding a cure for cancer. Sponsors include American Airlines, General Electric, Walgreens, Ford, Bank of America, New Balance, Yoplait, and Caterpillar Inc.

Cooperation among organizations is a common form of a workplace health promotion partnership. Organizational procedures, policies, and activities remain distinct and separate and are determined without

Table 6.1   Models of Partnerships (adapted from Skage, 1996)

Donation	Examples:
One-time contributions (financial or non-financial) to support an activity or event. Donors may expect public recognition or tax credits. Common among local small business, medical practices, human service organizations, and franchisees' neighbors.	• Community medical practice donating money to a community health fair • Local supermarket donating food and beverages to a community-wide violence prevention family activity event • Walmart store donating art supplies to summer camps that employees' children attend, particularly in areas with few summer activities and recreational opportunities
Sponsorship	Examples:
Giving financial support for a set time period or cycle of a program or providing a contribution for supporting an event or service program. Sponsors may expect public recognition in return for the support. Common among large corporations in the spirit of creating healthy neighborhoods and schools.	• Komen Million Dollar Council Elite • Bank of America Chicago Marathon • Ronald McDonald Houses
Cooperation	Examples:
Organizational procedures, policies, and activities remain distinct and separate and are determined without reference to the procedures and policies of the other agencies. The organizations are autonomous, function independently in parallel fashion, and work toward the identified goals of their respective programs, demonstrating a peaceful coexistence that is neither genuinely interactive nor interdependent.	• Employers Health Purchasing Corporation • Pacific Business Group on Health • Dallas/Fort Worth Business Group on Health • Florida Health Care Coalition
Coordination	Examples:
A multidisciplinary approach in which professionals from different organizations confer, share decision making, and coordinate their service delivery for the purpose of achieving shared goals and improving health care. Cooperation represents a sophisticated level of organizational interaction. It is a process of engaging in various efforts that alter or facilitate the relationships of independent organizations, staffs, or resources.	• Wishard-Eskenazi Health and Community Health Network • National Association of Community Health Centers • Small Business Assistance Program Community Health Advocates

reference to the procedures and policies of the other organizations. The organizations are autonomous, function independently in parallel fashion, and work toward the identified goals of their respective organizations. They come together, however, with the purpose of addressing employees' health needs and lowering the organizations' health costs. Such partnerships demonstrate a peaceful coexistence, but are neither genuinely interactive nor interdependent. Business groups focused on health, and which form partnerships at the local level, are models for cooperation in workplace wellness partnerships.

The final partnership model is coordination. It is a multidisciplinary approach in which professionals from different organizations confer, share decision making, and coordinate their service delivery for the purpose of achieving shared goals and improving health care. Coordination represents a sophisticated level of organizational interaction. It is a process of engaging in various efforts that alter or facilitate the relationships of independent organizations, staffs, or resources. Coordination is characterized by deliberate joint and often formalized relations for achieving shared or compatible goals. It involves establishing a common understanding of the services committed to (and provided by) each agency, and by determining each agency's accountability and responsibility to specific groups. An example of such a partnership is the Community Health Network and Health and Hospital Corporation of Marion County partnership between Wishard-Eskenazi Health and Community Health Network to place both systems and Indianapolis in the best possible position for health care reform and to improve access to quality care for all patients, particularly the indigent and underserved, including small businesses and community organizations (Community Health Network, n.d.).

Partnerships at the local level create a patchwork quilt of support for workplace health promotion programs. Ideally the various types of partnerships blend together to create opportunities for all employers and workplaces (large, midsized, and small). Table 6.2 shows such a patchwork of partnership support, with various sectors of the economy providing resources for it. Workplaces are one element contributing to the many partnerships existing in a community that address many issues including health. Partnerships face challenges being addressed by individuals, communities, employers and unions, the business community, media, faith leaders and congregants, and philanthropy and government officials at all levels to work together on promising strategies and solutions (Robert Wood Johnson Foundation, 2009). Recently the involvement of businesses in health and wellness partnerships has gained importance. And while the role of private business in health partnerships is changing, health agencies,

Table 6.2   Patchwork Quilt of Local Partnerships for Workplace Health Promotion (adapted from Robert Wood Johnson Foundation, 2009)

Community-based groups can adopt a "health lens" to view their communities by: • establishing farmers' markets and advocating for local supermarkets where none exist • ensuring streets are pedestrian- and bike-safe, and advocating for cross walks, bike paths, sidewalks, and security lighting • assessing and remediating hazardous conditions in housing	**Local and state governments** can lead by: • making early child development services a highest priority • offering financial incentives for grocery stores to locate in underserved neighborhoods • incorporating health-conscious designs into building codes and zoning and • adopting statewide smoke-free workplace and public spaces laws
Schools can provide a quality education to give students the best opportunity to achieve good health throughout life; promote healthy personal choices by students; and provide a safe and healthy physical and social environment by: • ensuring all school lunch and breakfast offerings meet the most current U.S. dietary guidelines; removing all junk food from cafeterias, vending machines and canteens • making daily physical activity one of the highest priorities	**The federal government** can lead by: • ensuring that the early developmental needs of children in low-income families are met • fully funding WIC and SNAP and ensuring that these programs are designed to support the needs of hungry families with nutritious food • funding research and evaluation of effective nonmedical and community-based interventions in all sectors that influence health; holding programs that receive federal support accountable for achieving results
Businesses and employers can exercise local leadership and promote employee health by: • making a visible commitment to increase physical activity at work • selecting health plans that include wellness benefits • implementing a comprehensive smoke-free workplace policy and offering proven tobacco-use treatment to smokers	**Philanthropies** can lead by: • supporting initiatives in disadvantaged communities that create opportunities for healthy living and healthy choices • identifying, supporting and championing innovative models of community building and design; joining with federal and state agencies and businesses as partners in supporting and rigorously evaluating place-based, multisector demonstrations
Health care providers, particularly those whose patients have lower incomes or live in disadvantaged communities, can help connect patients with community services and resources	**Governments** at all levels can provide incentives; seed assessments and plans; fund research and evaluations to identify effective approaches to improving health; and provide the foundation for collaborative efforts

and in particular public health agencies, historically have had relatively few formal partnerships with private business. Now it is recognized that both groups share an interest in ensuring a healthy population. Businesses have a financial interest in supporting organized public health efforts; in turn, business partnerships can increase the reach and effectiveness of public health. Such efforts benefit business and create opportunities for collaboration to improve the public's health (Simon & Fielding, 2006).

Collaborations Work at the Regional, State, National, and International Level

Collaborations are groups of interdependent organizations represented by individuals who share responsibility for specific outcomes across a region or state(s) working at the governmental and public policy level. Similar to teams and partnerships, the minimum defining features are shared responsibility and interdependence. Collaboration members use their organization's role and experience working with employees and employers, and a shared goal of helping and supporting to create resources and supports across a region or state(s), to address employee and employer health needs. For example, business and industry associations; business leader coalitions; health care advocacy organizations; hospital associations; health and safety organizations; state departments of business, commerce, and health; and unions can form a collaboration for planning, budgeting, and legislative actions to provide infrastructure to create and finance workplace health promotion programs and services. Similar to partnerships within large organizations, large organization collaborations frequently span states, regions, and nations.

As you gather information about the workplace's involvement with collaborations, assess the organization's appreciation and understanding of the role of collaborations. Collaborations provide access to a broad scope of knowledge and expertise for program and service planning, implementation, and evaluation. Collaborations help workplaces implement and sustain a complex change process to address health issues systemically, as part of a positive workplace climate to promote health. Collaborations provide a sustainable infrastructure for partnerships and capacity to provide resources and training for workplace wellness efforts. The collaborations facilitate large-scale social change that can only come from better cross-sector coordination rather than from the isolated intervention of individual organizations. Evidence of the effectiveness of this approach suggests that substantially greater progress can be made in alleviating many of our most serious and complex social problems if nonprofits, governments, businesses, and the public are together around a common agenda to create collective impact (Kania & Kramer, 2011).

A number of unique national public private collaborations to promote workplace health exist to plan, implement, and evaluate workplace health promotion programs. Most of these resources were developed in the past 25 years to address the range of health issues and problems that employers are asked to address. They can be used as models to compare and contrast with collaborations with which an organization is currently part of.

WELCOA—Wellness Council of America (http://www.welcoa.org/)

The Wellness Council of America (WELCOA) was established as a national not-for-profit organization in the mid-1980s through the efforts of a number of forward-thinking business and health leaders. Its mission is to serve business leaders, workplace wellness practitioners, public health professionals, and consultants of all kinds by:

+ Promoting corporate membership

+ Producing leading-edge worksite wellness publications and health information

+ Conducting trainings that help worksite wellness practitioners create and sustain results-oriented wellness programs

+ Creating resources that promote healthier lifestyles for all working Americans

National Business Group on Health (http://www.businessgrouphealth .org/)

The National Business Group on Health is the national voice of employers dedicated to finding innovative and forward-thinking solutions to the nation's most important health care issues. Its mission is to:

+ Provide practical solutions, including identifying and promoting best practices among employers. Where practical solutions do not exist, provide a forum for members and others to come together to create new solutions and learn from each other.

+ Be the national voice of employers so when new issues arise, create methods for employers to form a point of view, then represent that point of view to the public.

+ Link employers with lobbyists or federal government agencies to provide an ongoing and credible two-way information link between Washington, DC, policymakers and large employers on key health care issues.

- Drive enlightened national policy on health and productivity issues and to be an active player in key policy debates that impact health and productivity.

National Business Coalition on Health (http://www.nbch.org/)

The National Business Coalition on Health (NBCH) is a national, nonprofit, membership organization of purchaser-led health care coalitions. NBCH and its members are dedicated to value-based purchasing of health care services through the collective action of public and private purchasers. NBCH seeks to accelerate the nation's progress toward safe, efficient, high-quality health care and the improved health status of the U.S. population. NBCH's member coalitions and multi-stakeholder affiliates have been actively engaged in developing programs that foster the four pillars of value-based purchasing: standard performance measurement, public reporting of performance measurement results, health care delivery payment system reform, and informed and engaged consumer decision making.

Partnership for Prevention (http://www.prevent.org/)

The Partnership for Prevention is a nonpartisan organization of business, nonprofit, and government leaders working to make evidence-based disease prevention and health promotion a national priority. The partnership's unique blend of members and leaders helps unite diverse interests in support of strong prevention policies. Its members include corporations, trade associations, nongovernmental organizations, patient groups, associations of health professionals, health care delivery organizations, and government agencies.

Trust for America's Health (http://healthyamericans.org/)

Trust for America's Health (TFAH) is a nonprofit, nonpartisan organization dedicated to saving lives by protecting the health of every community and by working to make disease prevention a national priority. The Trust Workplace wellness initiative addresses how employers can support and promote community-based prevention-related efforts to healthy environments for their employees and their families at home. The States of Wellness is a TFAH national survey research project exploring the experiences, attitudes, and opinions of human resource professionals regarding worksite wellness. Included in the project is a nationwide online survey of human resource executives and separate regional polls in six states.

National Small Business Association (http://www.nsba.net/)

The National Small Business Association Inc. was established for the purpose of providing small business owners, their employees, and retirees access to innovative services, programs, information, and benefits that would help their businesses to succeed and improve the quality of their lives. The association is the longest-running small business advocacy organization in the United States, operating on a staunchly nonpartisan basis as a leader in health care policy. A key component of its health care platform is promoting the role that workplace wellness programs can play in keeping health care accessible and affordable for small-business owners and their employees.

Small Business Majority (http://www.smallbusinessmajority.org/)

Small Business Majority is an advocacy group founded and run by small business owners to focus on solving the biggest problems facing small businesses today. The group actively engages small business owners and policymakers in support of solutions that promote small business growth and drive a strong economy. It advocates for policies that create jobs and maximize business opportunities and cost savings in health care reform, clean energy, access to capital, and other areas.

Summary

Teams, partnerships, and collaborations take a socioecological approach to workplace health promotion. They address health concerns and problems. They work at the local level reflecting the commitment and investment of people and resources for the solution to local needs. Collaborations work on changes in practices and policies across a region, state, or states. Likewise they can work across large organizations. Workplace health promotion teams, partnerships, and collaborations that effectively address health concerns don't just happen. They are the result of strategic effort and commitment from many people and organizations. Gathering information about a workplace's health promotion teams, partnerships, and collaborations can help you to gain insight into current efforts as well as to make decisions about how each approach can best support workplace health promotion program.

For Practice and Discussion

1. Being a member of a team, partnership, and collaboration you will face conflict. It is a difficult process. Many people are uncomfortable with

conflict, but not dealing with it can paralyze your team. Below are five points to help you better manage conflict (Segal & Smith, 2011). Using the five points, discuss how you mange conflict. Do you agree with each of the points?

1. A conflict is more than just a disagreement. It is a situation in which one or both parties perceive a threat (whether or not the threat is real).

2. Conflicts continue to fester when ignored. Because conflicts involve perceived threats to an individual's well-being and survival, they linger until faced and resolved.

3. Individuals respond to conflicts based on their perceptions of the situation, not necessarily to an objective review of the facts. Perceptions are influenced by life experiences, culture, values, and beliefs.

4. Conflicts trigger strong emotions. If individuals are not comfortable with their emotions or able to manage them in times of stress, they won't be able to resolve conflict successfully.

5. Conflicts are an opportunity for growth. When individuals are able to resolve conflict in a relationship, it builds trust and the security of knowing that the relationship can survive challenges and disagreements.

2. Tour a workplace. During the tour ask about the different workplace teams. Identify the purpose and membership of the teams. Collect information about team activities, programs, and services.

3. Do a web search for workplace partnerships in your local community. Identify current members and their organizations. What are two other organizations that might strengthen and expand current services and programs?

4. One of the many benefits of belonging to and being active with a national workplace health promotion collaboration is attending their national meetings and conferences. Typically they have outstanding speakers, engaging workshops, and training opportunities, as well as ample time to network with conference participants about jobs, career development, programs, and resources. Investigate the conferences of the organizations listed in the chapter collaboration section. What speakers, workshops, and training are of most interest to you? Investigate conference cost including travel, conference fees, and lodging. Are there opportunities for students to volunteer at the conferences for a reduced admission fee? Will your school support student conference travel?

Case Study: Newly Promoted National Health and Safety Director—What Would You Do?

Mario Brown, the health and safety director for a large national corporation, worked for years as a safety inspector and director in each of the corporation's five manufacturing plants (each employing 500 to 700 machinist, technical, and administrative workers). Recently he was promoted to the national directorship with the mandate to combine the safety and health initiatives. His corporation has a strong safety culture. In fact every meeting regardless of level (e.g., factory floor, middle management, corporate office) starts with a safety briefing. His plan is to build a corporate health and safety team, form health partnerships, and be part of broad workplace health collaborations. Mr. Brown in his own words, however, is "looking at four office walls and a long list of unanswered emails. As I begin to plan our workplace program, I am one person given a title of national health and safety director. I am enthusiastic and energized but I really need to figure out what we are doing, what we want to do, and how we are going to do it, as well as how to evaluate it. I am thinking 'health and safety team formation' but there are already teams in the company. I am competing with people being part of teams for marketing, sales, plant health and safety, quality assurance, customer service, departments, unions, management, compensation and benefits, diversity, and staff development. I am not naïve about the task in front of me."

If you were Mario Brown, newly promoted to national health and safety director, what would you do?

KEY TERMS

Teams	Elements of collaboration
Partnerships	WELCOA—Wellness Council of America
Collaborations	National Business Group on Health
Socioecological approach	National Business Coalition on Health
Human resource teams	Partnership for Prevention
Organizational size	Trust for America's Health
Team membership	National Small Business Association
Partnership models	Small Business Majority
Partnership support and resource balance	

References

Community Health Network. (n.d.). *Community employer health.* Retrieved June 8, 2015, from http://www.ecommunity.com/s/community-employer-health /employee-wellness-services/com

Kania, J., & Kramer, M. (2011). Collective impact. *Stanford Social Innovation Review, 1*(9), 36–41.

Hewlett-Packard. (2015). *Living progress.* Retrieved from http://www8.hp.com /us/en/hp-information/global-citizenship/index.html?jumpid=reg_r1002_usen _c-001_title_r0001

Hunnicutt, D. (2007). 10 secrets of successful worksite wellness teams. *WELCOA's Absolute Advantage Magazine, 6*(3), 6–13.

Noe, R. A., Hollenbeck, J. R., Gerhart, B., & Wright, P. M. (2013). *Human resource management: Gaining a competitive advantage.* New York, NY: McGraw-Hill Irwin.

Robert Wood Johnson Foundation (2009, April). *Beyond health care: New directions to a healthier America.* Retrieved from http://www.rwjf.org/content/dam /farm/reports/reports/2009/rwjf40483

Segal, J., & Smith, M. (2011). *Conflict resolution skills.* Retrieved from http://www.helpguide.org/articles/relationships/conflict-resolution-skills.htm

Simon, P. A., & Fielding, J. E. (2006). Public health and business: A partnership that makes cents. *Health Affairs, 25*(4), 1029–1039.

Skage, S. (1996). *Building strong and effective community partnerships: A manual for family literacy workers.* Alberta, Canada: The Family Literacy Action Group of Alberta. Retrieved from http://en.copian.ca/library /learning/partner/partner.pdf

CHAPTER 7

ASSESSING EMPLOYEE HEALTH NEEDS AND TRANSITION TO IMPLEMENTATION

Employee Health Needs Assessment Data and Sources

Employee health needs vary by the workplace. Employee health needs assessments gather data (indicators) to accurately identify the scope and specificity of employee health needs. The data are specific pieces of information (or indicators) that can be used to make decisions related to the workplace health promotion program plan, implementation, and evaluation. Data sources can include but not be limited to the human resource management department, health promotion program staff, occupational health department, workers' compensation and benefits, and health insurance provider. The scope of the assessment refers to the range and variability of employee needs identified, whereas the specificity refers to the type and prevalence of identified needs. When feasible, health need assessments analyze as many of the following types of data as possible: demographic profiles, health status, health records, biometric screening, workers' compensation claims and costs, medical care claims and costs, and job productivity (Table 7.1).

Demographics

Demographics are sourced from human resource management to provide an overview of the workplace population. The gender, age, ethnicity, disability status, and job category (e.g., professional, clerical, technical, sales, labor) distribution shape and influence the health concerns that

LEARNING OBJECTIVES

- Identify employee health needs assessment data and sources

- Explain how to use needs assessment results to support and make program decisions

- Describe what to expect to know and to have at the conclusion of the planning process

Table 7.1   Examples of the Employee Health Needs Data, Source, Scope, and Specificity (adapted from Chenoweth, 2011, p. 23)

Data	Source	Scope	Specificity
Demographics	Human resource management	Age range 18 to 70 years Females 55% Management 10% Nonmanagement 90%	Average age 47 Median age 41
Health risk assessment	Health promotion program staff	8 of 10 lifestyle indicators rated poorly in > 70% of respondents	Five highest risk indicators: 1. Physical inactivity 2. Mental stress 3. Overweight or obesity 4. Existing musculoskeletal condition 5. Financial stress
Health records	Medical department	Utilization rankings Preemployment examination Job standard examination Risk exposure Accidents and injuries	Five highest concerns 1. Physical activity limitations 2. Stress 3. Substance usage 4. Lead exposure 5. Hearing and vision
Biometric screening	Occupation health department	Asthma 25% Diabetes 10% Hypertension 30% Migraine 10% Obesity 35%	75% of type-2 diabetes work in labor intensive jobs 33% of hypertensive cases are unmanaged
Workers' compensation claims and costs	Benefits manager/insurance provider	Compensation claims rising 5% each year	Factory floor musculoskeletal conditions account for 65% of all claims Number of injuries, percentage of employees with injuries, cost of injuries, days lost by types of injuries, time to return to work
Medical claims and costs	Benefits manager/insurance provider	Outpatient services costs rising 8% each year Inpatient costs rising 4% each year Prescription drug costs rising 7% each year	Diagnostic testing comprises 60% of all outpatient costs vs. 50% last year Average length of stay has dropped in 9 of 10 leading inpatient conditions
Productivity	Human resource management including benefits manager	Absenteeism 3% Presenteeism 15% Satisfaction 75 %	Self-reported presenteeism is 2 times higher among sedentary workers as in factory floor workers

a workplace health promotion program might address. For example, using the Healthy People 2020 initiative can identify potential health concerns that might be expected based on the demographics of a particular workplace.

Health Risk Assessments

Health risk assessments (HRAs) encourage employees to evaluate their current health and quality of life. They promote health awareness by reviewing employees' personal lifestyle practices and revealing health issues that could be impacted by personal choices. Examples of HRA health topic areas include health status, use of preventive health services, and health behaviors. HRAs focus on whether individuals are meeting public health standards or good health recommendations. These standards and recommendations come from government agencies and national and international health organizations. Harris and Fries (2002) note that although the term *health risk appraisal*, which connotes a goal of quantitative overall health risk computation (i.e., estimating odds of dying based on health status), was once commonly used, the preference slowly evolved to health risk assessment with its focus on triaging personalized interventions, assessing quality, measuring change, and meeting goals. Today HRAs are largely computerized, with many commercialized HRA tools in a variety of types and price ranges. HRAs can be found in self-scoring formats, computerized questionnaires forms with extensive outcome reports, phone-based tools, and interactive online versions. Some have added productivity-based questions in an attempt to simultaneously measure the effects of health risks on well-being and on-the-job productivity. Information can also be gathered on employees' interest, motivation, and community health engagement (e.g., access to parks and recreational facilities, recreational community sports team participation, and gym membership).

Examples of HRA Health Topic Areas (Centers for Disease Control and Prevention [CDC], 2013b)

*   **Health status**
    *   Self-perceived general health status (e.g., poor to excellent)
    *   Number of days per month impaired by poor physical/mental health
    *   Specific questions about diseases or health conditions (e.g., high blood pressure, high cholesterol, asthma, arthritis, stress)
*   **Use of preventive health services**
    *   Doctor visits
    *   Dental visits

- Flu vaccines

- Blood pressure and cholesterol checks

- Colonoscopies, mammograms, and Pap smears

- **Health behaviors**

  - Tobacco use—current smokers or other tobacco use, tobacco cessation

  - Diet and physical activity—weight and height (to calculate body mass index, or BMI); self-perceptions of weight; fruit/vegetable consumption; activity level at work; recent moderate/vigorous activity outside of the job

  - Alcohol consumption—drinks per week; drinks per sitting

  - Safety—seatbelt use

Making HRA mandatory for employee health insurance coverage may be appealing but not legal. Therefore to encourage employee participation, employers offer incentives and work to engage employees to be active in their health promotion. HRA design considers the number and type of questionnaire items, delivery mode (e.g., paper, web-based, personal report generation), time required to complete HRA, availability of risk-reduction follow-up (e.g., access to information and referrals), and costs (Chenoweth, 2011).

Using health informatics, the HRA results are aggregated without any employee names or personally identifying information, thereby protecting confidentiality but allowing employee population risk comparisons. The aggregated data are then compared and contrasted with any one of a number of aggregated data sets. These include previous organizational data from a prior year, aggregated data from other organizations in the region (e.g., county, section of state, or country), and industry. Other examples of common sources for good health comparisons (standards and recommendations) include the American Heart Association (AHA), American Cancer Society (ASC), American Diabetes Association (ADA), American Public Health Association (APHA), National Institutes of Health (NIH), Office of the Surgeon General, U.S. Food and Drug Administration (FDA), and World Health Organization (WHO).

Health Records

Employee health records are generated as the result of workplace-related employee physical examinations completed for preemployment, to determine individuals' fitness to medically and physically perform their roles (exam labels include job standard, regulatory, or compliance examinations), risk exposure (e.g., radiation and lead exposure), and employee wellness examinations. Preemployment physical exams may include health inquiries and physical examinations, including psychological tests, and physical or mental health assessments. To protect against discrimination in hiring, the physical examination should be required after a job is offered. The physical examination must be related to the job the applicant will be doing. There are several types of drug tests that candidates for employment may be asked to take. The types of drug tests, which show the presence of drugs or alcohol, include urine drug screen, hair drug or alcohol testing, saliva drug screen, and sweat drug screen. Physical ability tests measure the ability of an applicant to perform a particular task or the strength of specific muscle groups, as well as strength and stamina in general. The examination results, which become of the employee health record, are protected by federal legislation (HIPAA).

Biometric Screening

Biometric testing in the workplace is for screening rather than diagnosis or treatment. Included are measurements for total cholesterol, high-density lipoprotein (HDL), low-density lipoprotein (LDL), triglycerides, blood glucose, blood pressure, vision testing, BMI, and waist-to-hip ratio. The health records and screening results can help classify overweight and obese individuals and predict or detect cardiovascular problems and diabetes. They can also become part of the health risk assessment, which then triggers additional risk and health reporting. Other measures such as the percent of body fat, hemoglobin A1c, and high-sensitivity C-reactive protein may be collected but generally not recommended. The most difficult portion of most biometric testing is the blood draw, with finger stick technology being preferred. Generally for workplace health promotion programs less is better (Framer & Chikamoto, 2009). The results of the HRA in combination with the health record and biometric testing is aggregated and analyzed for the population. Consistent with the overall biometric testing purpose of screening (rather than diagnosis or treatment) disease risk factors and defining criteria are used to understand the health needs of the workplace population.

Workers' Compensation Claims and Costs

To help understand the cost of workers' compensation to a business, a number of benchmarks can be used (Workers Compensation Institute, n.d.). These include the benefit payment to the individual per claim with more than 7 days of lost time, the expense to the provider to provide the services to the individual per claim with more than 7 days of lost time (including medical and legal expenses), timeliness of knowing about the claim and payment to the individual, percentage of claims with more than 7 days of lost time, and medical utilization (e.g., costs, visits, and provider mix, by type of provider).

Looking at injury and workers' compensation data will allow for identifying causes of injury that should be targeted by an intervention program (CDC, 2013a). The Occupational Safety and Health Administration (OSHA) requires that injuries be reported for any organization with more than 10 employees. In addition to injuries sustained on-site, employers often collect data associated with near accidents and near misses. Accidents may or may not result in an injury. An analysis of injury data can examine patterns, rate changes, and trends over time. For example, are injuries more common among specific demographics groups (e.g., older adults or men); do they seem to occur at the same times (e.g., middle of the night in a 24-hour facility); are certain injuries related to specific job tasks; or which injuries are the highest cost (e.g., injuries resulting in knee replacement)?

Variables of interest when examining injury data include:

- Looking at the most common types of injuries (e.g., burns, cuts, sprains, bruises, fractures).

- Looking at the severity of injury and resulting workers' compensation or disability claims and costs, and the number of days the employee could not work.

- Looking at the most common areas of the body that were injured (e.g., hands, shoulders, head).

- Looking at the cause of injury (e.g., falls, slips, body position, struck by flying object).

- Looking at injury rates by shift (e.g., time of injury).

- Looking at the frequency of injury per shift, per day, and per employee. For example, the company has one injury resulting in medical attention every 45 days. Or the rate of near misses is one for every 50 employees over the past year.

- Looking at injury rates by sex, age, and job type.

- Review of OSHA or other logs of recorded accidents that resulted in injury or near misses that did not result in injury but may present a safety hazard.

Medical Claims and Costs

Assessing health claims and care costs by individual demographic characteristics (e.g., employment status, sex, age) and organizational demographic characteristics (e.g., unit or division, multiple sites in one organization) you can identify groups of individuals or workplaces with the highest health care costs, and results of those analyses can be used to identify priority populations or workplace health promotion programs. In order to assess health care expenditures, individual-level health claims data is obtained and aggregated from the health plan provider(s). Table 7.2 lists examples

Table 7.2   Potential Indicators of Health Claims Data Related to Workplace Health Promotion

Indicator	Data Elements Examples	
Use of preventive health (percentage of employees receiving)	Physical exam (annual)	Fasting lipid profile
	Colorectal cancer screening	Vision exam
	Mammography	Hearing screening
	Pap smear	Tobacco cessation
	Immunizations (influenza, pneumonia)	Counseling for obesity
	Screening for diabetes	Counseling for diabetes
Health claims (cost and percentage of employees receiving)	Health care visits	Breast cancer
	Heart disease	Colon cancer
	Diabetes	Lung cancer
	Diabetes complications	Prostate cancer
	Hypertension	Skin cancer
	High cholesterol	Depression
	Arthritis	Hearing loss
	Chronic obstructive pulmonary disease (COPD)	Influenza
	Reproductive health	Injury
	Oral health	Chronic liver disease, cirrhosis, and hepatitis
Medication use (number of patients and total costs for selected drug classes)	Anti-hypertensives	Asthma
	Diabetes (e.g., insulin)	Chemotherapy
	Antidepressants	Nonsteroid anti-inflammatory drug (NSAID)
	Antianxiety	Contraceptives
Quality of care: Screening (percentage of of adults age appropriate)	Colorectal cancer (CRC) screening	
	Mammogram in previous 2 years	
	PAP smear	
Quality of Care Diabetes (percentage of people with diabetes)	Percent receiving eye exam	
	Percent receiving foot exams	
	Percent receiving medication or insulin	

of information for each enrollee that might be considered when assessing medical claims data (http://www.cdc.gov/workplacehealthpromotion/assessment/claims_assessment/index.html).

Medical claim data is reported using medical claim codes. There are two main components of a medical claim: the International Statistical Classification of Diseases currently in its 10th edition (ICD-10) and Current Procedural Terminology (CPT) Codes maintained by the American Medical Association.

ICD-10 codes explain why the person sought medical attention. Every diagnosis, disease, and condition has its own ICD-10 code. As shown in Figure 7.1, the ICD-10 code for adult onset diabetes without complications is E11.9: If there were complications, such as blindness, then there would be a different code (E11.3). Specifications or complications of the general disease or condition (e.g., blindness associated with diabetes) build off the baseline code for the disease or condition. The ICD-10 code does not represent an expenditure or charge.

Each CPT code corresponds to a particular procedure, service, device, or treatment. Unlike the ICD-10 codes, CPT codes translate into direct medical costs. For instance, the diagnosis of diabetes is not a billable procedure, while the glucose test to diagnose the disease is.

Health care expenditures analysis can include health claims data for employees and employee dependents. Analyzing the data for employees and their dependents separately will assist in selecting the priority audience of the health promotion program. Health claims data for dependents can illuminate the health issues that contribute to an employee's absenteeism and time off.

Additional stratification of results by sex and age groups will also be helpful in identifying specific demographic groups with higher health care costs. Similarly, it is important to stratify results by place of service (e.g., emergency room [ER], inpatient services, outpatient services). This can both demonstrate the types of issues employees face and also the cost of these services. For instance, high costs from ER services each year may indicate an opportunity for preventive care policies and programs.

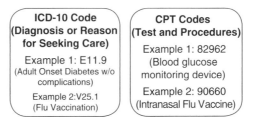

Figure 7.1   Medical Claim Codes

In order to identify major sources for health care expenditures, it is sufficient to look at the health care cost data from 1 year. However, depending on the sample size, more stable estimates would be obtained by combining health care claims data for 24 or more months.

When reporting the results, it is important to clarify the time period for which the costs are reported (e.g., 1- or 2-year period). It is also important to recognize employee retention and turnover rates when performing annual evaluations. For a company with a low turnover rate, data will likely remain the same and the population the team is evaluating will likely be the same population to receive the program at the workplace. However, for a company with a high turnover rate, it may be useful to focus on an evaluation for those employees considered "stable"—or likely to stay with the company for a longer period of time.

Productivity

Productivity measures can be a useful part of the health needs assessment. Examples include employee absenteeism, presenteeism, and satisfaction. This information is often available from a human resources (HR) representative. Both pre- and post-assessment of productivity measures and absenteeism can be conducted to assess program impact. Furthermore periodic climate/pulse check surveys can illustrate employees' understanding of:

- Company health-related policies

- Usage of company health-related programs

- Interest in particular programs or initiatives

- Quality of work life

- Highlight various areas of need

Employee engagement/climate surveys can also provide information about relationships in the workplace and highlight areas where improvements can be made. For example, surveys can be used to ascertain information about relationships among coworkers; assess the level of support provided by supervisors and colleagues; or determine who is most likely to provide employees information on the organization's health-related programs and policies (http://www.cdc.gov/workplacehealthpromotion/assessment/potential_data/attendance.html).

Use Needs Assessment Results to Support and Make Program Decisions

Workplace employee health needs assessment drives the decision making behind the program. The needs assessment data is used to make the business case for the program, stratify the employees' health needs, understand a health and safety problem, and set priorities. As part of priority setting, the data is used to analyze employees' health risks, prevalence of health problems, and adherence and participation in addressing health problems. Furthermore, as part of setting priorities, the data can be used to understand employees' health care choices and service utilization, which can clarify costs. Finally the needs assessment data is used to support the decision making of the health promotion program staff, and to lay the foundation for the program evaluation (to improve program performance and accountability).

Making the Business Case

Needs assessment data is used to make the business case for workplace health promotion programs. For small and midsized employers the business case often focuses on health concerns and problems among employees that are high and can be addressed, thereby lowering costs as well as improving productivity (i.e., healthy employees). For large organizations, making the business case might also focus on the organization's bottom line (i.e., profits and earnings). Essentially the data is used to argue that even though the workplace health promotion program costs money, in the long run the program will save money for the organization. As an example, a human resource manager and chief financial officer (CFO) at one large employer presented a business case to its executive team by estimating the company's total health-related costs (including medical, pharmacy, presenteeism, and absenteeism costs). The data showed that the employer was likely experiencing 8 days of lost health-related productivity (absenteeism and presenteeism) per full-time equivalent employee (FTE) per year, at a cost of $2,598 per employee. When multiplied by the number of FTEs in that workforce, the modeled health-related productivity costs for that employer totaled $153 million per year. With a workplace health promotion program, data showed that if the same employer could reduce health-related productivity loss by 1 day per FTE per year, it would add $18.8 million to the bottom-line earnings (Fireman, Bartlett, & Selby, 2004).

The National Business Group on Health (2014) to support businesses in their efforts to make a strong business case reported companies with highly effective workplace health promotion programs:

* Yield 20% more revenue per employee

* Demonstrate a 16.1% higher market value

* Deliver 57% higher shareholder returns

Have cost increases that are:

* 5 times lower for sick leave

* 4.5 times lower for longer disability

* 4 times lower for short-term disability

* 3.5 times lower for general health coverage

Stratify the Employees' Health Needs

As a prerequisite to establishing health care goals and programs, use the data to conduct a basic analysis of demographics, risk factors, and disease burden (the impact of health problems measured by indicators such as financial cost, mortality, and morbidity) to identify (stratify) employee populations that will benefit from specific programs. To stratify the employee population precisely requires the use of the medical and pharmacy claims data as well as the data on disability, workers' compensation and absence, HRA, and biometric data. The list below shows a four-level employee population health risk stratification to guide the selection of specific health promotion programs to impact the health problem, health care costs, and health-related productivity.

Four-Level Employee Population Health Risk Stratification
(Change Agent Work Group, 2009)

Level 1: High/Acute Risk. Medically unstable individuals (employees) who require frequent use of services and are noncompliant with evidence-based treatments. Many are candidates for case management. Also may include individuals who demonstrate high cardiometabolic risk due to recent biometric testing and/or family history.

Level 2: Chronic Risk. Less stable, evidence of noncompliance, poorly controlled disease state. Noncompliant/nonadherent individuals risk moving to level 1 without behavior change.

Level 3: Moderate Risk. Medically stable, compliant, and well controlled.

Level 4: Low Risk. Relatively healthy, undiagnosed, and exhibit healthy behaviors.

Assess Health and Safety Risks and Problems

Organizations need to assess and control risks in the workplace and comply with health and safety laws. A risk assessment is simply a careful

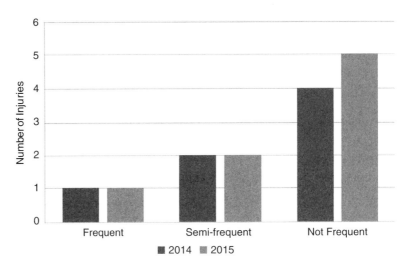

Figure 7.2   Injury Occurrence Associated With Routine and Nonroutine Work Tasks

examination of what, in the workplace, could cause harm to people, so that you can weigh whether you have taken enough precautions or should do more to prevent harm. Workers and others have a right to be protected from harm caused by a failure to take reasonable control measures. A hazard is anything that may cause harm, such as chemicals, electricity, working from ladders, an open drawer, and so forth. You can assess the risk by combining the chance (high or low) that these and other hazards will harm someone with an indication of how serious the harm could be. The risk assessment is a five-step process. The workers' compensation and injury data is a starting point for risk assessments. From such data it is possible to pinpoint hazards. For example, a manufacturing plant with high worker compensation claims identified that the frequency of injuries increased when workers completed nonroutine tasks (e.g., covering the area for an absent employee, assisting on a task for which the employee was not trained). Figure 7.2 illustrates that nonroutine tasks increased the probability of injury by four fold. Furthermore the data revealed the injury cause (Figure 7.3).

Such findings are used to take corrective actions and formulate safety and health promotion procedures and programs.

Five Steps to Risk Assessment (Health and Safety Executive, 2012)

Step 1. Identify the hazards.

Step 2. Decide who might be harmed and how.

Step 3. Evaluate the risks and decide on precautions.

Step 4. Record your findings and implement them.

Step 5. Review your risk assessment and update if necessary.

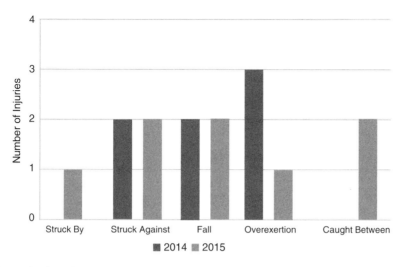

Figure 7.3 Injury Cause

Establishing Health Priorities

Needs assessment data is used to establish priorities in workplace health promotion programs for the employee populations identified through the employee health-risk stratification. Setting priorities is most likely a nominal group process or similar technique that is used to reduce the list of health problems to a manageable number of topics. Identifying the problems to address first requires that criteria (e.g., importance, feasibility for change, magnitude of problem, cost) be established and shared. These priorities provide justification for starting new programs and continuing or terminating existing programs. The following issues might be factors to consider in establishing program priorities at a workplace.

+ How many individuals are affected by the health problems?

+ Which problem has the greatest impact on disability and/or mortality?

+ What will be the consequences if the health problem is not corrected?

+ Would not correcting the problem cause other health-related problems?

+ What will be the potential impact on others in the community if the health problem is reduced?

+ How difficult will it be to correct the health problem?

+ How many resources will be required to solve the health-related problem?

+ How effective are available interventions in preventing or reducing the health-related problem?

- Do you have the expertise to resolve the health-related problem?
- What are the barriers (obstacles) to correcting the health-related problem?
- Do current laws permit the health-related program activities to be conducted?

As part of setting priorities the data is used to analyze employees' health risks, prevalence of health problems, and adherence and participation in addressing health problems. Furthermore the data can be used to understand employees' health program choices and service utilization, which contributes to clarifying costs.

The needs assessment provides a snapshot of the workplace employees' health risks (Table 7.3). Looking at that data identified through the HRAs,

Table 7.3   Risk Data Analysis Report

Top Five HRA-Identified Conditions		
High blood pressure (hypertension)	52	29.2%
High cholesterol	37	20.8%
Obesity (BMI of 30 or more)	37	20.8%
Low back pain (6 weeks or longer)	33	18.5%
Gastroesophageal reflux disease	32	18.0%
Participants with at least one condition	103	57.9%
Top Five Productivity-Related Risks		
BMI 27.5 or more	94	52.8%
Physical Activity <1 day per week	41	23.0%
Seatbelt—not all the time	22	12.4%
Current smoker (cigarettes, pipe, or cigar)	19	10.7%
Exceeds weekly alcohol consumption	17	9.6%
Participates with at least three productivity-related risks	31	17.4%
Top Five Areas Indicated as Ready to Change		
Diet	155	87.1%
Stress	105	59.0%
Exercise, strength	89	50.0%
Exercise, cardio	67	37.6%
Lose weight	40	22.5%
Participants ready to change at least one area	173	97.2%

Table 7.4 Chronic Condition Prevalence

Chronic Condition	Current Year	Previous Year
Asthma	8.6%	8.4%
Depression	12.3%	11.7%
Diabetes	5.3%	5.2%
Hyperlipidemia	17.4%	16.9%
Hypertension	18.4%	18.1%
Lower Back Pain	19.2%	16.5%

medical records, and biometric screenings, we can know the top health conditions and productivity risks that need to be addressed as part of a program. In addition, using HRA questions based on Transtheoretical Model Health Stages allows for the collection and assessment of employees' readiness to make changes to address health risks. Furthermore drawing from the medical claims data, chronic condition prevalence among the population management data is calculated and compared over time (Table 7.4).

The data can be compared and contrasted with previous periods to show participation and adherence in the health promotion program. For example, Table 7.5 shows comparisons for participation in the HRA and preventive care. The data contribute to understanding the adherence of employees in the improvement of their health as well as providing feedback on where the program perhaps needs to focus its efforts. A desired participation level target (e.g., 80%) can be included to provide additional feedback and to gauge progress.

The data is used to understand employees' health care service and utilization choices. The goal of such analysis is utilization of services that is transparent and maximizes effectiveness for both the employee's health outcomes and health care costs (Baicker, Cutler, & Song, 2010; O'Donnell, 2015).

Table 7.6 shows utilization of health care by care delivery platforms. There is a cost associated with each delivery platform. Workplace health promotion programs can develop strategies and initiatives to encourage employees' use of the most cost-effective delivery platforms. Table 7.7 illustrates the use of the data to understand lost time at work due to incidental absences, short-term disability, and workers' compensation. Comparing and contrasting the data over 2 years allows you to understand where you need to focus efforts, and highlights as well the impact of current efforts in these areas. Figure 7.4 shows the utilization of the Employee Assistance Program (EAP). Similar to the other data analyses, this data

Table 7.5   Participation and Adherence Comparison

HRA Participation	$n = 41,915$	40,262	
	Current Year	**Previous Year**	**Target**
% Group health members completing HRA:	61.2%	60.4%	80%

Preventive Care

Cancer Screening Compliance	Current Year	Previous Year
Breast cancer screening	72.4%	69.8%
Cervical cancer screening	70.4%	67.6%
Colorectal cancer screening	58.3%	58.3%

	Current Year	Previous Year
Periodic Health Exam (within last 3 yrs.)	58.6%	64.2%

Clinical Lab Improvement

Risk	Current Year	Previous Year
Weight (BMI $\geq$ 25)	58.0%	57.7%
Glucose (F $\geq$ 100; NF $\geq$ 140)	4.8%	4.6%
Total cholesterol ($\geq$ 200)	32.1%	32.3%
LDL cholesterol ($\geq$ 130)	13.8%	32.7%
HDL cholesterol (m $\leq$ 39; f $\leq$ 49)	7.0%	8.3%
High blood pressure ($\geq$ 120/80)	41.6%	40.5%
Triglycerides ($\geq$ 150)	23.8%	24.7%

Table 7.6   Utilization by Care Delivery Platform

	Visits/1,000	
Platform	**Current Year**	**Previous Year**
e-Visits	2.5	2.6
On-site Clinic Visits	52.9	30.2
Retail Clinic Visits	14.4	22.2
PCP Visits	1,745.3	1,772.8
Ambulatory Care Center Visits	279.4	239.5
Wellness Visits	887.1	873.5
Specialist Visits	2,926.7	2,824.4
ED Visits	238.0	235.1

Table 7.7 Lost Time at Work Due to Incidental Absences, Short-Term Disability, and Workers' Compensation

Lost Work Time Category	Estimated. Cost/Employee		% of Employees. Absent/Day		Estimated Productivity Loss	
	Current Year	Previous Year	Current Year	Previous Year	Current Year	Previous Year
Incidental Absence	$572	$575	1.3%	1.3%	$32,247,286	$28,861,952
Short-Term Disability	$459	$382	1.1%	0.9%	$25,889,520	$19,168,320
Workers' Compensation	$91	$98	0.2%	0.2%	$5,106,024	$4,897,704
Totals	$1,121	$1055	2.6%	2.4%	$63,242,830	$52,927,976

Number of Days in a Transitional Restricted Capacity

	Current Year	Previous Year
Short-Term Disability	33,274	30,686
Workers' Compensation	42,532	39,049

Return to Work Claim Percentage

	Current Year	Previous Year
Short-Term Disability	11.6%	15.1%
Workers' Compensation	16.3%	17.6%

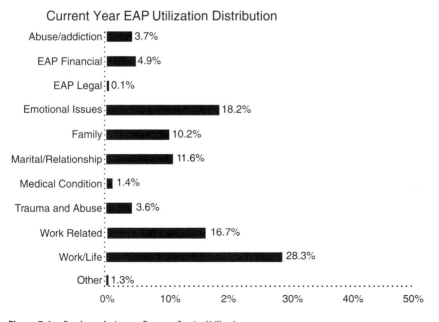

Current Year EAP Utilization Distribution

- Abuse/addiction: 3.7%
- EAP Financial: 4.9%
- EAP Legal: 0.1%
- Emotional Issues: 18.2%
- Family: 10.2%
- Marital/Relationship: 11.6%
- Medical Condition: 1.4%
- Trauma and Abuse: 3.6%
- Work Related: 16.7%
- Work/Life: 28.3%
- Other: 1.3%

Figure 7.4 Employee Assistance Program Service Utilization

help to set priorities as to where to focus programmatic efforts related to the EAP.

Support Health Promotion Program Staff Decision Making

Highly effective workplace health promotion program staff members are knowledgeable of the employee health needs assessment. Staff may or may not be involved with making the business case, stratifying the population, or setting program priorities. However, staff members' knowledge of the needs assessment data contributes to their understanding of how the program design meets employees' health needs and the implications of the data for decisions related to program operation (Table 7.8).

Laying the Foundation for Evaluation

The needs assessment data lay the foundation for program evaluation. Ongoing analytics are performed on the common drivers of employee health status and health care costs. Evaluations analyze metrics associated with specific programs along with a comprehensive set of metrics for overall health management performance. (For example, what impact is the disease management vendor having on costs associated with diabetes? How successful has a health coaching service been in directing at-risk employees to their doctors or producing healthy behavior changes?) In addition to measuring the impact of programs on medical cost trends, analytics should measure their impact on incidental absence, short-term disability, long-term disability, and workers' compensation. The needs assessment is part of the overall program evaluation cycle of asking and answering questions that provides stakeholders (i.e., employers and employees) information and data to improve the program and to provide program accountability (Perales, Fourney, MkNelly, Mamary, 2010).

The data collected as part of the needs assessment process reflect that the ACA for workplace health promotion programs raised a higher degree of accountability for program quality, appropriateness, and efficiency, as well the need to improve program outcomes. The expectations are now for workplace health promotion programs, as well as all health care providers and services, to use evidence-based interventions and practices, reduce variability in strategies, methods, and resource use that cannot be clinically justified, and increase coordination of programs through the use of information technology and team-based initiatives, all the while emphasizing prevention and disease management and giving individuals (employees) a stronger voice in their own health and health care and in defining what matters. The needs assessment is part of the process by which

Table 7.8   Examples of the Health Promotion Program Staff Decision-Making Implications Drawn From Health Needs Data, Source, Scope, and Specificity (adapted from Chenoweth, 2011, p. 23)

Data	Source	Scope	Specificity	Implications
Demographics	Human resource management	Age range 18 to 70 years Females 55% Management 10% Nonmanagement 90%	Average age 47 Median age 41	Most workers are approaching middle age Programs need to reach wide range of ages
Health risk assessment	Health promotion program staff	8 of 10 lifestyle indicators rated poorly in > 70% of respondents	Five highest risk indicators: 1. Physical inactivity 2. Mental stress 3. Overweight or obesity 4. Existing musculoskeletal condition 5. Financial stress	Workforce needs program regarding: Total mind-body wellness Stress management
Health records	Medical department	Utilization rankings Preemployment examination Job standard examination Risk exposure Accidents and injuries	Five highest concerns 1. Physical activity limitations 2. Stress 3. Substance usage 4. Lead exposure 5. Hearing and vision	Worker preparation and training expansion to include health and physical activity and stress management
Biometric screening	Occupation health department	Asthma 25% Diabetes 10% Hypertension 30% Migraine 10% Obesity 35%	75% of type-2 diabetes work in labor intensive jobs 33% of hypertensive cases are unmanaged	Assess real impact of diabetes on productivity Hypertension case management program is needed
Workers' compensation claims and costs	Benefits manager/ insurance provider	Compensation claims rising 5% each year	Factory floor musculoskeletal conditions account for 65% of all claims Number of injuries, percentage of employees with injuries, cost of injuries, days lost by types of injuries, time to return to work	Assess the factory floor machinery ergonomics that need to be addressed
Medical claims and costs	Benefits manager/ insurance provider	Outpatient services costs rising 8% each year Inpatient costs rising 4% each year Prescription drug costs rising 7% each year	Diagnostic testing comprises 60% of all outpatient costs vs. 50% last year Average length of stay has dropped in 9 of 10 leading inpatient conditions	Asses factors that are driving more testing
Productivity	Human resource management including benefits manager	Absenteeism 3% Presenteeism 15% Satisfaction 75%	Self-reported presenteeism is 2 times higher among sedentary workers as in factory floor workers	Need to explore options to motivate sedentary workers to become more physically active

organizations demonstrate their compliance with the law and commitment to promoting employees' health.

What to Expect to Have and to Know at the Conclusion of the Planning Process

At the conclusion of the entire planning process (i.e., upon preparing program mission statements and goals, setting objectives, and making decisions on program priority areas as a result of the employee needs assessment), you can expect to have concrete details on the program design. Expect consensus (agreement among the stakeholders) on what the program will be. In large and midsized organizations, program vendors and service providers for employee health promotion are selected (Chen, Sheu, & Chen, 2010). As part of the planning, reports are generated that detail program implementation including logic models and Gantt charts as well as budgets. Expect to know the program inputs (e.g., staffing, materials, equipment), activities, interventions, goals, timelines, and resources (funding). During planning you have created the initial program structures and operations (Breny Bontempi, Fagen, & Roe, 2010).

At the conclusion of the planning process, you can also expect to know a lot about the organization as a result of the planning process data collection. And information about the organization is critical to the program implementation. For different sized organizations the expectations for what you should know at this point differs. The employees' health priorities that are to be addressed are unique to an organization and flow from the employee needs assessment. Equally important is the organizational data gathered during the program planning.

In large organizations it might be expected to have the workplace health promotion program operated as part of strategic human resource management with assigned staff, and well-developed and functioning teams, partnerships, and collaborations. A high level of readiness and capacity would be in place with a proven track record of previous successful workplace health promotion activity. Program champions and advocates are active. And the organizational culture and climate promote employee health. Policy, procedures, and legal requirements are current and support employees' healthy behavior choices. If these are not present, that information can be used to shape and design the program efforts. The data provide insights to help you assess and direct actions to implement the workplace health promotion program.

In midsized organizations a team may or may not be present. An individual who may have many administrative duties is often tasked with the employee workplace health promotion program operation. Similar to what happens in the large organization, the data generated during the planning process directs the actions and expectations for what is possible within the organization. With small employers it is mostly a business owner, who is doing many different types of tasks and making many different types of decisions, who will make the decisions on the employee health promotion program as well. As with any size organization, knowing its readiness, capacity, culture, climate, partnerships, and collaborations shapes what a program can and will do.

Data and Information Generated During Program Planning

- Workplace readiness
- Workplace capacity
- Champions and advocates
- Workplace culture and climate
- Policy and procedures
- Legal issues and procedures
- Teams
- Partnerships
- Collaborations
- Employee needs assessment
  - Demographics
  - HRAs
  - Health records
  - Biometric screening
  - Workers' compensation claims and costs
  - Medical claims and costs
  - Productivity

Program planning is about making decisions on mission, goals, objectives, interventions, outcomes, policies, and procedures and achieving acceptance and support for the program in the workplace. Furthermore planning a workplace health promotion program is about installing the program with a focus on creating structural supports necessary to initiate it. At the conclusion of the planning there is a transition to program implementation. The program begins to operate.

Program operation varies by program priorities. A lot of activity might happen within strategic human resources management. For example, activities might focus on the wellness team, benefit package design, health and safety, and workers' compensation. Perhaps the initial program operations engage workers in a 6-week diabetes prevention program at different company factories and offices using site-based instructors and online activities.

At the conclusion of planning a program is built to reflect the workplace's readiness, capacity, culture, climate, partnerships, and collaborations; it ensures the availability of funding streams, human resource strategies, and supportive policy, and creates as well referral mechanisms, reporting frameworks, and outcome expectations. While the program is installed additional resources may be needed to realign current staff, hire and train staff members, secure appropriate space, or purchase needed technology (e.g., cell phones or computers). These activities and their associated startup costs are necessary first steps in beginning a new workplace health promotion program (Fixsen, Naoom, Blase, Friedman, & Wallace, 2005).

Summary

Workplace employee health needs assessments drive program decision making. Employee health needs assessments gather data (indicators) to use to make decisions related to the plan, implementation, and evaluation of the workplace health promotion program. The data sources can include but may not be limited to the human resources management department, health promotion program staff, occupational health department, workers' compensation and benefits, and health insurance provider. When feasible, employee health need assessments analyze and use as many of the following types of data as possible: demographic profiles, health status, health records, biometric screening, workers' compensation claims and costs, medical care claims and costs, and job productivity. At the conclusion of the planning process (i.e., program mission statements, goals, and objectives as well as decisions on program priority areas as a result of the employee needs assessment) expect to have concrete details on the program design. And expect to know a lot about the organization as a result of the planning process data collection. This latter information is critical to the program installation and implementation.

For Practice and Discussion

1. Compare and contrast the seven examples of employee health needs data, source, scope, and specificity as seen in Table 7.1. What are the pros and cons of each data source? What is the reliability and validity of each data source?

2. Table 7.1 lists potential program implications of each employee health needs data source. Propose changes in the scope and specificity examples listed in the table. What is the impact of the changes on the program implications?

3. Discuss the impact of the organization's size (e.g., large, midsized, small) on using the data collected as part of program planning. Compare and contrast the ease you might expect to when making decisions about program details and implementation among different sized organizations.

4. It is not usual for a business to work with a number of health promotion program vendors. Typically a vendor will collect and then report "its" data to the business. One of the challenges for a business is to be able to compare and contrast and ultimately use the data (reports) from a number of different vendors. Suggest strategies for a business to manage and use the information from its health promotion program vendors.

5. Talk with a small business owner to find out what information would be the most persuasive and helpful to motivate the owner to implement a workplace health promotion program for employees. What data and information would make the most sense and be most helpful to the owner making the decision to do the program?

Case Study: Employee Participation in HRA and Biometric Screening—What Would You Do?

Encouraging employees to complete a health risk assessment (HRA) and biometric screening makes sense. Companies may subsidize as much as 90% of the employees' health insurance premiums. They have the fiduciary need to push employees toward better health through risk identification and risk awareness tools based on HRA-and biometric screening. Looking at HRA results together with medical and pharmacy claims data, health care service utilization summaries, and biometric data presents a major opportunity to identify, educate, and motivate those most likely to provide program ROI.

The vice president of human resources at a large food service operator in the Midwest wants a creative, engaging, and supportive engagement strategy for the company HRA and biometric screening. The VP has the goal of increasing employee participation from its current level of 26% to 35% next year and 45% in three years. Currently the company uses a web-based HRA and an on-site screening vendor at company-sponsored health fairs and health education programs. Jordon Taylor, the director of benefits planning and design, is charged with the task to make it happen. What would you do?

KEY TERMS

Demographics	Productivity
Health status	Business case
Health risk assessment (HRA)	Employee health needs stratification
Health records	Health and safety problem
Physical examinations	Health priorities
Biometric screening	Health risks
Workers' compensation claims and costs	Health problem prevalence
Medical care claims and costs	Adherence and participation
International Statistical Classification of Diseases (ICD-10)	Health care choices and service utilization
Current Procedural Terminology (CPT)	Program evaluation

References

Baicker, K., Cutler, D., & Song, Z. (2010). Workplace wellness programs can generate savings. *Health Affairs (Millwood)*, 29(2), 304–311.

Breny Bontempi, J. M. B., Fagen, M. C., & Roe, K. M. (2010). Implementation tools, program staff and budget. In C. Fertman & D. Allensworth (Eds.), *Health promotion programs: From theory to practice* (pp. 153–175). San Francisco, CA: Jossey-Bass/Wiley.

Centers for Disease Control and Prevention. (2013a). *Workplace health promotion: On-the-job injuries data*. Retrieved from http://www.cdc.gov /workplacehealthpromotion/assessment/potential_data/injuries.html

Centers for Disease Control and Prevention. (2013b). *Workplace health promotion: Workplace health model*. Retrieved from http://www.cdc.gov /workplacehealthpromotion/model/index.html

Change Agent Work Group. (2009). *Employer health asset management*. Retrieved from http://www.aon.com/attachments/improving_health.pdf

Chen, W. W., Sheu, J.-J., & Chen, H.-S. (2010). Making decisions to create and support a program. In C. Fertman & D. Allensworth (Eds.), *Health promotion programs: From theory to practice* (pp. 121–150). San Francisco, CA: Jossey-Bass/Wiley.

Chenoweth, D. H. (2011). *Worksite health promotion* (3rd ed.). Champaign, IL: Human Kinetics.

Fireman, B., Bartlett, J., & Selby, J. (2004). Can disease management reduce health care costs by improving quality? *Health Affairs, 23*(6), 63–75.

Fixsen, D. L., Naoom, S. F., Blase, K. A., Friedman, R. M., & Wallace, F. (2005). *Implementation research: A synthesis of the literature.* Tampa, FL: University of South Florida, Louis de la Parte Florida Mental Health Institute, The National Implementation Research Network (FMHI Publication #231).

Framer, E., & Chikamoto, Y. (2009). The assessment of health and risk: Tools, specific uses, and implementation processes. In *ACSM's worksite health: A guide to building healthy and productive companies* (2nd ed., pp. 140–150). Champaign, IL: Human Kinetics.

Harris, J. S., & Fries, J. (2002). The health effects of health promotion. In *Health promotion in the workplace* (pp. 1–19). Toronto, ON: Delmar Thompson Learning.

Health and Safety Executive. (2012). *Five steps to risk assessment.* Retrieved from http://www.hse.gov.uk/pubns/indg163.pdf

National Business Group on Health. (2014, January). *Staying@Work Survey Report 2013/2014, United States: The business value of a healthy work-force.* Towers Watson/National Business Group on Health. Retrieved from https://www.businessgrouphealth.org/benchmarking/surveyreports.cfm

O'Donnell, M. P. (2015). What is the ROI for workplace health promotion? It really does depend, and that's the point. *American Journal of Health Promotion, 29*(3), v–viii.

Perales, D., Fourney, A., MkNelly, B., & Mamary, E. (2010). Evaluating and improving a health promotion program. In C. I. Fertman & D. D. Allensworth (Eds.), *Health promotion programs: From theory to practice* (pp. 259–290). San Francisco, CA: Jossey-Bass.

Workers Compensation Research Institute. (n.d.) *About WCRI.* Retrieved May 8, 2015, from http://www.wcrinet.org/about.html

PART THREE

IMPLEMENTATION

WORKPLACE HEALTH PROMOTION PROGRAM IMPLEMENTATION HEALTH PRIORITY: PHYSICAL HEALTH

Program Implementation: Physical Health Priority

Most individuals would define physical health as being free from pain, physical disability, chronic and infectious diseases, and bodily discomforts that require the attention of a physician. The workplace health promotion program implementation health priority, physical health, focuses on anything that has to do with our bodies as a physical entity—our ability to perform daily activities and duties without any problem.

The Physical health priority is rooted in medicine, involving the largest number and range of medical professionals and services of all workplace health promotion programs. Physical health problems are assessed in terms of the number and variety of diseases (morbidity), number and variety of deaths (mortality rates), office visits to clinicians, hospitalizations, medication prescriptions, lifespan, and health care expenditures. These numbers are used to understand the specific needs or current physical health status of a workforce. The physical health priority is not only about primary care but also considers how to give the employees opportunities and encouragement to improve on their current physical health state.

LEARNING OBJECTIVES

- Discuss program implementation focused on a physical health priority

- Identify evidence-based physical health policies, practices, interventions, and services

- Explain physical health workplace program challenges

- Describe advocacy partnerships and organizations

Evidence-Based Physical Health Policies, Practices, Interventions, and Services

Physical health priority–focused program implementation is rooted in evidence-based medicine: the conscientious, explicit, and judicious use of current best evidence in making decisions about the care of individuals. The practice of evidence-based medicine means integrating individual clinical expertise with the best available external clinical evidence from systematic research (Sackett, Rosenberg, Gray, Haynes, & Richardson, 1996). A report from the Joint Commission on Accreditation of Healthcare Organizations (2002) that focused on strategies at a system level in support of organizations (i.e., workplaces) fueled the demand for evidence-based medicine and the development of evidence-based physical health policies, practices, interventions, and services.

Concerns about medical costs drive the mix and type of programs developed for the workplace through the physical health priority efforts to reduce health care costs. The company-owned health clinics of the late 1800s, established to treat injuries stemming from dangerous work conditions, high accident rates, and often remote locations with little access to health care outside the company, have transformed into sophisticated physical health programs built to address employee physical health and to reduce employee health care costs. The business case for all the following physical health programs is that organizations will save money (reduce employee health care cost) by implementing the programs (Russell, 2009).

Primary Care Centers

With roots in the company-owned health clinics of the late 1800s, workplace primary care centers offer a custom approach to routine medical care, available to employees at the workplace. These employee health centers are designed to meet the personal health care needs of workers and, if applicable, their families. Elements of primary care centers can be customized to best suit each employer's needs. The scope of care can be limited to urgent and episodic care for conditions such as flu, minor injuries, and allergies, or can be expanded to provide care for chronic medical conditions such as hypertension and diabetes. Outside referral to a specialist might also be available when necessary. Table 8.1 shows common services that are offered in a workplace primary care center. Centers operated by Walmart Corporation are one example. The centers began to operate in Texas stores that charge their own employees $4 a visit if they are covered by Walmart's health insurance. Nurse practitioners staff the clinics. They will perform lab tests, treat basic illnesses such as flu and strep throat, and manage care

Table 8.1 Workplace Primary Care Center Services (Sisters of Mercy Urgent Care, 2014)

Preventive Care

Physical examinations
- Post-offer/Pre-placement
- Annual
- Return-to-work
- Department of Transportation (DOT)
- Workers' comp

Medical Review Officer services

OSHA-mandated services
- Hepatitis B vaccinations
- Post-exposure treatment and documentation

Drug testing/specimen collection
- Non-DOT drug testing
- DOT drug testing
- Preemployment
- Post-accident
- Random
- Periodic

Special clinical testing
- EKGs
- Pulmonary function screening
- Audiometric testing
- FIT testing (respirator)

Breath alcohol testing

Additional services
- Wellness assessments
- Immunizations
- Body fat analysis (BMIs)
- X-rays

Workplace Education Programs

- CPR
- First aid
- Simple wound care
- Removal of foreign bodies from eyes

- Blood-borne pathogens
- Establishing and providing backup for standard procedures
- Burn care

Immediate Care

- Cuts
- Strains and sprains
- Broken bones
- Colds
- Ear infections
- Cough or sore throat
- Sinus pain
- Flu
- Fever

- Mild asthma
- Mild allergic reactions
- Digestive issues (nausea, vomiting, diarrhea)
- Urinary tract infection
- Skin irritations
- Animal bites
- Minor burns

of chronic conditions like diabetes, asthma, and high blood pressure. The clinic will also refer patients to specialists.

One benefit of employee primary care centers is they offer comprehensive and preventive health care on-site—making access to primary care physicians more convenient. Employees receive the treatment they need, when they need it, ensuring time and cost savings for the employee and the employer. The primary care center staff helps employees manage their health and well-being, returning them to work and productivity faster. Increasingly as part of disability management, rehabilitation services such as physical and occupational therapy are being offered within the centers as well.

Disease Management

Disease management is offered to employees with costly chronic conditions (e.g., asthma, diabetes, congestive heart failure, coronary heart disease, atrial fibrillation, end-stage renal disease) and focuses on improving medication adherence, self-care knowledge and abilities, monitoring individual's health status, and encouraging/prompting regular preventive health screening. Completion of a disease management program typically requires 6 to 9 months, during which participants have a series of calls with a nurse that average 15 to 25 minutes per call. Completion of a program occurs when the participant is successfully managing his or her condition. Programs are tailored to individuals based on a specific disease(s). Table 8.2 lists examples of tailored disease management program content.

The use of information technology tools such as remote monitoring, self-testing, email communication, and computer-generated patient (employee) reports are used to increase the individual's engagement with their health. Home monitoring assists with the ongoing supervision of employees' health status and timely adjustment of treatment plans leading to both enhanced clinical outcomes and reduced rates of hospitalization.

Disability Management (Workers' Compensation Management)

Disability management as part of workplace health promotion programs addresses the needs of employees receiving workers' compensation. Workers' compensation benefits are paid for, in some way or another, by the employers and therefore add to the organization's health care expenses. Workers' compensation systems vary from state to state, but employers pay for workers' compensation typically in one of three ways: premiums to a state-run insurance program, payments to an insurance company, or payments directly to workers.

Table 8.2   Tailored Disease Management Program Content (National Committee for Quality Assurance, 2014)

Management of People With Heart Failure	Management of People With Ischemic Vascular Disease
• Influenza vaccination	• LDL-C screening
• Pneumococcal vaccination	• LDL-C control
• Assessment of tobacco use	• Aspirin or other antithrombotic use
• Assistance with tobacco cessation	• Persistence of beta-blocker treatment after a heart attack
	• Influenza vaccination
	• Pneumococcal vaccination
	• Assessment of tobacco use
	• Assistance with tobacco cessation

Management of People With COPD

• Influenza vaccination

• Pneumococcal vaccination

• Assessment of tobacco use

• Assistance with tobacco cessation

Management of People With Asthma

• Appropriate medication use

• Influenza vaccination

• Pneumococcal vaccination

• Assessment of tobacco use

If an employee is receiving workers' compensation benefits, the company from which the worker receives the workers' compensation benefits may or may not be the employee's employer. It may instead be the state government, the insurance company, the employer, or a third party administrator hired by the employer to be responsible for administering the employer's workers' compensation claims. Regardless of who is managing the workers' compensation, disability management seeks to increase engagement in prevention and wellness programs by individuals receiving workers' compensation. Given the structure of workers' compensation, information gaps often exist between the treating provider and the disability management process. Disability management is designed to overcome these gaps, building a bridge between disability management and health benefits, in order to increase employee involvement in addressing serious, chronic health conditions and reduce disability duration and recidivism. Disability management considers the state regulations, health plan design, employee needs, and culture of the organization to develop a course of action for addressing complex situations and obtaining resolution (Disability Management Employer Coalition, 2014).

Return-to-work strategies can differ across employers and even between administrators within a company. Pransky et al. (2005) identify four basic models of disability management and prevention: medical model, physical rehabilitation model, job-match model, and managed-care model. The medical model places the responsibility on the physician to determine physical status and possible job limitations. The physical rehabilitation model gives rehabilitation professionals the power to communicate the importance of rehabilitation in returning to work and normal activities. The job-match model relies on the ability of employers to accurately communicate physical job requirements in an effort to prevent work-related injuries. The managed-care model uses acceptable standards for medical treatment and duration of work absence as criterion for returning to work.

Absence Management

Absence management programs are an evolving model that couples disability management, workers' compensation, and absence programs (e.g., Family Medical Leave Act [FMLA], intermittent absences, short-term disability) making the argument that the model improves tracking, ensures regulatory compliance, and enhances a company's productivity and bottom line. There is a growing need for employers to be consistent in their approach to absence management regardless of the cause. There is increasing employer compliance risk due to tighter regulations associated with the FMLA, the Americans with Disabilities Act (ADA), and the ever-changing state workers' compensation systems. Employers must comply with FMLA and ADA regulations while employees are off work with occupational and nonoccupational illnesses and injuries. For companies that use separate outside vendors to manage disability, workers' compensation, and leave of absence benefits, the information is not easily shared or integrated between all parties. With multiple processes and vendors to oversee, managing the details of each benefit can become a challenging task for an employer's risk management, human resource, and legal teams, as well as the employee's direct supervisor. The coupled model uses a team approach to handle the clinical steps such as evaluation and duration management, stay-at-work and return-to-work planning, job accommodation, and vocational rehabilitation. For long-term disability cases, integrated services include return-to-work planning, case management, and Social Security assistance (Sedgwick, 2014).

Pharmacy Benefit Management

Historically, a pharmacy benefit manager (PBM) is a third-party administrator of prescription drug programs. PBMs are primarily responsible for developing and maintaining the formulary, contracting with pharmacies, negotiating discounts and rebates with drug manufacturers, and processing and paying prescription drug claims. For the most part, they work with self-insured companies and government programs striving to maintain or reduce the pharmacy expenditures of the plan while concurrently trying to improve health care outcomes. The list below has the five largest PBMs.

Increasingly, PBMs offer programs to help control prescription costs. Some of these areas include information about tablet splitting, lower-cost therapeutic alternatives, tiered trials of specific medications in a therapeutic class, evaluating clinical programs for large populations, medication therapy management programs, and mail-order service (Pharmacist.com, n.d.). Examples of PBMs include Express Scripts, CVS Caremark, Medco, Catalyst Rx, and Magellan Rx Management.

PBMs offer a core set of services to manage the cost and utilization of prescription drugs and improve the value of plan sponsors' drug benefits. Some offer additional tools, such as disease management for priority populations. It is up to the client of the PBM, however, to determine the extent to which these tools will be employed.

PBM Core Set of Services

- Pharmacy networks—Networks of retail pharmacies, known as preferred pharmacy network, to provide consumers convenient access to prescriptions at discounted rates. PBMs monitor prescription safety across all of the network pharmacies, alerting pharmacists to potential drug interactions even if a consumer uses multiple pharmacies.

- Mail-service pharmacies—PBMs provide mail-service pharmacies that supply home-delivered prescriptions without the face-to-face consultation provided by a pharmacist.

- Formularies—PBMs specify particular medications that are approved to be prescribed under a particular insurance policy. PBMs use panels of independent physicians, pharmacists, and clinical experts to develop lists of drugs approved for reimbursement based on efficacy, safety, and cost-effectiveness of drugs.

- Plan design—PBMs advise their clients on ways to structure drug benefits to encourage the use of lower-cost drug alternatives (such as generics), when appropriate. This is done by setting plans up with different copay tiers; in this case the client will apply a lower copay for generic drugs than it would for brand drugs.

- Electronic prescribing (e-prescribing)—PBMs use e-prescribing to electronically transmit a new prescription or renewal authorization to a community or mail-order pharmacy.

- Clinical management—PBMs use a variety of tools such as drug utilization review and disease management to encourage the best clinical outcomes for individuals.

- Pharmacy discount cards—PBMs are able to offer discounts that can save between 10% and 75% on prescription medication.

Medical-Second Option

Second-opinion medical services can be an effective benefits cost-containment tool for employers' payment of treatment costs for complex cases such as cancer and back injuries. The services are available to fully insured and self-insured employers, regardless of size, and can be purchased either on a case-by-case basis or under a contractual arrangement in which the employer pays a per-employee fee each month. The argument for having a medical second option as part of a workplace health promotion program is that the service will more than pay for itself given the nominal cost—usually less than $1,000 per case—compared with the cost of treatment for many complex cases. According to recent data collected by three major second-opinion medical service providers, misdiagnoses are discovered in up to 20% of medical cases and treatment changes are recommended in more than half of them. As the cost of health care rises for employers of all sizes, there is more interest among smaller and midsized employers who pay $2 to $3 per employee per month for a second-opinion service (Wojcik, 2011).

Medical-second option vendors market their product as a service to save money but also to alleviate the fear that often accompanies a serious diagnosis. Furthermore the service can corroborate a diagnosis for an employee who faces a complicated surgery. It can relieve the employee's concern, and confirm that the treating physician is a good one and there is no need to change physicians.

Health Advocates and Concierges

Workplace health advocates and concierges provide employees with personal health advocates (PHAs), typically registered nurses supported by medical directors and administrative experts. PHAs help employees navigate the health care system and resolve clinical, insurance, and administrative issues. Other services might include a wellness advocate, who provides a menu of wellness solutions that complement PHA recommendations to help employees adopt healthier behaviors. Likewise PHAs can work as a benefits integrator, enrollment advocate, FMLA support, and independent appeals administrator. Standard PHA services offered to an individual include (Health Advocate, 2007):

- Provider and facility referrals
- Appointment and transportation scheduling
- Exam preparation and results explanation
- Record, x-ray, and lab result transfer facilitation
- Post-discharge patient care and home-care arrangements
- Claim and billing support
- Drug switch and mail order assistance

There are two main types of decision assistance PHAs provide. *Shared decision making* is a process that helps employees (patients) make choices based on their values and belief systems, and *mediation* (or conflict resolution) helps families make difficult decisions related to their loved ones' care.

An important part of any PHA's work is helping employees make decisions about their health and medical needs. While it would seem a fairly simple explanation to say a decision specialist provides pros and cons and lets an employee decide, that underestimates the real skill this kind of advocacy requires, and the gravity of importance it holds for an employee. Shared decision making is a defined process that first uncovers an employee's beliefs and value system, then helps the individual use those beliefs and values to make the best decision for him or herself—regardless of what the doctor suggests, and regardless of the standard of care. For example, consider a situation where a 40-year-old employee who has had hip pain for 10 years, probably from an old football injury. He may be able to do physical therapy, or even acupuncture to relieve the pain, but both of those require ongoing, perhaps lifelong, dedication. Or he can choose surgery, which will replace his hip but expose him to additional problems, like infections. Further, since hip replacements typically last 20 years, he'll likely have to repeat that surgery at least once (American Association of Hip and Knee Surgeons, 2015).

When difficult health care decisions need to be made by more than one person, and those parties don't agree, they may call on a health care mediator (PHA) to help them. This form of health advocacy facilitates difficult discussions among individuals (i.e., employee and family members) and helps them resolve the conflict that arises from these sorts of tough decisions. For example, consider the employee family who must decide that their mother needs to be moved to a nursing home, but the oldest brother, who lives across the country, refuses to sign the paperwork.

Value-Based Benefit Design

Value-based benefit design (VBBD) addresses the way health benefits are structured and utilized by employees. It alters the design of insurance benefits with the intention to lower health care costs for employers and employees. Three VBBD models exist (Table 8.3). Each model is coupled with inducements to encourage appropriate health-seeking behavior. Although there are incentives such as copay reductions or waivers, premium reductions, and health-saving contributions, not all incentives are financial. Employers use VBBD strategies to change behaviors by aligning incentives that lead to:

- Appropriate use of high-value services including preventive care

- Adherence to treatment regimens

- Utilization of high-performance providers (doctors, nurse practitioners, pharmacists, hospitals, retail health clinics) who adhere to evidence-based treatment guidelines

- Adoption of healthy behaviors

VBBD is also called "value-based incentive design," or "value-based insurance design," or "evidence-based benefit design." No matter what it

Table 8.3   Models of Value-Based Benefits with Associated Examples

Individual health competency	Incentives most often through cash equivalent or premium differential • Health risk assessment • Biometric screening • Health coaching
Condition management	Incentives most often through copay/coinsurance differential or cash equivalent • Adherence to evidence-based guidelines • Adherence to chronic medications • Participation in a disease management program
Provider guidance	Incentives most often through copayment or co-insurance differential • Utilization of an ambulatory care clinic versus an emergency room • Care through a "center of excellence" • High performance providers

Table 8.4   High- and Low-Value Services

High-Value Services	Low-Value Services
Age-appropriate cancer screenings	Early elective C-sections
Eye and foot exams for diabetics	MRI for low back pain (with no red flags)
Medications for chronic heart disease, asthma, diabetes, and hypertension	Sleep studies
	Annual EKG/cardiac screening for low-risk patients
Transplant drugs	Bone density test for low-risk women under 65
Defibrillators for certain patients with congestive heart failure	

is called, the purpose is the same: to encourage the consumer to utilize high-value services that produce better health and lower health care costs (Table 8.4).

Although many of the early adopters of VBBD have been large companies, more and more smaller organizations are now adopting value-based strategies that use a set of common incentives. Today the opportunity to utilize new and unique benefit designs is no longer limited to large employers. The strategies remain the same regardless of the size of the organization.

Commonly Used Incentives in Value-Based Benefits Programs

- Cash or gift cards
- Copayment reductions
- Premium reductions
- Eligible for broader benefit plan
- Access to benefit (often used as an disincentive)

Factory Floor- and Office-Level Evidence-Based Physical Health Interventions and Practices

Workplaces have factory floor- and office-level physical health interventions and practices to address their particular workforce health needs. From small and midsized organizations to large national employers, these engage employees at the workplace (factory floor and office), and are lower cost and practical, with fairly easy administration. Outside vendors both national and local compete for contracts to offer the interventions. Examples of widely implemented evidence-based interventions and practices are:

- **Truck driver preemployment physicals and drug testing:** The Federal Motor Carrier Safety Administration (FMCSA) and Truckload

Carriers Association (TCA) require every first-time driver to undergo a preemployment physical exam that includes testing for controlled substances as well as for alcohol abuse. The alcohol abuse testing also includes a blood alcohol test to determine if the applicant is under the influence of alcohol during the test, if this is determined to be necessary (U.S. Department of Transportation, FMCSA, 2014).

    • **Police and Fire service qualification examinations:** The International Association of Directors of Law Enforcement Standards and Training require every law enforcement applicant to undergo a physical fitness assessment, a drug test for use of controlled substances, as well as a standard medical exam. The standard medical examination evaluates the candidates' physiological readiness to learn. It also determines the relative risk that their health will compromise their ability to perform the frequent and critical tasks assigned to them. The physical fitness assessment includes testing of physical conditioning, fitness, and agility. The drug testing is required due to the need for the officers to enforce the law regarding the use and possession of these illegal controlled substances. If the officers themselves are using these substances, the validity of their enforcement is compromised.

    • **Back-health programs:** Programs geared to promote healthy backs use integrative medicine that includes evidence-based, alternative therapies within the context of conventional medicine. These programs can include treatments such as acupuncture, mind-body interventions, and stress management, which all have shown benefits for back pain reduction (Kimbrough, Lao, Berman, Pelletier, & Talamonti, 2010). Peer-based low-back pain information and reassurance programs for employees are other back-health programs that have been shown to decrease negative consequences such as the amount of sick leave days. Odeen et al. (2013) showed that this type of program is effective in reducing low-back pain related sick days as well as in reducing faulty beliefs about low-back pain among workers.

    • **Prenatal care programs:** Programs for prenatal care consist of medical care, support, and advice for pregnant women, information about health insurance, and other services for pregnant women and their babies. One recent example of this type of program is Text4baby, the largest national mobile health initiative and one that has reached over 555,000 mothers since its launch in 2010. This free, mobile information service is sponsored by Johnson & Johnson along with others to provide expecting mothers with three informational text messages a week, timed with their expected due date (National Healthy Mothers, Healthy Babies Coalition, 2012).

- **Flu shots and vaccinations:** Workplace health promotion programs within both large and small corporations focus on increasing vaccination rates among employees and their families to ensure their health and safety. Ofstead et al. (2013) showed that introducing workplace interventions to increase influenza vaccination rates is effective in increasing the number of employees who are vaccinated. Another example of an influenza vaccination program uses the opt-in versus opt-out condition as a promoter for getting vaccinated. This model gives the employee the option to opt-out of a vaccination, thus making getting the vaccination the default condition versus the alternative, by which setting the default as opting-out of the vaccination makes the employee actively pursue or opt-in to the vaccination (Chapman, Li, Colby, & Yoon, 2010).

- **Automated external defibrillator programs:** An automated external defibrillator (AED) is a computerized medical device. An AED can check a person's heart rhythm. It can recognize a rhythm that requires a shock. And it can advise the rescuer when a shock is needed. The AED uses voice prompts, lights, and text messages to tell the rescuer the steps to take. A workplace AED program determines the type, number, and location of AEDs required for optimal response, employee AED responder training, AED responder activation, and coordination with local EMS organizations. The AED Programs represents an efficient method of delivering defibrillation to persons experiencing out-of-hospital cardiac arrest; its use by both traditional and nontraditional first responders appears to be safe and effective (Marenco, Wang, Link, Homoud, & Estes, 2001).

Physical Health Priority Implementation Challenges

Health care costs are a major driver in the implementation within the physical health arena. However, challenges exist that create a gap between proposed savings and benefits and realistic program implementation. These challenges include issues of access, privacy, infrastructure communication disconnection, and using all of the physical health service options. Before talking about how to engage and support employee participation, these challenges need to be addressed so employees believe their participation will make a difference in their health status and future well-being.

Access

Access issues for workplace physical health promotion programs can be broken up into five main elements: coverage, services, timeliness, workforce, and compliance. Coverage considers a person's health insurance and their ability to access health-related goods and services. In workplaces that offer health insurance as well as workplaces that do not, the challenges are the same for employers who need and want healthy employees. Oftentimes the amount of coverage a person has, either too much or not enough, determines the treatment and care that is available to them regarding their physical health. When thinking about access issues, one must also consider the services that are being provided to each person. This refers to the consistency of the source of care a person has and its effects on their health outcomes. Primary care providers are usually an important piece of stability in a person's physical health services, as they provide appropriate care on the foundation of constant patient-provider trust and communication. In addition to primary care services, it is important to consider both the basic and advanced emergency care services that are available to an individual; they provide a crucial link to the maintenance of physical health, especially in the later years of life. The challenge of access also includes timeliness, which refers to the ability of one to receive quality care quickly after a need arises. Waiting times in doctors' offices and emergency departments, as well as delays for test results, directly affect a person's physical health. Prolonged waiting times affect a person's satisfaction with the service and can cause medically significant delays in treatment. The available medical workforce affects a person's access. Recently there has been a decrease in the number of primary care physicians available to promote the stability of service that was described earlier. Finally, there is the ability to support an individual's treatment compliance: the ability to complete the prescribed activities and tasks, such as fill prescriptions, attend physical therapy, complete additional testing and examinations (U.S. Department of Health and Human Services, 2015).

Confidentiality and Privacy

Confidentiality and privacy are a large challenge when promoting physical health in the workplace. It is important to recognize and identify each employee's specific physical health needs while still maintaining proper confidentiality of information. Laws that affect information collected in medical records include HIPAA and ADA. Individual states also have laws about the privacy and confidentiality of personal medical records. In particular according to HIPAA, employers have access to some pro-tected health information if the disclosure is required to comply with laws relating to workers' compensation. HIPAA also allows disclosure per the requirements of state or federal laws and regulations. Workplace health clinicians regularly keep personal health information (e.g., medi-cal conditions not related to work). They generate medical records that document care of work-related illnesses and injuries or those that are specific to workplace requirements. These records may include medical and employment questionnaires, job descriptions, pre-placement examinations, medical surveillance examinations, biological and other screening results, occupational exposure evaluations, and workers' compensation medical records. When documenting or observing the physical health of an employee, one must consider the level of exposure of these records to ensure proper confidentiality (U.S. Department of Labor, n.d.).

Infrastructure Communication Disconnection

Implementing the physical health priority results in a patchwork quilt of providers, organizations, vendors, partnerships, and collaborations working together and interacting with employees. It is not unusual for disconnections to occur between and among all of the parties (other than employees) involved in implementing the physical health priority. The organizations may see themselves in competition to provide large portions of services and receive large contracts. In other words, they may share the same priority population (employees) but have different goals and objectives based on their service and contract. It is the responsibility of the health promotion program leadership to develop and support infrastructure communication to keep all part of the workplace health promotion program up to date on infrastructure changes (e.g., new staff, products, service hours, location, telephone numbers, e-mail addresses). Training for all staff (regardless of organizational affiliation) is an effective strategy to prevent disconnection. If providers are disconnected they are limited in their abilities to meet the needs of employees.

Physical Health Services Continuum Utilization

A continuum of physical health service options now exists. A driving force in the development of service options is costs. The high cost of individuals seeking treatment at hospital emergency rooms has fueled the growth of lower cost, efficient, and innovative options such as ambulatory care centers, telemedicine, medical technology, and home health care services. In particular ambulatory care centers located in the community can offer routine workplace physical health care services without the need for appointments at lower costs than the primary physician or emergency room. However, for a workplace health promotion program to take advantage of ambulatory care centers as well as other innovative approaches, employees need to be aware of them and encouraged to use them.

Advocacy and Resource Partnerships and Organizations

Through advocacy and resource partnerships and organizations, workplace physical health can be addressed in additional ways. These partnerships and organizations direct their attention to the physical health of the U.S. workforce. Some focus on specific physical health problems that affect worker's health every day and cause financial stress on employers.

Workplace Solutions American Cancer Society
(http://www.acsworkplacesolutions.com/)

The American Cancer Society's Employer Initiative Workplace Solutions programs are customized to fit the specific needs of every company and have a positive impact on the company's bottom line. Workplace Solutions provide evidence-based health and wellness programs that help reduce employee risk of cancer and other serious illnesses as well as opportunities to participate in well-known community events such as the American Cancer Society Relay for Life and Making Strides Against Breast Cancer. For employers and employees involved in Workplace Solutions, many programs are offered to help implement comprehensive wellness programs and provide information and high-quality support for cancer screening and care.

U.S. Preventive Services Task Force
(http://www.uspreventiveservicestaskforce.org/)

The U.S. Preventive Services Task Force (USPSTF) is an independent panel of nonfederal experts in prevention and evidence-based medicine and is composed of primary care providers (e.g., internists, pediatricians, family physicians, gynecologists/obstetricians, nurses, and health behavior specialists). The USPSTF conducts scientific evidence reviews of a broad range of clinical preventive health care services (e.g., screening, counseling, preventive medications) and develops recommendations for primary care clinicians and health systems. These recommendations are published in the form of "Recommendation Statements."

Health and Productivity Management Toolkit
(hpm.acoem.org/about.html)

The Health and Productivity Management Toolkit is a resource created by the Health and Productivity section of the American College of Occupational and Environmental Medicine (ACOEM).

ACOEM's mission is to promote healthier, more productive workplaces. The Toolkit helps individuals understand the concepts of Health and Productivity Management and the value of a healthy workforce. It was designed for physicians, nurses, health resource and health benefits professionals, insurers, employers and others who deal with health and wellness issues in the workplace.

The National Quality Forum (http://www.qualityforum.org)

The National Quality Forum (NQF) is a not-for-profit, non-partisan, membership-based organization that leads national collaboration to improve and catalyze health and health care quality. NQF convenes working groups to foster quality improvement in both public and private sectors; endorses consensus standards for performance measurement; ensures that consistent, high-quality performance information is publicly available; and seeks real time feedback to ensure measures are meaningful and accurate.

Institute for Health and Productivity Studies (http://hip.emory.edu /about/partners/ihps.html)

The Institute for Health and Productivity Studies (IHPS), a collaborative project established between the Rollins School of Public Health's Department of Health Policy and Management at Emory University and the health care business of Thomson Reuters, conducts empirical research on the relationship between employee health and well-being, and work-related productivity. Studies performed by the IHPS help inform decision makers in both the private and public health sectors on issues related to the health and productivity cost burden of certain health risk factors and common disease conditions, and the impact that innovative health, safety, and productivity management programs have on medical, safety, and productivity-related outcomes.

Disability Management Employer Coalition (http://dmec.org)

Disability Management Employer Coalition (DMEC) is dedicated to knowledge, education, and professional networking in integrated disability, absence management, and return-to-work solutions. DMEC and its network of local chapters provide companies with trusted information, strategies, tools, and management resources to minimize lost work time and improve workforce productivity. DMEC formed an alliance in 1994 with the Insurance Educational Association (IEA) to develop the Certified Professional in Disability Management (CPDM) course of study.

Summary

Reducing employee health care spending is the driving force for the workplace health promotion program implementation in regard to the physical health priority. Primary care centers, disease management, disability management (workers' compensation management), pharmacy benefit management, medical second option, health advocates and concierges, value-based benefits design, and evidence-based programs and practices propose to lower health care costs and seek to engage employees as active decision makers in their health and health care. Challenges that mitigate efforts to implement the physical health priority include the employee's access to the programs, employee concerns with confidentiality and privacy, disconnection among the many programs, providers and vendors who are potentially involved with an employer's health promotion program, and employees' use of the now available range of physical health services.

For Practice and Discussion

1. Reflect on your own or family members' and friends' health care experience to identify situations that might be considered a duplication of service and tests, limited use of information systems, medical errors, medication mismanagement (e.g., not using a medication as prescribed), miscommunication among providers, and violation of an individual's privacy. As part of a workplace health promotion program implementation, how would you address the situations?

2. Compare and contrast vendors who offer physical health priority programs. Who are the vendors and what do they offer the organizations they are seeking to contract with to provide their services? Identify vendors who offer multiple services (e.g., primary care centers, disease management, pharmacy benefit management, medical second option, value-based benefit design). Compare these vendors to those who specialize in one service (e.g., pharmacy benefit management, medical second option).

3. A consequence of the increased importance of the physical health priority implementation to lower the cost of health care for employers and employees is the creation of businesses (commonly known as vendors) that design and sell physical health programs (products). These products include disease management, disability management,

second options, pharmacy benefit management, health advocates, and concierges. Select a vendor of a particular product to research. What are the organization's history, mission, staff, programs, services, and fees? What evidence is provided to support the product's effectiveness to improve employees' health status and lower employer health costs?

4. Prepare a 1,000-word review of the literature of current evidence-based workplace physical health interventions and practices reviewed in the *Journal of Occupational and Environmental Medicine* (http://journals.lww.com/joem/Pages/default.aspx). Describe the workplace population, physical health concern, intervention, and results. Can you find examples of similar interventions and practices across employers (i.e., small, midsized, large) as well as industry (e.g., manufacturing, service, mining, transportation, education)?

Case Study: Walmart Corporation Health Centers—What Would You Do?

Sarah Brown, M.D., a medical director of a large big-box retailer, is being asked to respond to the Walmart Corporation health care centers in Texas stores that will charge their own employees $4 a visit if they are covered by Walmart's health insurance. The charge for everyone else, including customers, is $40. Walmart reports about 1.1 million of its employees and family members are covered by its health care plans. Nurse practitioners staff the centers. They will perform lab tests, treat basic illnesses such as flu and strep throat, and manage care of chronic conditions like diabetes, asthma, and high blood pressure. The centers will also refer patients to specialists.

Walmart's push into primary care centers for their employees and customers isn't a shock. The company has spent several years dropping hints that it would make a play for the care delivery market. Walmart's move keeps with the broader trend of retailers, big-box stores, and other nontraditional competitors charging into health care delivery. And Walmart's entry into the market could push hospitals and doctors to up their game. Health systems and physicians groups have to understand that if there's a Walmart clinic open 15 hours a day, that's the standard they may have to meet.

For Dr. Brown, Walmart's new centers highlight one aspect of the emerging trend of employee health care. Her corporation wants to respond to Walmart's actions. What would you do?

KEY TERMS

Physical health

Evidence-based medicine

Evidence-based policies, practices, interventions, and services

Primary care centers

Disease management

Disability management

Absence management

Pharmacy benefit management

Medical second option

Health advocates and concierges

Value-based benefit design

Evidence-based practices and programs

Access

Confidentiality and privacy

Infrastructure communication

Physical health service continuum

References

American Association of Hip and Knee Surgeons. (2015). *Total hip replacement.* Retrieved from http://www.aahks.org/care-for-hips-and-knees/do-i-need-a-joint-replacement/total-hip-replacement/

Chapman, G. B., Li, M., Colby, H., & Yoon, H. (2010). Opting in vs opting out of influenza vaccination. *Journal of the American Medical Association, 304*(1), 43–44. doi:10.1001/jama.2010.892

Disability Management Employer Coalition. (2014). *History.* Retrieved from http://dmec.org/about-dmec/history/

Health Advocate. (2007). *Guide to workplace wellness.* Retrieved from http://healthadvocate.com/downloads/whitepapers/WorkplaceWellnessGuide.pdf

Joint Commission on Accreditation of Healthcare Organizations (2002). Weaving the fabric: Joint Commission strategic initiatives and national health care priorities. Retrieved from http://www.jointcommission.org

Kimbrough, E., Lao, L., Berman, B., Pelletier, K. R., & Talamonti, W. J. (2010). An integrative medicine intervention in a Ford Motor Company assembly plant. *Journal of Occupational and Environmental Medicine, 52*(3), 256–257. doi:210.1097/JOM.1090b1013e3181d09884.

Marenco, J. P., Wang, P. J., Link, M. S., Homoud, M. K., & Estes, N. M., III. (2001). Improving survival from sudden cardiac arrest: The role of the automated external defibrillator. *Journal of the American Medical Association, 285*(9), 1193–1200.

National Committee for Quality Assurance. (2014). *DM technical specifications.* Retrieved from http://www.ncqa.org/HEDISQualityMeasurement/PerformanceMeasurement/DMTechnicalSpecifications.aspx

National Healthy Mothers, Healthy Babies Coalition. (2012). *About Text4baby.* Retrieved from https://www.text4baby.org/index.php/about

Occupational Safety & Health Administration. (n.d.). *Clinicians.* Retrieved May 15, 2015, from https://www.osha.gov/dts/oom/clinicians/

Odeen, M., Ihlebaek, C., Indahl, A., Wormgoor, M. E., Lie, S. A., & Eriksen, H. R. (2013). Effect of peer-based low back pain information and reassurance at the workplace on sick leave: A cluster randomized trial. *Journal of Occupational Rehabilitation, 23*(2), 209–219. doi: 10.1007/s10926–013–9451-z

Ofstead, C. L., Sherman, B. W., Wetzler, H. P., Dirlam Langlay, A. M., Mueller, N. J., Ward, J. M.,. . . Poland, G. A. (2013). Effectiveness of worksite interventions to increase influenza vaccination rates among employees and families. *Journal of Occupational and Environmental Medicine, 55*(2), 156–163. doi:110.1097/JOM.1090b1013e3182717d3182713.

Pharmacist.com. (n.d.). *Pharmacy benefit management.* Retrieved from http://www.pharmacist.com/sites/default/files/files/Profile_24_PBM_SDS_FINAL_090707.pdf

Pransky, G., Gatchel, R., Linton, S.J., & Loisel, P. (2005). Improving return to work research. *Journal of Occupational Rehabilitation. 15*(4) 454–457.

Russell, L. (2009). Preventing chronic disease: An important investment, but don't count on cost savings. *Health Affairs, 28*(1), 42–45. doi:10.1377/hlthaff.28.1.42

Sackett, D. L., Rosenberg, W., Gray, J., Haynes, R. B., & Richardson, W. S. (1996). Evidence based medicine: What it is and what it isn't. *British Medical Journal, 312*(7023), 71–72.

Sedgwick (2014). *Sedgwick White Paper: Integrated disability management.* Retrieved from https://www.sedgwick.com/news/Documents/Studies/IntegratedDisabilityManagementWhitePaper.pdf

Sisters of Mercy Urgent Care. (2015). *Business and industrial services: All services.* Retrieved May 28, 2015 from http://www.urgentcares.org/en/business_services.php

U.S. Department of Health and Human Services, Office of Disease Prevention and Health Promotion. (2015). *Healthy People 2020.* Retrieved from http://www.healthypeople.gov/2020/default.aspx

U.S. Department of Transportation, Federal Motor Carrier Safety Administration. (2014, April 18). *Pre-employment testing.* Retrieved from http://www.fmcsa.dot.gov/faq-pre-employment-testing

Wojcik, J. (2011). Firm seeks medical second opinions. *Business Insurance, 45*(47), 6. Retrieved from http://www.businessinsurance.com/article/20111204/NEWS05/312049987

WORKPLACE HEALTH PROMOTION PROGRAM IMPLEMENTATION HEALTH PRIORITY: MENTAL AND BEHAVIORAL HEALTH

Program Implementation: Mental and Behavioral Health Priority

Mental health encompasses a person's emotional, psychological, and social well-being. Emotional well-being refers to such things as life satisfaction, cheerfulness, happiness, and a sense of peace. Psychological well-being includes self-acceptance, feeling open, hopeful and optimistic, and having a sense of control and purpose in life. Social well-being depends on feeling socially accepted, useful to society, and being part of something larger than oneself. This notion of well-being is captured in the 1999 Surgeon General's Report on Mental Health, in which mental health is defined as "successful performance of mental function, resulting in productive activities, fulfilling relationships with other people, and the ability to change and to cope with adversity" (National Institute of Mental Health, 1999). Similarly and more recently, the World Health Organization defined mental health as "a state of well-being in which every individual realizes his or her own potential, can cope with the normal stresses of life, can work productively and fruitfully, and is able to make a contribution to his or her community" (World Health Organization, 2010). Thus, being mentally healthy doesn't just mean that you don't have a mental health problem.

LEARNING OBJECTIVES

- Discuss program implementation focused on a mental and behavioral health priority

- Identify evidence-based mental and behavioral health policies, practices, interventions, and services

- Explain mental health and behavioral workplace program challenges

- Describe advocacy partnerships and organizations

It is a positive state in which you can play a full part in your family, workplace, community, and among friends. You can meet the demands of everyday life.

An individual's mental health status can be influenced by biological factors, such as genes or brain chemistry; life experience, such as trauma or abuse; and a family history of mental health problems. Certain societal conditions need to be in place to support mental health: adequate housing, safe neighborhoods, equitable jobs and wages, quality education, and equal access to quality health care. When these are not in place, individuals' mental health can suffer. Mental health problems, then, refer to a wide range of mental disorders that can develop when any of these facets of an individual's well-being are impaired or disrupted by any of these factors. Mental health problems can range from everyday worries to serious long-term conditions; they affect all age, ethnic, gender, and socioeconomic groups. The most common form of mental illness is depression, a mood disorder. Anxiety disorders, stress management problems, family/work-life conflicts, substance abuse, eating disorders such as anorexia and bulimia, and psychotic disorders such as schizophrenia are other types of mental health problems.

Recently, the term "behavioral health" has come to be used interchangeably with mental health. As when discussing mental health programs, behavioral health deals with the prevention, diagnosis, intervention, and treatment of mental illness. Behavioral health also addresses problems that arise from an individual's choices and actions, such as addictive disorders like substance abuse and gambling. In this text, the use of the terms "mental health" and "behavioral health" apply to workplace health promotion programs that are intended to foster employees' well-being and that provide support and treatment when needed.

Evidence-Based Mental and Behavioral Health Policies, Practices, Interventions, and Services

Employers understand the need for workplace mental and behavioral health programs, both out of concern for employees' well-being and in the recognition that organizational performance is directly related to the mental health of their workers. Mental health and behavioral disorders have a direct impact on workplace absenteeism, presenteeism (attending work when sick), accidents, turnover, productivity, and health care costs. Estimates of the costs to employers of employee mental illness range from $79 billion to $105 billion per year. To meet this need, employers offer a range of programs. A number of the common and effective mental and behavioral health workplace programs are highlighted in this section.

Employee Assistance Programs

An employee assistance program (EAP) is a voluntary workplace benefit for employees and their family members through which they can receive free and confidential referrals, short-term counseling, and follow-up services across a broad range of issues that can be accessed in a variety of ways to accommodate individual needs and preferences (Table 9.1). The type and number of services provided by an EAP varies depending on the employer. EAP services may address substance abuse, mental health, finances, legal matters, violence, trauma, illness, family matters, sexual harassment, grief, or any other issue that impacts one's ability to be productive in the workplace or that disrupts the work/life balance. EAPs may provide wellness or retirement services, or programs that help employees deal with difficult peers and supervisors. Some employee assistance programs offer assistance with child and elder care issues; legal matters, such as estate planning, wills, contract disputes, and divorce; and financial planning. EAP staff members

Table 9.1 Employee Assistance Program Services

Typical issues addressed:

- substance abuse
- stress
- divorce
- grief
- anger management
- child care and elder care
- health concerns
- financial problems
- legal concerns
- family and work relationship conflicts
- workplace trauma
- return-to-work post mental health illness and recovery support
- medication management
- veterans assistance and affairs

Many ways to access services:

- 24-hour hotlines
- face-to-face counseling
- smartphone and web-based resources and tools

offer educational workshops that can be tailored to a particular topic of interest to workplace staff, such as stress management, hypertension management, or coping with depression. The EAP staff members are licensed mental and behavioral health professionals.

Supervisor training is a major component of EAP implementation that focuses on employee identification, the EAP referral process, and employee support and rights. EAP counselors will work with employers to educate employees about the availability of employee assistance programs. They also work closely with administrators to address employee needs, either for a group or an individual. They can consult with supervisors and managers to provide guidance on handling staff issues and in making referrals. Supervisors and managers may be trained in how to identify employees in need of assistance. They also receive training on making referrals to the EAP when decreases in job performance are documented. Counselors can work with employers in preventing or coping with emergency situations and in developing written policies and procedures for developing programs or handling specific situations.

EAP service structures vary. Internal EAPs are housed and operated within the company. The staff are company employees. Many employers like internal EAPs for their responsiveness and understanding of the organization's culture and climate. External EAPs are operated by an external organization (i.e., vendor) through a contract with the employer. This separate relationship is frequently perceived as providing enhanced employee privacy and confidentiality. However, the relationship may be limited in its ability to directly address workplace conditions and issues that impact mental health. Midsized and small employers often form partnerships to collaborate and link with local community behavioral health providers for services similar to large corporation EAPs.

The number of organizations (vendors) offering external EAP programs is growing (Table 9.2). In 2011, Magellan Health Services, OptumHealth, and ValueOptions were the top three providers of EAP services. Together, these three vendors represent around 35% of the 2011 market, compared to almost 51% of the market in 2002 (Morgan et al., 2012). External EAPs generally offer two types of programming. First they offer programs to serve the entire workplace employee population providing services that promote mental and behavioral health (e.g., stress management, mindfulness, positive psychology) as well as counseling, support, and referral for mental and behavioral health problems and concerns. The second is to offer to individual employees, on a per diem basis only, counseling, support, and referral for mental and behavioral health problems and concerns.

Table 9.2   Ten Largest EAP Vendor Organizations (Morgan et al., 2012)

1	Magellan Health Services, Inc.
2	OptumHealth
3	ValueOptions Inc.
4	ComPsych Corporation
5	Aetna Behavioral Health
6	Workplace Benefits, LLC
7	CIGNA Behavioral Health, Inc.
8/9	LifeCare
	WellPoint, Inc.
10	Ceridian

Family/Work-Life Programs

Family/work-life programs assist employees to effectively manage their professional and personal interests and responsibilities. While many programs refer to work/life "balance," in reality people often face uneven and often unpredictable demands on their time from the many roles they play—employee, spouse, community member, son or daughter, parent, aunt or uncle, and so forth. Competing and unresolved conflicts among these roles can directly impact an individual's well-being and mental health. Employers are increasingly inclined to offer a wide range of options to assist employees in juggling these demands on their time, while still being productive in the workplace, by suggesting alternative ways to structure work time, providing resources to support family needs, and implementing workplace policies. Some workplaces are instituting a new framework, career customization, to respond to the realities of the current workforce and the shortcomings of more traditional flexibility options (Table 9.3). Transparency and clear communication are critical to the success of family/work-life programs to avoid tension and resentment among colleagues so that those without children, for example, are not assuming the workload of those leaving early for soccer games and pediatrician appointments. Employers who offer a range of family and work-life options gain a competitive advantage in attracting, motivating, fostering loyalty in, and retaining productive employees.

Table 9.3   Features of a Family/Work-Life Program

Traditional Family/Work-Life Options	Career Customization Program
Ways to structure work time: • flex-time schedules • part-time schedules • compressed work week • sabbatical leaves • job sharing • work from home • telecommuting	Provides an alternative to traditional work/life options, responding to current workforce trends: • shrinking skilled labor pool • changing family structures • increasing number of women • changing expectations of men • evolving expectations of Gen X and Gen Y • increasing impact of technology
Resources to support employee needs: • time off for births and adoptions for mothers and fathers • lactation rooms • on-site child care • emergency backup child care • resources for raising special-needs children • teen driving courses • college counseling • time off for extended family caregiving • time off for community service • pet care • concierge services • elder parent and family care and support • home health care and end-of-life support	Allows employees to "dial up" and "dial down" their career path, along four dimensions: • pace • workload • location/schedule • role (from individual contributor to leader) At four work-life points: • career years 0–3 • career years 4–7 • career years 8–14 • career years 15+
Workplace policies: • reduced work travel • ability to say no to overtime without career penalty • no email outside normal business hours • no weekend business use of laptops or cell phones • sensitivity to needs of cultural groups, employees with disabilities, LGBT employees	Responds to shortcomings of flexible work arrangements: • adaptations in work schedule often made at times of personal/family crisis • focus on current job vs. long-range career path • assume norm of continuous, full-time employment throughout a career • can sideline or derail employee advancement • may be viewed by men primarily as options for women

Stress Management Programs

Job stress should not be confused with job challenge. A challenge is energizing and motivating, and a worker feels positive and satisfied when the challenge is met. Job stress develops when a person is unable to cope with the pressures and demands of the job, and it produces harmful responses that can lead to physical and mental illness. Job stress is associated with high levels of absenteeism, turnover, accidents, and burnout. Effective workplace stress management programs have a dual focus: interventions to improve the coping skills of individual employees and workplace modifications to reduce stressful job conditions (Table 9.4). While stress management techniques can improve an individual's ability to cope with a stressful workplace, the benefits are often short-lived unless the root causes of stress are addressed in the work environment. Since the demands of each job vary widely, it is essential that every workplace assess the stressors particular to its employees.

Table 9.4 Features of a Stress Management Program

Interventions for Individuals	Workplace Modifications
Awareness and education	Assessment
• employee personal stress self-assessment	• employee surveys to identify levels and sources of workplace stress
• stress management quiz about sources of stress and stress management strategies	• focus groups
• posters with stress management tips displayed in cafeterias, restrooms, break rooms, other areas	• data analysis of absenteeism, illness, turnover, performance
• regular e-mail messages with stress management tips	• training for managers to identify employees suffering from stress
• paycheck inserts with stress reduction strategies	Job redesign
• workshops and guest speakers	• clarify expectations
• newsletters	• simplify work roles
Workplace stress management options	• reduce workload
• yoga, tai chi, aerobics classes	• increase work breaks
• relaxation sessions—meditation, deep breathing	• increase worker decision making
• mindfulness training	• increase social support from coworkers and supervisors
• stress management coaches	• provide training to improve skills and lead to advancement
• support groups	Environmental changes
• conflict resolution training	• reduce noise
• walking groups during breaks	• increase privacy
• regular stretch breaks	• reduce air pollution
• quiet or relaxation room for employees	• increase safety
	• improve ergonomics

Depression Prevention and Treatment Programs

Depression impacts employee production and teamwork, and it will rank second only to heart disease as the leading cause of disability worldwide by the year 2020. Depression affects almost 20% of adults in the United States at some point in their lives and costs employers 200 million lost workdays annually. Depression contributes (comorbidity) to the severity of heart disease, diabetes, and stroke. Workplace depression programs span primary, secondary, and tertiary prevention including awareness, assessment, integration, treatment, support, and workplace policies and procedures (Table 9.5). For instance, Beyond Blue, a workplace depression prevention

Table 9.5   Features of a Depression Prevention and Treatment Program (Langlieb & Kah, 2005; Unützer & Park, 2012)

Features of a Depression Prevention and Treatment Program	Implementation Strategies
Awareness A broad-based informational campaign helps employees recognize the signs and symptoms of depression and become aware of the help available to them. Managers learn to understand the signs of depression, know what to expect, and develop skills in approaching employees about depression.	**Employees** • newsletters • brochures • confidential self-assessments • information displayed in cafeterias, break rooms, bulletin boards • First Aid Kit for the Mind distributed at new employee orientation • Nurse Care Line: telephone resource to inform employees about available services **Managers** • books • training programs • Mental Health First Aid: 8-hour certification course to prepare managers and others to recognize and respond to signs of mental illness
Assessment Early and accurate diagnosis of depression by a trained mental health clinician is a critical step in helping employees begin treatment before needing hospitalization. Employees might be reluctant to divulge their need for help.	• in-house employee screening • absenteeism data analysis to identify employees who might need referral or treatment
Integration Employees are often seen first by their primary care physician (PCP). Yet PCPs accurately diagnose depression only 19% of the time compared to 90% accurate diagnoses by trained mental health clinicians. Effective programs combine care from primary care physicians and psychiatrists through careful coordination and communication.	• incentive reimbursements to PCPs for depression screening • consultations for PCPs with 24/7 on-call psychiatrists • free web-based continuing medical education courses about depression • care managers who coordinate medical and mental health treatment • integrating depression treatment with physical activity

(continues)

Table 9.5   (*Continued*)

Features of a Depression Prevention and Treatment Program	Implementation Strategies
Treatment Treatment for depression includes antidepressant medication, individual psychotherapeutic counseling, or a combination of these approaches.	• in-person psychotherapy • structured psychotherapy over the telephone for individuals reluctant to enter treatment
Support Employees often need support to adhere to their medication and therapy regimens.	• care planner telephones regularly to encourage compliance with treatment • work schedules are altered to permit participation in treatment • treatment is offered in the evening to accommodate work schedule
Workplace Policies and Procedures Senior management commitment and participation are central to the development and implementation of workplace policies and procedures promote employee mental health.	Surveys identify workplace conditions leading to depression • climate • coworker and supervisor conflict • time pressures • physical demands of the job • lack of control and decision making • lack of advancement opportunities and mentoring • lack of workplace recognition Responses to survey findings • job skills training • communication skills training and procedures • conflict resolution training • standards of conduct for employees and supervisors

program from Australia, offers its National Workplace Program to increase the knowledge and skills of staff and managers to address mental health (depression) conditions in the workplace. The program consists of five workshops (Table 9.6). Many workplace depression programs are based on cognitive behavioral therapy (American Psychiatric Association, 2006) that helps individual correct inaccurate dysfunctional beliefs, including defeatist expectancies ("it won't be fun"), low self-efficacy ("I always fail"), anomalous beliefs ("spirits will harm me"), and ageist beliefs ("I'm too old to learn"), that interfere with goal-directed activities. An example of a program for adults in the workplace is Beating the Blues (2014), a web-based depression program developed in England, that uses cognitive behavioral therapy.

Table 9.6   Beyond Blue National Workplace Program to Prevent Depression (Beyond Blue, 2015)

1. **Senior executive briefing:** Highlights the importance of mental health in the workplace to senior executives. The presentation incorporates a business case for tackling the most common mental health problems in the workplace and leadership strategies to address mental health in the workplace.

2. **Organizational awareness:** Increases awareness among staff members about depression and anxiety and their impact, and support for mental well-being.

3. **Employee awareness to action:** Increases awareness among general staff members about the most common mental health conditions and their impact on the workplace. Uses case studies and structured discussions to increase staff member confidence to approach a colleague they may be concerned about.

4. **Manager awareness, impact, and action:** Educates managers on the impact of common mental health conditions on individuals, the workplace environment and the organization as a whole. Present the principles and planning required to approach an employee they may be concerned about as well as to develop management strategies to address mental health within their organization.

5. **Strategies and solutions for HR professionals:** Specifically geared to enable HR professionals to promote mental health awareness and to meet the challenge of addressing depression, anxiety, and related disorders in the workplace. Participants will be guided through the fundamentals of mental health problems in the workplace, including an examination of prevention strategies at an organizational level, how to develop appropriate policies and procedures, and how to advise managers on addressing mental health problems with their staff.

Tobacco Cessation Programs

Tobacco products have always existed in several traditional forms including cigars, pipes, cigarettes, hookahs (or water pipes), small cigars, *bidis* (small, thin hand-rolled cigarettes imported to the United States primarily from India and other Southeast Asian countries), chewing tobacco, and snuff. Now there are even more tobacco options such as electronic cigarettes, mists, vapors, and smokeless tobacco. The two major purposes of tobacco cessation programs in the workplace are encouraging tobacco users to quit, and reducing employees' exposure to second-hand smoke. Nicotine addiction is often severe and may require multiple quit attempts before the tobacco user can quit permanently. Tobacco cessation should be structured to provide support for multiple quit attempts.

Workplace program interventions aimed at individual workers cover group therapy, individual counseling, self-help materials, nicotine replacement therapy, and social support (Cahill & Lancaster, 2014). Employee programs are frequently provided on-site at the workplace. Programs will identify employees who use tobacco, such as through the use of an employee health survey or by screening employees for their tobacco status, and then provide follow-up counseling and treatment (Paul, 2013). Approaches may include referral to outside organizations or quitlines (state-based or self-contracted) that offer these services, or bringing a health educator or tobacco cessation counselor on-site. A critical part of any workplace health promotion program is a tobacco-free workplace policy that combines tobacco cessation campaigns and referral programs (World Health Organization, 2007). Such programs emphasize that a tobacco-free environment protects everyone—tobacco users and nonusers alike. Many studies have shown that smoking bans and restrictions are effective strategies to reduce exposure to second-hand smoke, a preventable cause of significant illness and death. Creating tobacco-free buildings and campuses requires more than nonsmoking signs. The integration of multiple approaches—such as communications/media campaigns, classes, smoking bans and restrictions, clinics, and telephone and quitline referrals—is recommended (Cahill & Lancaster, 2014; Stolz et al., 2014). The list below includes a sample of available workplace tobacco cessation tools and resources.

Workplace Tobacco Cessation Tools and Resources

- *Leading by Example: Creating Healthy Communities through Corporate Engagement* published in 2011 by the Partnership for Prevention features 19 businesses and business groups who are providing leadership and reaching out to improve the health and wellness of their communities, providing many benefits to their organizations.

- *Leading by Example: The Value of Worksite Health Promotion to Small- and Medium-sized Employers*, published in 2011 by the Partnership for Prevention, provides best practices and strategies for creating or enhancing a workplace health promotion program as well as workplace health program descriptions from almost 20 small employers.

- The Centers for Disease Control and Prevention (CDC) has developed a brochure titled *Save Lives, Save Money: Make Your Business Smoke Free*, which provides guidelines and a business case for developing tobacco-free campus policies.

- The American Cancer Society's Workplace Solutions (http://www.acsworkplacesolutions.com/) has developed *Strategies for Promoting and Implementing a Smoke-free Workplace*, adapted from the CDC's comprehensive guide *Making Your Workplace Smokefree: A Decision Maker's Guide*, to assist employers in creating a safe, healthful environment for employees.

- The Partnership for Prevention has published *Investing in Health: Evidence-Based Health Promotion Practices for the Workplace*, which contains multiple tips for controlling tobacco use at the workplace. These include implementing tobacco-free policies, adding tobacco cessation benefits, and improving access to tobacco cessation quitlines.

Factory Floor- and Office-Level Evidence-Based Mental Health Interventions and Practices

Workplaces have factory floor- and office-level mental health interventions and practices to address their particular workforce health needs. From small and midsized organizations to large national employers, these engage employees at the workplace (factory floor and office) and are lower cost and practical, with fairly easy administration. Outside vendors both national and local compete for contracts to offer the interventions. Examples of widely implemented evidence-based interventions and practices are:

Mental health first aid: An adult public education program used to improve workplace supervisors' knowledge of, and modify their attitudes and perceptions about, mental health and related issues, including how to respond to individuals who are experiencing one or more acute mental health crises (e.g., suicidal thoughts and/or behavior, acute stress reaction, panic attacks, and/or acute psychotic behavior) or are in the early stages of one or more chronic mental health problems (e.g., depressive, anxiety, and/or psychotic disorders, which may occur with substance abuse).

The intervention is delivered by a trained, certified instructor through an interactive 12-hour course (Mental Health First Aid, 2015). The course introduces supervisors to risk factors, warning signs, and symptoms for a range of mental health problems, including comorbidity with substance use disorders; builds supervisors' understanding of the impact and prevalence of mental health problems; and provides an overview of common support and treatment resources for those with a mental health problem.

Sleep hygiene programs: Sleep hygiene is a variety of different practices that are necessary to have normal, quality nighttime sleep and full daytime alertness. Sleep plays a major role in employees' work habits (CDC, 2009). Employees may be unable to fall asleep due to work or personal reasons, which may lead to a reduced quality of life and an increased likelihood of getting sick. This may also lead to greater monetary costs to employers. Therefore, many employers offer programs on how employees can get the best sleep they can by reducing stress and falling asleep easier. Research suggests that both educating employees and giving them individual sleep therapy allows workers to get better rest. For example, ProjectZ (2015) uses a three-step approach of clinically screening employees, creating individual plans, and continuing treatment and ongoing engagement with employees for their sleep habits. Fatigue management tracker websites (Health Improvement Solutions, 2015) track sleep patterns and help set realistic and specific goals for individuals' sleep to ensure that employees get a better night's rest. Companies that used workplace health programs that educated employers on proper sleep hygiene and allowed employees to speak one-on-one with educated professionals about their sleep habits saw less tired employees during the workday, resulting in healthier employees overall. (Nishinoue et al., 2012).

Mindfulness training: Mindfulness training is a systematic procedure to develop enhanced awareness of moment-to-moment experience of perceptible mental processes. The approach assumes that greater awareness will provide more veridical perception, reduce negative affect, and improve vitality and coping. Mindfulness workplace training focuses on the degree to which individuals are mindful in their work setting (Dane & Brummel, 2014). Through mindfulness training employees can improve stress management, create greater mental clarity and focus, enhance creativity, gain a greater sense of effective emotional regulation and resilience, become better empathizers, and be able to manage change better (Grossman, Niemann, Schmidt, & Walach, 2004). Programs, such as Organisational Mindfulness (http://www.organisationalmindfulness.com/), combine information about mindfulness, goals, and effective leadership training that benefits employers and employees. Kudesia (in press) used a workplace mindfulness program to bolster employees' creativity. Online mindfulness training has created opportunities to reach a wide range of employees. Researchers report that online programs have resulted in employees being happier in their work environments, less stressed, and more resilient to mental fatigue (Aikens et al., 2014; Mask, Chan, Cheung, Lin, & Ngai, 2015).

Suicide prevention and postvention programs: Employers and employees are affected when coworkers, family members, clients, vendors, and others who surround the workplace attempt suicide or die by suicide (Hempstead & Phillips, 2015). Workplace suicide prevention programs include a range of activities (Milner, Page, Spencer-Thomas, & Lamotagne, 2015): for example, educating managers and supervisors about the warning signs of suicide and appropriate actions. Likewise, programs focus on increasing awareness among employees of the warning signs and how to intervene by reaching out to the person in distress. Postvention programs provide psychological first aid, crisis intervention, and other support after a suicide to affected individuals or the workplace as a whole to alleviate possible effects of a suicide death (Carson J Spencer Foundation, 2013).

Mental and Behavioral Health Priority Implementation Challenges

Employers recognize the value of workplace mental health programs, adopt best program practices, and realize benefits from the programs for their organizations and employees. However, establishing comprehensive, evidence-based, effective mental health programs in the workplace faces challenges of employer reluctance and employee resistance and mental health stigma. Furthermore the Mental Health Parity and Addiction Equity Act of 2008 requires health insurance plans to have parity between mental health and substance use disorder benefits and medical/surgical benefits with respect to financial requirements and treatment limitations. This law is very detailed and contains many complex concepts that may be difficult for employers to implement.

Employer Reluctance

There is both a philosophical and financial basis for employer reluctance to build comprehensive mental health services into a workplace health promotion program. First, there are conflicting beliefs about the locus of responsibility for addressing mental health issues in the workplace. One position holds that it is in the employer's interest to promote and sustain the well-being of employees both physically and mentally. Conversely, some employers believe that worker safety is their responsibility but that worker mental and physical health is the responsibility of the individual. Even among some employers who believe that supporting worker physical health is an appropriate workplace strategy, there exists a general wariness about mental illness that makes them reluctant to tackle the problem. Employers may not consider how the work environment affects workers' emotional and mental well-being.

Second, many employers lack information about the direct and indirect costs of mental illness in the workplace and hold misperceptions about the cost-effectiveness of treatment. For example, employers may not be aware that 25% of people of working age experience mental illness or substance abuse problems in any given year; more than 70% of people diagnosed with depression are employed; more workers are absent from work because of stress and anxiety than because of physical illness or injury. The direct cost to employers of medical care for workers' mental illness is substantial. Workers with untreated mental illness use inpatient and outpatient services three times more than those receiving treatment; Individuals with depression consume 2 to 4 times the health care resources of workers without depression; mental illness short-term disability claims are growing by 10% annually. In one study (Donohue & Pincus, 2007) of the impact of modifiable health risk factors (e.g., smoking, overweight, hypertension, high stress, and depression), depression predicted the largest increase in medical costs, a 70% increase compared with 46% for the condition associated with the next largest increase in cost. Indirect costs are even higher. Mental illness ranks near the top of the list for lost productivity due to absence and disability; employees with depressions cost employers $44 billion per year in lost productive time.

Employee Resistance and Mental Health Stigma

There are many barriers that interfere with employees seeking mental health services: feeling ashamed, thinking the problem can be handled without treatment, not knowing where to go for services, not having time, feeling that treatment would not help the problem, fear of being involuntarily committed or forced to take medication, cost and accessibility of services, lack of confidentiality, and stigma. In particular, stigma is a cluster of negative attitudes and beliefs that motivate the general public to fear, reject, avoid, and discriminate against people with mental illness. Stigma is a key problem for individuals with mental illness, as it may prevent them from seeking treatment (Regier et al., 1993; Wang et al., 2007) and contribute to negative interactions with friends, peers, employers, landlords, and law enforcement (Wahl, 1999; Wright, Gronfein, & Owens, 2000). Thus, reducing the stigma associated with mental illness is a critical step for workplace mental health programs that promote the prevention of and early intervention in mental disorders and the improvement of the quality of life at work for individuals with mental illness. A number of programs that aim to reduce the stigma and discrimination associated with mental illness have been launched both in the United States and worldwide (Corrigan, 2012). These stigma and discrimination reduction initiatives can involve a variety of components, such as training, education, media campaigns, contact with people with mental illness, or combinations of these strategies (Collins, Wong, Cerully, Schultz, & Eberhart, 2012; Knifton, Walker, & Quinn, 2009).

Mental Health Parity and Addiction Equity Act

Mental health research, the information/technology economy, and improved treatment options are creating an environment in which the importance of workplace mental health programs is increasingly apparent to employers. Those employers who will now be inclined to offer mental health benefits will find their plans governed by a strengthened Mental Health Parity and Addiction Equity Act. While Congress passed the act in 2008 to establish equality between mental and other medical care, insurance companies often treated mental health and physical health benefits differently. In 2013 it was clarified that while the act does not require insurance plans to offer coverage for mental illnesses or substance use disorders, if mental health benefits are offered, they must have the same levels of coverage (e.g., copays, deductibles, visit limits) as those for medical/surgical conditions. This will eliminate insurance discrimination against employees with mental health needs. Employers concerned about the cost of adding mental to their employee benefits can make the most of their investment by carefully avoiding duplication of services across programs, making sure they are offering the most effective services, and joining or forming community employer coalitions to leverage market power (Milliman, n.d.).

Advocacy and Resource Partnerships and Organizations

Many business and nonprofit groups provide ongoing research, materials, and advocacy for the best, evidence-based practices that support and maintain workforce mental health. Among those groups are:

The American Psychiatric Foundation Association Partnership for Workplace Mental Health (http://workplacementalhealth.org/)

The Partnership for Workplace Mental Health is a program of the American Psychiatric Foundation. The Partnership works with businesses to ensure that employees and their families living with mental illness, including substance use disorders, receive effective care. The Partnership reviews the research, identifies trends, and highlights innovative employer strategies through its publications: *Mental Health Works* (quarterly journal), *Eupdate* (monthly electronic newsletter), *Research Works* (literature reviews), *Surveys* (collaborations with other organizations). The Partnership also provides resources to support business mental health programs including case examples of best practices.

Families and Work Institute (http://www.familiesandwork.org/)

Families and Work Institute (FWI) is a nonprofit, nonpartisan research organization that studies the changing workforce, family, and community. FWI workplace mental health projects focus on the effective workplace, impact of the current economy on employers and their policies, workplace and career flexibility, health of the American workforce, low-wage workforce and upward mobility, and working in retirement.

National Alliance on Mental Illness (NAMI) (http://www.nami.org/)

NAMI is the nation's largest grassroots mental health organization dedicated to building better lives for the millions of Americans affected by mental illness. It provides an array of support and education programs, advocates for a wide range of public policy initiatives, and disseminates information about promising mental health practices. There are more than 1,000 local NAMI Affiliates across the country.

National Council for Community Behavioral Healthcare (http://
www.thenationalcouncil.org/)

> The National Council for Community Behavioral Healthcare
> is the oldest and largest national community behavioral health
> care advocacy organization in the country. It was formed in 1970
> and represents the interests of community behavioral health care
> organizations nationwide. The National Council conducts federal
> advocacy activities, representing the industry on Capitol Hill and
> before federal agencies, and offers a national consulting service
> program, publications, and annual training conference.

**Substance Abuse and Mental Health Services Administration
(SAMHSA)** (http://www.samhsa.gov/)

> SAMHSA is the agency within the federal Department of
> Health and Human Services that leads public health efforts to
> advance the behavioral health of the nation. As a government
> agency, SAMHSA has an enormous array of programs, grants,
> publications, data, and information about behavioral health. The
> Division of Workplace Programs provides resources for businesses,
> including such guides as *A Mental Health Friendly Workplace*.

Employee Assistance Professionals Association (EAPA) (www
.eapassn.org)

> A membership organization for employee assistance pro-
> fessionals, the Employee Assistance Professionals Association
> (EAPA), provides education, training, a code of ethics, and advo-
> cacy. EAPA publishes the *Journal of Employee Assistance*, hosts
> the annual World EAP Conference, and offers online training.
> EAPA offers a Certified Employee Assistance Professional creden-
> tial (CEAP®) for professionals in the EAP field.

Summary

Employers understand the need for workplace mental and behavioral health
programs, both out of concern for employees' well-being and in recognition
that organizational performance is directly related to the mental health
of their workers. The costs of employee mental health and behavioral
concerns and problems have a direct impact on workplace absenteeism,
presenteeism, accidents, turnover, and productivity. Employee assistance
programs, family/work-life programs, stress management, depression prevention and treatment, and tobacco cessation are examples of mental
and behavioral health priority programs implemented in the workplace.

Challenges that hamper efforts to implement the mental and behavioral health priority include employer reluctance and employee resistance and mental health stigma. Those employers who are inclined to offer mental health and behavioral programs have recently found support and challenges from the Mental Health Parity and Addiction Equity Act.

For Practice and Discussion

1. Reflect on your own (as well as family members' and friends') mental health experience to identify situations that might be barriers to seeking help for a mental health concern or problem. As part of a workplace health promotion program implementation, how would you address the situations?

2. Table 9.2 lists the 10 largest vendors offering employee assistance programs in the United States. Investigate the range and types of services being offered. Is there a set of common EAP services and activities offered by all the vendors? Can you identify unique services offered by companies that might provide them a competitive edge when competing to be a workplace service provider? Large organizations have workplaces in many communities and employ individuals with diverse ethnic, cultural, and language backgrounds. How do the vendors present their capacity to offer their services in different languages and locations?

3. What are your recommendations for the implementation of an evidence-based stress management program for middle-level female managers working in the technology field at remote locations around the southwest United States? The women are home-based in El Paso and Austin, both in Texas, and in Phoenix, Arizona in Albuquerque, New Mexico, and in San Diego, California, providing hardware and software support for small and midsized education and medical clients in their areas. As part of middle managers' responsibilities they oversee and manage technical staff members who work on-site at the client offices.

4. Compare and contrast workplace nicotine cessation program approaches and modalities both medical and nonmedical. How do these programs compare with workplace efforts to address alcohol and other drug use and abuse, as well as disordered eating, among employees?

5. Manufacturer's Association of North Texas based in Fort Worth, Texas, is requesting a proposal for its member education and training program on the topic of reducing mental health stigma at the

workplace. The request for proposal states "to avoid workplace stigma and discrimination, employees with mental health problems will usually go to great lengths to ensure that coworkers and managers do not find out about their illness, including avoiding employee assistance programs and shunning effective treatment options. Indeed, the majority of employees who have mental health problems will fail to receive appropriate treatment. Yet, the majority of those who are appropriately treated will manifest improved work performance and reduced disability days sufficient to offset employer costs for treatment." What approach do you recommend for the Association to be proactive in identifying and managing mental health problems among employees and in fostering an organizational cultures that promote mental health?

Case Study: Employer and Employee Mental Health Promotion—What Would You Do?

Talking with directors of human resource departments of large organizations, they all know that employees at risk of, struggling with, or deeply troubled and disabled by stress-related illness are an organizational reality. The well-being of these individuals can affect organizational outcomes. Preparing leaders and professionals with the skills necessary to address all aspects of the mental health continuum effectively, as early as possible, and with an understanding of systemic effects, is essential to ensure long-term organizational health and stability. For example employees with depression is an area of increasing concern. When an employee is depressed, it can affect not only that employee's productivity and happiness, but the entire mood of his or her coworkers and their productivity, too. Luckily, depression in the workplace is not inevitable or hopeless. Steps can be taken to help someone who is depressed. Many employees who suffer untreated depression are doing so because they fear retribution or loss of their job if they report their problems. As well, many do not recognize that depression is treatable. Yet most people can be treated successfully and will miss little, if any, time from work.

Small and midsized workplaces have been slower to address employees' mental health concerns. Often the employers have less available resources and staff experience in the area. Teresa Bradbury, who works with small and midsized workplaces, is being asked to create a small business employer and employee mental health promotion program. If you were Ms. Bradbury, what would you do for the program design, implementation, and evaluation?

KEY TERMS

Mental health

Behavioral health

Employee assistance program (EAP)

Family/work-life program

Stress management

Depression prevention

Beyond Blue

Beating the Blues

Tobacco cessation programs

Mental health first aid

Sleep hygiene

Mindfulness training

Suicide prevention

Employer reluctance

Employee resistance and mental health stigma

Mental Health Parity and Addiction Equity Act

References

Aikens, K. A., Astin, J., Pelletier, K. R., Levanovich, K., Baase, C., Park, Y. Y., & Bodnar, C. M. (2014). Mindfulness goes to work: Impact of an online workplace intervention. *Journal of Occupational & Environmental Medicine*, *56*(7), 721–731.

American Psychiatric Association. (2006). Treatment of patients with major depressive disorder. In *American Psychiatric Association practice guidelines for the treatment of psychiatric disorders*. Arlington, VA: American Psychiatric Publishing.

Beating the Blues. (2014). *Beat depression and anxiety*. Retrieved from http://www.beatingtheblues.co.uk/

Beyond Blue. (2015). *National workplace program*. Retrieved from http://www.beyondblue.org.au/about-us/programs/workplace-and-workforce-program/programs-resources-and-tools/national-workplace-program

Cahill, K., & Lancaster, T. (2014). Workplace interventions for smoking cessation. *Cochrane Database of Systemic Reviews*, *2014*(2), CD003440.

Carson J Spencer Foundation. (2013*). A manager's guide to suicide postvention in the workplace: 10 action steps for dealing with the aftermath of suicide*. Denver, CO: Carson J Spencer Foundation.

Centers for Disease Control and Prevention. (2009). Perceived insufficient rest or sleep among adults: United States. *Morbidity and Mortality Weekly Report*, *58*(42), 1175–1179.

Collins, R. L., Wong, E. C., Cerully, J. L., Schultz, D., & Eberhart, N. K. (2012). *Interventions to reduce mental health stigma and discrimination: A literature review to guide evaluation of California's Mental Health Prevention and Early Intervention Initiative*. Santa Monica, CA: RAND Corporation.

Corrigan, P. W. (2012). Where is the evidence supporting public service announcements to eliminate mental illness stigma? *Psychiatric Services, 63*(1), 79–82.

Dane, E., & Brummel, B. J. (2014). Examining workplace mindfulness and its relation to job performance and turnover intention. *Human Relations, 67*(1), 105–128.

Donohue, J. M., & Pincus, H. A. (2007). Reducing the societal burden of depression. *Pharmacoeconomics, 25*(1), 7–24.

Health Improvement Solutions. (2015). *Our products and services.* Retrieved from http://www.healthimprovementsolutions.com/services.html

Grossman, P., Niemann, L., Schmidt, S., & Walach, H. (2004). Mindfulness-based stress reduction and health benefits: A meta-analysis. *Journal of Psychosomatic Research, 57*(1), 35–43.

Hempstead, K., & Phillips, J. (2015). Rising suicide among adults aged 40–64 years: The role of job and financial circumstances. *American Journal of Preventive Medicine, 48*(5), 491–500.

Knifton, L., Walker, A., & Quinn, N. (2009). Workplace interventions can reduce stigma. *Journal of Public Mental Health, 7*(4), 40–50.

Kudesia, R. S. (in press). Mindfulness and creativity in the workplace. In J. Reb & P. W. B. Atkins (Eds.), *Mindfulness in organisations.* Cambridge, UK: Cambridge University Press.

Langlieb, A. M., & Kahn, J. P. (2005). How much does quality mental health care profit employers? *Journal of Environmental Medicine, 47*(11), 1099–1109. Retrieved from http://www.workpsychcorp.com/QualityMentalHealthCare.pdf

Mask, W., Chan, A., Cheung, E., Lin, C., & Ngai, K. (2015). Enhancing web-based mindfulness training for mental health promotion with the health action process approach: Randomized controlled trial. *Journal of Medical Internet Resource, 17*(1), e8.

Mental Health First Aid. (2015). *Mental health first aid programs.* Retrieved from http://www.mentalhealthfirstaid.org/cs/

Milliman. (n.d.). *Mental Health Parity & Addiction Equity Act.* Retrieved from http://www.milliman.com/Solutions/Services/Mental-Health-Parity-and-Addiction-Equity-Act/#

Milner, A., Page, K., Spencer-Thomas, S., & Lamotagne, A. (2015). Workplace suicide prevention: A systematic review of published and unpublished activities. *Health Promotion International, 30*(1), 29–37.

Morgan, P. J., Collins, C. E., Plotnikoff, R. C., Cook, A. T., Berthon, B., Mitchell, S., & Callister, R. (2012). The impact of a workplace-based weight loss program on work-related outcomes in overweight male shift workers. *Journal of Occupational and Environmental Medicine, 54*(2), 122–127. doi:110.1097/JOM.1090b1013e31824329ab.

National Institute of Mental Health. (1999). *Mental health: A report of the Surgeon General.* Rockville, MD: U.S. Department of Health and Human Services.

Nishinoue, N., Takano, T., Kaku, A., Eto, R., Kato, N., Ono, Y., & Tanaka, K. (2012). Effects of sleep hygiene education and behavioral therapy on sleep quality of white-collar workers: A randomized controlled trial. *Industrial Health, 50*(2), 123–131.

Paul, C. L. (2013). Implementation of personalized workplace smoking cessation program. *Occupational Health, 63*(8), 568–574.

ProjectZ. (2015). *ProjectZ: How it works.* Retrieved from http://www.optisom .com/project-z/

Regier, D. A., Narrow, W. E., Rae, D. S., Manderscheid, R. W., Locke, B. Z., & Goodwin, F. K. (1993). The de facto US mental and addictive disorders service system: Epidemiologic catchment area prospective 1-year prevalence rates of disorders and services. *Archives of General Psychiatry, 50*(2), 85–94. doi:10.1001/archpsyc.1993.01820140007001

Stolz, D., Scherr, A., Seiffert, B., Kuster, M., Meyer, A., Fagerström, K. O., & Tamm, M. (2014). Predictors of success for smoking cessation at the workplace: A longitudinal study. *Respiration, 87*(1), 18–25.

Unützer, J., & Park, M. (2012). Strategies to improve the management of depression in primary care. *Primary Care, 39*(2), 415–431.

Wahl, O. F. (1999). Mental health consumers' experience of stigma. *Schizophrenia Bulletin, 25*(3), 467.

Wang, P. S., Simon, G. E., Avorn, J., Azocar, F., Ludman, E. J., McCulloch, J., . . . Kessler, R. C. (2007). Telephone screening, outreach, and care management for depressed workers and impact on clinical and work productivity outcomes: A randomized controlled trial. *JAMA, 298*(12), 1401–1411.

World Health Organization. (2007). *Protection from exposure to second-hand tobacco smoke: Policy recommendations.* WHO Tobacco Control Papers. Retrieved from http://escholarship.org/uc/item/0nb6z24q

World Health Organization. (2010, September). *Mental health: Strengthening our response.* Fact sheet N 220.

Wright, E. R., Gronfein, W. P., & Owens, T. J. (2000). Deinstitutionalization, social rejection, and the self-esteem of former mental patients. *Journal of Health and Social Behavior*, 68–90.

WORKPLACE HEALTH PROMOTION PROGRAM IMPLEMENTATION HEALTH PRIORITY: PHYSICAL ACTIVITY

Program Implementation: Physical Activity Priority

Physical activity is any body movement that stimulates a person's muscles and requires more energy than resting. Walking, running, dancing, swimming, yoga, and gardening are a few examples of physical activity. Exercise is a type of physical activity that is planned and structured. Lifting weights, taking an aerobics class, and playing on a sports team are examples of exercise. The technical measure of physical activity is metabolic equivalent of task (MET), or simply metabolic equivalent, which defines the energy cost of physical activities.

In 2008 the U.S. Department of Health and Human Services released the *2008 Physical Activity Guidelines for Americans*, a comprehensive resource that provides guidance on the importance of being physically active. Although the workplace is not the only place where physical activity can occur, the fact that people spend a large amount of time at work makes the setting an ideal one in which to promote an individual's physical activity. When we think about the workplace and getting people physically active, the emphasis is to increase an individual's activity level (Table 10.1). With an increase in activity level comes increases in health benefits. The total amount of time spent participating in physical activity does not need to be done at one time. Performing several 10-minute bouts of

LEARNING OBJECTIVES

- Discuss program implementation focused on a physical activity priority
- Identify evidence-based physical activity policies, practices, interventions, and services
- Explain physical activity workplace program challenges
- Describe advocacy partnerships and organizations

Table 10.1   Total Weekly Amounts of Aerobic Physical Activity (Centers for Disease Control and Prevention, 2012)

Levels of Physical Activity	Range of Moderate-Intensity Hours a Week (defined by MET units)	Summary of Overall Health Benefits	Comment
Inactive	No activity beyond baseline	None	Being inactive is unhealthy
Low	Activity beyond baseline but fewer than $2\frac{1}{2}$ hours a week	Some	Low levels of activity are clearly preferable to an inactive lifestyle
Medium	$2\frac{1}{2}$ hours to 5 hours a week	Substantial	Activity at the high end of this range has additional and more extensive health benefits than activity at the low end
High	More than 5 hours a week	Additional	Current science does not allow researchers to identify an upper limit of activity, above which there are no additional health benefits

physical activity of any type provides benefits and is better than not moving at all (Centers for Disease Control and Prevention [CDC], 2012).

Evidence-Based Physical Activity Policies, Practices, Interventions, and Services

Implementation of the physical activity priority spans the workplace and community. Small and midsized workplaces and many large workplaces do not have physical activity space or facilities (e.g., fitness center, gym, pool, walking trails, bike path, showers, changing area, equipment storage, and maintenance) but rather use existing facilities in the surrounding workplace communities and employee neighborhoods. Partnerships and collaborations for workplace physical activity are a mainstay of the physical activity priority implementation.

The local weather and climate conditions, shift work patterns (e.g., operate 24 hours a day, with three shifts), decentralized (e.g., home-based virtual work stations), and multiple locations all impact workplace physical activity programming. Depending on the occupation, employees may be active because of the physical nature of the work they perform. Restaurant wait staff may walk several miles in the course of a shift, and construction workers may lift hundreds of pounds of material over the course of a day. However, an active job does not guarantee that the employees will achieve the moderate to vigorous level of aerobic and/or muscle-strengthening activities they need to meet the recommended physical activity guidelines. Implementation considers all of these factors and builds from the types of physical work employees perform.

Health and Fitness Centers

A health and fitness center can be at the workplace or in the community. A center is defined as any business or entity that provides an opportunity for individuals to engage in activities that may reasonably be expected to involve placing stress on one or more of the various physiological systems, such as cardiovascular, muscular, or thermoregulatory (American College of Sports Medicine [ACSM], 2012). Fitness centers ordinarily charge a fee, usually monthly, to their members for access to the facilities and programs. According to the International Health, Racquet, and Sports Club Association (IHRSA), the health and fitness industry consists of 30,500 health clubs in the United States in 2012, which accounted for 50.2 million members and $21.8 million in revenue (IHRSA, 2013). Facilities within a workplace, and those made available by partnering with community and neighborhood facilities external to the workplace, share four characteristics that are important to consider when implementing a physical activity program. When working with a health and fitness center assess the facility for these four specific characteristics and be able to identify how the center can best serve the population (employees) in your program.

First, the foundation of any health and fitness facility is the programs and activities that it offers. Many different options exist that include group exercise classes, wellness programs, senior fitness classes, personal training, aquatics instruction, indoor cycling, fitness incentive programs, intramural sports, youth programs, and programs for people with special medical considerations. Some facilities may also offer outdoor education and adventure team-building programs for youth, adults, and corporate employee teams. The availability of these programs to members will differ greatly between each health and fitness facility. Members may be required to pay extra to participate or these classes may be included in their existing membership. It is important to be aware of the available programs and activities in a facility to be able to utilize them through a health promotion program. Because many facilities have programs and activities already available to members, it may be easy to include these in a workplace health promotion program.

Second, every health and fitness facility offers a variety of options that can be utilized by its members. These options may include a general fitness floor, gymnasium, locker rooms, sport court areas (basketball, tennis, volleyball, etc.), pools, outdoor recreation areas, exercise classrooms, running tracks, fitness testing areas, and more. A fitness floor may include a variety of options that include free weights, resistance training machines, cardiovascular training equipment, and floor mat areas. In addition to these common facility options, some facilities may offer specialty options such as spa areas, youth supervision centers, or physical therapy services.

Third, while it is evident that each facility requires individual regulations catered to its unique facility options, it is important to understand that basic safety standards exist among all health and fitness facilities. The ACSM lists recommended standards that provide minimum requirements a fitness facility needs to meet to ensure a safe environment in which physical activity and exercise programs can occur. The general standards categories are described below. The standards represented here are merely general and do not provide the detail necessary to implement them successfully. For more information about these standards, visit http://www.acsm.org. In addition to these recommended standards, ACSM in collaboration with NSF International (an independent public health and environmental organization that provides standards development) are currently working to create a voluntary certification for health and fitness facilities based on a version of the ACSM standards. It is anticipated that the certification would positively impact the health and fitness industry if widely adopted.

ACSM Health and Fitness Facility Standards

- *Preactivity Screening*—A facility must offer each adult member a preactivity screening (e.g., PAR-Q) that is appropriate to the physical activities to be performed by the member.

- *Orientation, Education, and Supervision*—Once a new member or prospective member has completed the preactivity process, operators of the fitness facility must provide the user with a general orientation of the facility and provide a means by which the user can obtain assistance or guidance with their physical activity program.

- *Risk Management and Emergency Policies*—A facility must have practices and systems in place to reduce the risk of having an employee, member, or user experience an event that could result in individual harm or harm to the business itself.

- *Professional Staff and Independent Contractors for Health/Fitness Facilities*—All fitness and health care professionals must have the necessary competencies for fulfilling their various roles and responsibilities, which usually involves some combination of education, training, certifications, and hands-on experience.

- *Health/Fitness Facility Operating Practices*—Although several successful operating practices exist, a facility must have formalized operating practices to ensure the consistent delivery of its products and services in the desired manner.

- *Health/Fitness Facility Design and Construction*—While a facility may offer a wide variety of fitness and multipurpose spaces, they must, to the extent required by law, adhere to the standards of building design as detailed by the Americans with Disabilities Act (ADA) as well as be in compliance with all federal, state, and local building codes.

- *Health/Fitness Facility Equipment*—Facility equipment can be broken up into four categories: cardiovascular equipment, variable-resistance and selectorized resistance equipment, free weight equipment, and fitness accessory equipment. A facility may offer any combination of these types of equipment. However, the facility must provide proper maintenance, equipment reinvestment, and safety equipment pertaining to the equipment. The aquatic and pool facilities must provide proper safety equipment according to state and local codes and regulations.

- *Signage in Health/Fitness Facilities*—A facility must post appropriate signage alerting users to the risks involved in their use of those areas of a facility that present potential increased risk(s).

Finally the staff within a health and fitness facility is an important resource that may be useful when implementing a physical activity program. There are many different people who have unique duties within a health and fitness facility, but each has an important role in the common goal of making a facility run smoothly, effectively, and safely. As one of the ACSM standards states, each facility must have "professional supervision of all physical activity areas and programs" (Pronk, 2012). The supervision of physical activity areas and programs includes supervision of program content, program staffing, or the programming space. These supervisory staff positions may include a fitness director, aquatics director, and group exercise coordinator. A fitness director usually holds a four-year college degree in a health/fitness-related field and is responsible for the fitness floor, fitness programs, fitness program instructors, and personal trainers.

City and County Parks and Recreation Departments

City and county parks and recreation departments are potential partners and allies for workplace programs focused on promoting employees' physical activity. Most cities or counties have a parks and recreation department that commonly is in charge of park maintenance as well as conservation, community programming, recreation centers, senior centers, aquatics centers, and more. The employees of these departments are government employees who report to their respective level of government. Ordinarily, parks and recreation directors work under the city or county executive to oversee operations in or involving public spaces. Working under a parks and recreation director may be specific directors of (for instance) parks, aquatics, and recreation centers. In bigger cities and towns, several levels of management may exist within the parks and recreation department. The National Recreation and Park Association (NRPA) is the accreditation, educational, and resource association for these departments and ensures quality throughout parks and recreation professionals and departments throughout the country (https://www.nrpa.org/).

Paralleling the local governmental parks and recreational infrastructure are the state and national parks and recreational governmental systems, including state and national park systems. Each has its internal state infrastructure and partnership opportunities. For example the National Association of State Park Directors (http://www.americasstateparks.org /NASPD) is devoted to helping state park systems effectively manage and administer their state park system, including partnerships to promote physical activity. The U.S. Park Service (http://www.nps.gov/index.htm) offers similar opportunities for health promotion.

Workplace capacity assessments also consider community programming and its public facility capabilities. Most local parks and recreation departments have a website or web page on the local government's website with current information about programming, events, schedules, and more. These resources are especially helpful when determining the scope of an individual area's community programs and the recreation services that may be available to employees. Being active with the local government officials and participating in local planning activities are instrumental in the decision-making process for the development, maintenance, and support of facilities offering recreational and leisure-time activity. Employers and employees as part of the local economy are a constituency that can have a voice in government decisions affecting employees and, in particular, employee health (e.g., physical activity).

Community Recreational Associations and Organizations

Community recreation associations and organizations develop independent of the governmental park and recreation infrastructure. The associations and organizations reflect the unique characteristics, culture, history, and preferences of the individuals and families that live in communities and neighborhoods. The community associations and organizations are potential partners and allies for workplace health promotion programs offering employees (and their families) opportunities for physical activities. As part of implementing the workplace physical activity priority, the community associations and organizations provide the opportunity to tailor programmatic efforts to the specific employees' interest, abilities, locale (e.g., climate), social support, and schedule (e.g., work, family responsibilities). The employees to their fullest extent self-determine their participation and thereby require the workplace program to be creative in how best to promote and build upon individuals' engagement in physical activity. Physical activity programs create opportunities for an organization (workplace) to partner with the local community. Local organizations are eager to collaborate on activities that benefit the community. These can be one-time events or long-term relationships (Table 10.2).

Organizations can also exist at the grassroots level, with individuals interested in particular sports or activities, such as soccer, biking, running, cross country skiing, that are self-sustaining and change based on individuals' interest, time, and energy, local conditions, and access to a field or area to engage in the activity (e.g., field, trails, pools). Frequently, the grassroots

Table 10.2   Partnering With Your Community Recreation Associations and Organizations (adapted from Centers for Disease Control and Prevention, 2012)

Whom it affects: Partnering with the community recreation associations and organizations affects all employees and family members who choose to actively participate with the associations and organizations.

Why it works: Your workplace is able to:

Tap into or expand employees' existing social connections.

Demonstrate corporate citizenship and social leadership.

Promote the health of the community.

What it takes: Get to know the associations and organizations. Become more knowledgeable about the community and its economic conditions, political structures, norms and values, demographic trends, history, and experience with business engagement efforts. Some of this knowledge can be gleaned by simply talking to other businesses or nonprofit businesses in the community. Connect with local hospitals and health agencies to understand community health issues and what community efforts already exist to promote physical activity in the community.

Evaluation: Consider evaluating how many new partnerships are established with community recreation associations and organizations because of reaching out to the community. Determine how much time was dedicated to community outreach and document what the results of these efforts have been for promoting physical activity among employees and within the community. Share the results with employees and other key stakeholders in the community. Use this as an opportunity to share your corporate citizenship and social leadership.

organizations have no formal infrastructure or means to sustain themselves beyond the individuals currently participating with the group. When implementing a workplace physical activity priority, however, consider how the local grassroots organizations can support employees that are engaged locally on the weekends in running and biking fund raising events, soccer tournaments, and golf outings. Paying event fees, being listed as a sponsor on the back of an event garment, and in-kind support (e.g., healthy snacks) are examples of contributions that are low cost but offer intrinsic value that adds value to the employees' physical activity engagement.

Personal Trainers

The professional focused on physical activity in workplace health promotion frequently is a personal trainer with the goal to support and engage the employees in physical activity. A personal trainer works with apparently healthy individuals as well as those with health challenges who are able to exercise independently to enhance quality of life, improve health-related physical fitness and performance, manage health risk, and promote lasting, healthy behavior changes. A personal trainer conducts basic pre-participation health screening assessments, submaximal cardiovascular exercise tests, and muscular strength/endurance, flexibility, and body composition tests (ACSM, 2012). Personal trainers work with health and fitness centers, in personal training studios, and as private contractors in a variety of venues. They work one-on-one or with a small group of people to assess health and fitness needs, design exercise programs, and implement for their clients the exercise programs that are safe, effective, and based in scientific evidence.

It is expected that personal trainers hold a professional degree and certification to ensure they are recommending and prescribing safe exercises and movements to their clients. Most personal trainers complete a bachelor's or master's degree in a health- and fitness-related field such as kinesiology, exercise science, physical therapy, athletic training, and strength and conditioning. Personal trainer certifications are offered by a variety of organizations but most notably are the American College of Sports Medicine and the National Strength and Conditioning Association, which both offer various levels of certifications for fitness professionals and personal trainers. Certifications vary on the amount of training and education required, from short online exams to undergraduate and graduate level education. Often personal trainers will specialize in an area of physical activity, kinesiology, or medical conditions to better serve a specific population's needs (e.g., athletics, geriatric considerations, muscle activation therapy, rehabilitation). Professional specialization often requires additional certifications or trainings in conjunction with the basic certifications.

It is common for a personal trainer to meet with a client two or three times a week, and in some cases more often. Personal training sessions usually last from 30 to 60 minutes but can also vary greatly based on the client's needs and schedule. During the session, the trainer will lead the client through a personally designed workout for that day that addresses their unique health and fitness goals. These sessions are usually based on progression to goals, set by the client and the trainer, based on the client's physiological needs. A personal trainer must ensure that all movements and exercises being performed by clients are pertinent to the successful achievement of their goals and safe for the clients to perform in their current physical state.

Factory Floor- and Office-Level Evidence-Based Physical Activity Interventions and Practices

Workplaces have factory floor- and office-level physical activity interventions and practices to address their particular workforce health needs. For small- and midsized organizations as well as large national employers, the interventions and practices engage employees at the workplace (factory floor and office), are low cost and practical with fairly easy administration. Outside vendors both national and local compete for contracts to offer the interventions. Examples of widely implemented evidence-based interventions and practices are:

Sitting Reduction Programs: Many people today are sitting for very long periods throughout their daily routine at work and home. High amounts of daily sitting time has been linked to chronic diseases such as obesity and type II diabetes. Workplace sitting reduction strategies have typically had a beneficial impact on productivity, absenteeism, and injury costs. Below are five sitting reduction programs, four of which are distinct strategies and one that uses a combination of strategies. The most widely used strategies are increasing the number of breaks and implementing strategies around postural change (Dunstan, Howard, Healy, & Owen, 2012).

- Increasing the number of breaks from sitting time
- Implementing strategies around postural change
- Focusing on ergonomic changes to the individual workspace
- Altering the built design of the broader workplace
- Using multiple strategies (combinations of the strategies outlined above).

Walking Campaigns: Walking campaigns are popular. They are an easy, effective, and inexpensive way to promote physical activity using the resources within any workplace. A workplace walking campaign usually consists of the organization of walking groups, routes around the office or within easily accessible areas around the workplace, and some type of incentive to participate in the program. Employees benefit from being active throughout the day, receive a break from daily work, and become healthier individuals. Benefits from workplace walking programs have been well established. Gilson et al. (2013) showed that the Walk@Work program increased workday walking by 25% overall using various delivery methods over a 6-week period. In addition, Warren, Maley, Sugarwala, Wells, and Devine (2010) found a mean increase of 1,503 daily steps among women in rural workplaces throughout a 10-week period.

Aerobic Fitness—Stairwell Usage Programs: While aerobic activity in an office or workplace is often impractical, a health promotion program may be able to use the existing stairwells to increase the amount of daily aerobic activity employees complete. Many times, health promotion programs can focus solely on increased daily use of the stairwells rather than elevators or escalators. Swenson & Siegel (2013) showed that the use of stairwell decorations and interactive paintings such as maps, story boards, and wish lists would encourage the employee use of stairwells. Daily stair and elevator usage were measured before and after the implementation of the environmental intervention. After the implementation of the program, a significant increase of employee stairwell usage was recorded and sustained over a 6-week period.

Weight Training: Weight training or resistance training is a form of physical activity that is designed to improve muscular fitness by activating a muscle or a muscle group against external resistance. This type of exercise is commonly achieved through lifting free weights, using resistance machines, using body weight, bands, and much more. The benefits of regular resistance training include increased muscular fitness, prevention of osteoporosis, decreased risk for heart disease by reducing body fat, decreasing blood pressure, improving cholesterol, and more (ACSM, 2012). The ACSM recommends prescribed resistance training two to three times per week for all major muscles groups (ACSM, 2012). Weight training can be utilized within workplace health promotion programs through various avenues, such as traditional in-house programs, gym membership incentives, job specific weight training, injury prevention programs, and personal trainers.

Physical Activity Priority Implementation Challenges

While the workplace is not the only venue where physical activity can occur, the fact that people spend a large amount of time at work makes the setting an ideal one in which to promote physical activity participation. When thinking about the workplace and getting people physically active, the emphasis is to increase an individual's activity level. With an increase in activity level comes increases in health benefits. Challenges to getting people physically active include issues of built environment, the virtual workplace, unchanged physical activity levels, and adapted physical activity.

Built Environment

In general, a built environment is defined as the part of the physical environment that is constructed by human activity (Saelens & Handy, 2008). When considering a built environment it must be first understood that some places are physical activity–friendly by nature or design, such as playgrounds, health clubs, open spaces, stairs, sidewalks, and trails. Other places predispose sedentary behaviors, such as movie theaters, classrooms, offices, and elevators (Sallis, 2009). The evaluation of these aspects of a workplace environment, and whether they are within easy access of the employees, is important to understanding the reality of workplace physical activity promotion. A built environment within a community generally reflect aspects of urban design, land use, transportation infrastructure, and patterns of human activity within the environment, all of which affect how people will utilize the environment for physical activity participation (Handy, Boarnet, Ewing, & Killingsworth, 2002). Similarly, a workplace built environment can positively and negatively affect the physical activity levels of employees. The physical built environment within and around the workplace can include shared space within a building, physical activity supporting facilities (e.g., changing and shower rooms), and access to gym and outdoor facilities. Some workplaces may offer many different facilities and have access to various physical activity friendly environments, while some may have none. When initiating a health promotion program, the assessment of the workplace environment and physical access must be understood and addressed. An example of an organization that assesses the built environment is the Walking and Bicycling Suitability Assessment (WABSA) Project. The WABSA Project provides step-by-step instructions to help assess the suitability of your sidewalks for walking and roads for bicycling, and then to help develop a plan for improvements (http://www.unc.edu/~jemery/WABSA/). A walkability assessment can help plan or strengthen a walking program, one of the easier physical activity programs to implement.

Virtual Workplace

Not all workplaces contain all employees. In fact, it is more and more common to find businesses of all sizes spread across multiple locations. Therefore we need to be certain to include all work locations and employees. If you establish a health and fitness center at headquarters, be sure to offer similar equipment in other locations, or at least subsidize fitness center memberships for those located elsewhere. Ensure that information from lunch-and-learn programs is shared through intranet, wellness pages, or e-mail for easy access by all employees.

Think of how to use multiple workplace locations (including employees working from home) as a way to foster interest in physical activity through interoffice competitions. Have each location create their own wellness committee and encourage them to create their own programs. Walking clubs may not be effective in offices located in the North during the winter months, but may be very possible for locations in the South and Southwest. Create programs that encourage the different offices to compete against each other. If the company is able to come together occasionally during the year (for business meetings or retreats), find ways to foster the interoffice programs and recognize individuals and teams from all locations.

Unchanged Physical Activity Levels

American Life, an annual publication from the Bureau of Labor Statistics, documents how Americans spend their time (Table 10.3). In 2012, employed people worked for about 7.7 hours each day, spent two hours on household chores, and spent between 5 and 6 hours on leisure activities, with close to 3 of those hours spent viewing television. Watching TV was the leisure activity that occupied the most time (2.8 hours per day), accounting for about half of leisure time, on average, for those age 15 years and over (Bureau of Labor Statistics, 2015).

Time spent watching TV has inched upward with every passing year, and although Internet use is slowly replacing TV time, the web has yet to take up a large portion of Americans' time. The latest survey found both men and women spend less than 30 minutes of leisure time per workday on the computer. Regardless, both Internet and TV use fall into the same category of activity: sedentary behavior. The challenge to promote physical activity in the workplace is less about the amount of leisure time spent

Table 10.3   What Americans Do (Bureau of Labor Statistics, 2015)

	Working	
7.7 HOURS	Employed persons worked an average of **7.7 hours** on the days they worked. More hours were worked, on average, on weekdays than on weekend days—**8 hours** compared with **5.7 hours**.	
8.5 HOURS	Among full-time workers (those usually working 35 hours or more per week), men worked longer than women—**8.5 hours** compared with **7.9 hours**.	
	Household Activities	
WOMEN 82%	On an average day, **82 percent** of women and **65 percent** of men spent some time doing household activities such as housework, cooking, lawn care, or financial and other household management.	MEN 65%
WOMEN 2.6 HOURS	On the days they did household activities, women spent an average of **2.6 hours** on such activities, while men **spent 2 hours.**	MEN 2 HOURS
	Leisure Activities	
MEN 6 HOURS	On an average day, nearly everyone age 15 years and over (96 percent) engaged in some sort of leisure activity, such as watching TV, socializing, or exercising. Of those who engaged in leisure activities, **men spent more time in these activities** (6.0 hours) **than did women** (5.2 hours).	WOMEN 5.2 HOURS
2.8 HOURS	**Watching TV** was the leisure activity that occupied the most time (**2.8 hours per day**), accounting for about half of leisure time, on average, for those age 15 years and over.	

in front of a screen and more about the fact that virtually all aspects of Americans' daily life take place while sitting—and the workplace does not escape blame. In the workplace, our jobs have changed so that we have much more sedentary work.

Adapted Physical Activity

More than 6 million U.S. workers have one or more disabling conditions (U.S. Department of Labor, n.d.). Workplace health promotion programs support workers with disabilities and chronic health conditions to be physically active. A chronic health condition is defined as any illness, disease, disorder, or disability of long duration or frequent recurrence, including asthma, diabetes, serious allergies, epilepsy, and obesity. Workplaces establish policies that allow full participation by all employees in physical activity.

The Americans with Disabilities Act (ADA) requires that newly constructed or altered governmental, public, and commercial facilities to be accessible, and usable by, individuals with disabilities. The ADA Accessibility Guidelines (ADAAG) provides standards for compliance with these requirements. Specific requirements exist for recreation facilities such as exercise facilities and swimming pool areas. These requirements ensure consistency and usability of the facility for individuals with a disability. These are minimum requirements and it is encouraged to exceed the minimum requirements.

In the case of workplace health promotion programs, persons with disabilities may benefit greatly from well-designed and thoughtful programs that fit their specific needs. The U.S. Department of Labor's Office of Disability Employment Policy (ODEP) provides recommendations to ensure the engagement of employees with any type of disability in a wellness program. The ODEP suggests working directly with each individual to develop and design wellness programs to ensure accessibility for them specifically. Furthermore the ODEP encourages that any promotion program or facility design be accessible and inclusive to any employee, and that incentives and rewards associated with a health promotion program be given to those with varying ability levels. ODEP advises making necessary accommodations to allow full participation by any individual in any health promotion program (U.S. Department of Labor, n.d.).

Advocacy and Resource Partnerships and Organizations

Through advocacy and resource partnerships and organizations, workplace physical health can be addressed in additional ways and resources. These partnerships and organizations direct their attention to the physical health of the U.S. workforce. Some focus on specific physical health problems that affect worker's health every day and cause financial stress on employers.

National Coalition for Promoting Physical Activity (http://www .ncppa.org/about-us)

The mission of the National Coalition for Promoting Physical Activity (NCPPA) is to unite the strengths of public, private, and industry efforts into collaborative partnerships that inspire and empower all Americans to lead more physically active lifestyles. It is a policy consortium that promotes all sectors of American society working together to improve the public's health and prevent and manage chronic diseases through increased levels of physical activity. NCPPA supports a broad spectrum of policies that promote physical activity.

American College of Sports Medicine (http://www.acsm.org/)

The American College of Sports Medicine (ACSM) is the largest sports medicine and exercise science professional membership organization. The organization's mission is to make advances and integrate scientific research to provide educational and practical applications of exercise science and sports medicine. The ACSM is a leading authority in the world of health and fitness, sports medicine, and exercise science. This organization provides leading health and fitness certifications, recommendations, industry standards and guidelines, education, and collaborations.

Adventure Cycling Association (http://www.adventurecycling.org/)

The Adventure Cycling Association is a nonprofit organization whose mission is to inspire and empower people to travel by bicycle. This organization is the premier bicycle-travel organization in North America, with more than 35 years of experience and 46,500 members. The organization offers guided tours, routes and maps, membership, the *Adventure Cyclist* magazine, online resources, a store, and more. The Adventure Cycling Association works to encourage physical activity through cycling as a lifestyle. It provides resources for group rides and guided tours including self-contained, inn-to-inn, van-supported, fully-supported, "Family Fun," and educational tours.

American Heart Association—Wellness in the Workplace (http://www.startwalkingnow.org/home.jsp)

The American Heart Association addresses workplace physical health promotion through a variety of programs that offer employees ways to improve their physical fitness and reduce their risk for medical problems, chronic diseases, and illness. Some of these programs include:

- Fit Friendly Workplace Recognition
- Heart at Work Newsletter
- National Walking Day
- Snacking Well in the Workplace
- My Activity Tracker

National Institute for Health and Care Excellence (http://www.nice.org.uk/getinvolved/contact_us.jsp)

The National Institute for Health and Clinical Excellence (NICE) in London, England, produces public health guidance on how to encourage employees to be physically active. The guidance is for employers and professionals in small, midsized, and large organizations who have a direct or indirect role in, and responsibility for, improving health in the workplace. These recommendations support their ongoing guidance generally regarding physical activity and the environment, and workplace smoking and obesity. Recent NICE recommendations are in the areas of policy and planning, implementing a physical activity program, components of a physical activity program, and supporting employers.

Summary

Physical activity is any body movement that activates a person's muscles and requires more energy than the resting state. Walking, running, dancing, swimming, yoga, and gardening are a few examples of physical activity. Exercise is a type of physical activity that's planned and structured. In thinking about the workplace and getting people physically active, the emphasis is to increase an individual's activity level. Implementation of the physical activity priority spans the workplace and community. Partnerships and collaborations for workplace physical activity are a mainstay of implementing the physical activity priority. Small and midsized workplaces and many large workplaces do not have physical activity space or facilities (e.g., fitness center, gym, pool, walking trails, bike path, showers, changing area, equipment storage, and maintenance) but rather use existing facilities in the surrounding workplace communities and employee neighborhoods. You therefore need to be able to leverage the employees as a group of potential customers for local facilities to demand high quality, safe, and well-managed facilities to maximize the health outcomes for employees. Furthermore you need to engage and partner with the local community parks and recreational organizations, as well as health promotion professionals who work with the employee in physical activity programs where employees work, live, and play.

For Practice and Discussion

1. Using the U.S. Department of Health and Human Services *Physical Activity Guidelines for Americans* as a reference, talk with your family members about their current level of physical activity. How active are they? What aspects of their daily lives encourage them to be physically active? What aspects of their daily lives are barriers to be physically active? Can they remember a time in their lives when they were more physically active?

2. Review the American College of Sports Medicine (ACSM) Facility Standards and Guidelines and the ADA Accessibility Guidelines

(ADAAG). The standards and guidelines provide the minimum requirements that a fitness facility needs to meet to ensure a safe environment for which physical activity and exercise programs can occur. Once you are familiar with the ACSM and ADAAG standards and guidelines, arrange an informational meeting and tour with the director of a local fitness facility. As you meet the director and tour the facility assess how the present standards and guidelines might suggest actions for the facility to improve its services and programs. Check to see if the facility director and staff are aware of the standards and guidelines.

3. With increasing number of employees working virtually at varied sites, forming partnerships and collaborations in employees' communities and neighborhoods for workplace physical activity is a mainstay of implementing the physical activity priority of a workplace health promotion program. In your own neighborhood, identify potential partners and resources for physical activity. Identify whom you would talk with at the organization. Imagine you were a business owner with 50 employees. What types of physical activity services that are not currently offered by the business might be of interest for your employees?

4. Walking campaigns are a popular workplace physical activity. Talk with a few supervisors and managers of local businesses (e.g., neighborhood retail stores, food markets, fast food restaurants, big-box retailers) in your community. Ask if they have ever done or considered doing a walking campaign with their employers? Inquire about what they consider the pros and cons of an employee walking campaign. Compare and contrast your answers. What are differences among the answers when you consider the business type (e.g., neighborhood retail stores, food markets, fast food restaurants, big-box retailers)?

Case Study: Encouraging Employees' Physical Activity—What Would You Do?

Employees at a small medical supply company in Cleveland with 44 employees went the extra miles last year to earn additional paid time off. And they want to do the same this year. Employees at the firm got one extra hour of paid time off for every 33,000 steps they take during the first 3 months of the year, for up to 3 extra days of paid leave. Many employees did laps around the parking lot at lunch and took extra walks after work at home. Earning time off with pay was a great motivator to get people moving.

Fran Williams, the company owner, wants to keep his staff moving. He is looking for creative, fun ideas to encourage his employees to be physically active. If you were Mr. Williams, what would you do?

KEY TERMS

Physical activity

Metabolic equivalent of task (MET)

Physical Activity Guidelines for Americans

Health and fitness center

ACSM Facility Standards and Guidelines

City and county parks and recreation

departments

Community recreational associations and organizations

Personal trainer

Built environment

Virtual workplace

American Time Use Survey

Adapted physical activity

ADA Accessibility Guidelines

References

American College of Sports Medicine. (2012). *ACSM's health/fitness facility standards and guidelines* (4th ed.). Champaign, IL: NIRSA Education & Publication Center Human Kinetics.

Bureau of Labor Statistics. (2015). *American time use survey*. Retrieved from http://www.bls.gov/tus/

Centers for Disease Control and Prevention. (2012). *Steps to wellness: A guide to implementing the 2008 physical activity guidelines for Americans in the workplace.* Retrieved from http://www.cdc.gov/nccdphp/dnpao/hwi /downloads/Steps2Wellness_BROCH14_508_Tag508.pdf

Dunstan, D. W., Howard, B., Healy, G. N., & Owen, N. (2012). Too much sitting—a health hazard. *Diabetes Research and Clinical Practice, 97*(3), 368–376.

Gilson, N. D., Faulkner, G., Murphy, M. H., Meyer, M., Washington, T., Ryde, G. C. & Dillon, K. A. (2013). Walk@Work: An automated intervention to increase walking in university employees not achieving 10,000 daily steps. *Preventive Medicine, 56*(5), 283–287.

International Health, Racquet, and Sports Club Association. (2013). *About the industry*. Retrieved from http://www.ihrsa.org/about-the-industry/

Pronk, N. P. (2012). A best practice resource for worksite health practitioners: The IAWHP online certificate course. *ACSM's Health & Fitness Journal, 16*(5), 40–42. doi:10.1249/FIT.1240b1013e318264cc318210

Handy, S. L., Boarnet, M. G., Ewing, R., & Killingsworth, R. E. (2002). How the built environment affects physical activity: Views from urban planning. *American Journal of Preventive Medicine, 23*(2), 64–73.

Saelens, B. E., & Handy, S. L. (2008). Built environment correlates of walking: A review. *Medicine and science in sports and exercise, 40*(7 Suppl.), S550–566.

Sallis, J. F. (2009). Measuring physical activity environments: A brief history. *American journal of preventive medicine, 36*(4), S86–S92.

Swenson, T., & Siegel, M. (2013). Increasing stair use in an office worksite through an interactive environmental intervention. *American Journal of Health Promotion, 27*(5), 323–329.

U.S. Department of Labor. (n.d.). Retaining employees in your worksite wellness program. Retrieved from http://www.dol.gov/odep/research/WellnessToolkit.pdf

Warren, B. S., Maley, M., Sugarwala, L. J., Wells, M. T., & Devine, C. M. (2010). Small steps are easier together: A goal-based ecological intervention to increase walking by women in rural worksites. *Preventive Medicine, 50*(5–6), 230–234.

WORKPLACE HEALTH PROMOTION PROGRAM IMPLEMENTATION HEALTH PRIORITY: NUTRITION

Program Implementation: Nutrition Priority

In the United States, the workplace food environment (culture) is often fraught with temptations that are sometimes worse than the ones at home. Danish pastries, muffins, and cakes are standard fare at morning meetings and conference breaks. Office birthday parties bring more cake. Vending machines are usually filled with high-calorie drinks, chocolate, and salty snacks. Fast-food restaurants seem to surround the workplace premises with the offer of unlimited sugary drinks and fried potatoes every day of the week. Just a meal or two a week at one such restaurant can lead to serious weight gain (Kruger, Greenberg, Murphy, Difazio, & Youra, 2014). Coworkers order pizza or greasy sandwiches for delivery, and the odor fills the room. On top of this, many workers feel pressure to skip lunch, grab a 10-minute lunch, or stay at their desks to eat—the so-called desktop dining or SAD (stuck at desk) café phenomenon. For example, the American Dietetic Association (2011) found in 2003 that 62% of workers eat lunch at their desks and 50% snack there during working hours. For many employees, eating a meal is just another task to juggle during a busy workday of e-mails, phone calls, texts, meetings, and deadlines. And as more employees opt to multitask their way through breakfast, lunch, and even dinner, "desktop dining" has quickly become a mainstay of corporate culture. A missed or incomplete meal can lower worker productivity, increase stress, and ultimately lead to snacking (Sommer, Stürmer, Shmuilovich, Martin-Loeches, & Schacht, 2013).

LEARNING OBJECTIVES

- Discuss program implementation with a nutrition priority focus

- Identify evidence-based nutrition policies, practices, interventions, and services

- Explain nutrition workplace program challenges

- Describe advocacy partnerships and organizations

The goal of implementing a workplace health promotion program with a focus on the nutrition priority is to engage and support employees to eat well. Healthy eating is defined by a diet focusing on foods and beverages that help achieve and maintain an ideal body weight, promote health, and prevent disease. A healthy diet can reduce the risk of major chronic diseases such as heart disease, diabetes, osteoporosis, and some cancers (U.S. Department of Agriculture [USDA] & U.S. Department of Health and Human Services, 2010).

Less discussed but critical to the implementation of nutrition priority–focused programs is recognition that workers' diets and eating reflect larger societal dynamics related to food and nutrition (Henderson, Coveney, & Ward, 2010). Program implementation requires exploring and recognizing that what we eat and the way we eat it express our social identities (as members of social classes, ethnic groups, religions, etc.). It should be understood how preparing and consuming (or *not* consuming) food reproduces gender roles. Furthermore the economic system for producing and marketing food affects what (and how much) we eat and how food is an object of politics (e.g., a target for government regulation such as the USDA and the Food and Drug Administration), a subject of politics (e.g., agriculture, food industry lobby groups), and an economic force employing millions of workers (e.g., food service, agriculture and food production, restaurant and fast food, food marketing industries).

Evidence-Based Nutrition Policies, Practices, Interventions, and Services

The nutrition priority–focused program implementation is carried out from an ecological perspective that workplace programs are one intervention point in an unfolding multipronged strategy to address workers' diet and eating. This approach is supported by the 2015 Dietary Guidelines (USDA, 2015) with their emphasis on food and nutrient intake, dietary patterns, foods and nutrients and their health outcomes, individual diet and physical activity behavior change, food environment and settings, and food sustainability and safety. Recognized as part of implementation is that the workplace environment contributes positively or negatively to the diet of the employees. The diet of employees can be positively influenced by such programs as making healthy food options available, reducing the price of healthful food choices in cafeterias, offering healthful food choices in vending machines, and providing nutrition education through e-mails and texts. But workers' diets, nutrition, and eating at work are linked to influences beyond the workplace: family, ethnicity, economics, and community.

Workplace programs balance healthy dietetic practice and dietary habits within a supportive environment that is respectful of workers' family, ethnic, economic, and community influences. Furthermore programs increasingly are raising awareness to challenge employers and employees to think critically about issues and dilemmas involving food production, food consumption behaviors, and nutritional outcomes as controversies in contemporary society. Nutrition priority–focused program implementation increasingly has the potential to make significant contributions to workers' understanding of the context within which the production and consumption of food and beverages takes place.

Nutrition and Weight Management Education

Nutrition and weight management education is a common way to make positive changes in the diets of employees. *Nutrition and weight management education* is a broad term used to indicate that some type of information about nutrition and health eating is being given to a worker. Programs typically use social media platforms and can include brochures, e-mails, text messages, Twitter campaigns, blogs, handouts, seminars, questionnaires, websites, videos, and Lunch and Learn sessions. The main goal of this modality is to educate the workers on diet and proper eating, which will hopefully correlate with improved dietary behaviors among employees and contribute to a healthier life. It also educates workers about diets for individuals with a chronic disease, disordered eating behavior, and other medical issues. Sometimes the information being provided is specific to each person, and at other times will address general concerns by providing information to the entire employee population. One advantage of using nutrition and weight management education is the little time it takes for the workers to receive it and process its content when compared to more aggressive forms of dietary intervention. Examples of program topics include:

- Understanding the basics
- Weight management and body image
- Fad diets
- Fats and cholesterol
- Salt reduction
- Planning balanced meals for the whole family
- Aging well
- Making smart choices while grocery shopping and reading food labels
- Programs for specific health conditions (diabetes, heart conditions, etc.)
- Healthy eating on the run

- Ethnic food recipes and preparations
- Vegetarian eating
- Food production
- Genetically engineered foods
- Federal Drug and Food Administration Resources

Dietitian Services

A dietitian is a health professional who has university qualifications consisting of a 4-year bachelor's degree in nutrition and dietetics or a 3-year science degree followed by a master's degree in nutrition and dietetics, including a certain period of practical training in different hospital and community settings. A dietitian is an expert in prescribing therapeutic nutrition. As part of a workplace health promotion program dietitians consult with the food services on food selection, preparations, and menu. Furthermore they provide to workers diet and nutrition screenings, assessments, and interventions.

Diet and nutrition interventions help individuals acquire the skills, motivation, and support they need to develop healthy eating and food preparation habits. The interventions include strategies for self-monitoring, overcoming barriers to selecting healthy foods, goal-setting, shopping and food preparation, role playing, and social support.

An important concern that workplace dietitians address is eating disorders such as anorexia, bulimia, and binge eating. Extreme emotions, attitudes, and behaviors surrounding weight and food issues are also considered. Eating disorders are serious emotional and physical problems that can have life-threatening consequences for females and males. Eating disorders are also important in individuals with specialized dietary concerns, such as people with diabetes. The availability of screening for eating disorders is crucial for catching the problem and taking the first steps to help a person (employee) with an eating disorder. The National Eating Disorders Association (NEDA) provides the public with a low-pressure online eating disorder screening tool (www.mybodyscreening.org). This screening tool provides an anonymous questionnaire to determine if the individual indeed has an eating disorder.

Food Services and Food Services Industry

It is common for companies to work with outside vendors to offer food services within their company. These vendors will usually be in charge of distribution, supply, and staffing of the food services venues such as cafeterias, dining rooms, or food courts within the workplace. Large vendors hire staff to control everything from the factory to preparation of the food. Vendors work by charging the company a fee for their services. Some notable food service vendors in the United States are Sysco, Sodexo, UniPro Foodservice, and Performance Food Service. These vendors play an important role in the nutrition of the employees because the menus are often predetermined or limited in some way. It is important to understand what vendor a company is using and what options they offer as far as healthy food choices before beginning a nutrition program. Each is marketing its own healthy eating program as a strategy to capture and maintain its market share.

Workplaces are in a unique position to promote healthy dietary behaviors and help ensure appropriate food and nutrient intake among their workers. There are increasing number of resources to support workplace food services, such as offer brochures, handouts, menu and recipe ideas, a toolkit, and nutrition standards that can be used by any organization for the purpose of making their program and employees healthier (Harvard School of Public Health, 2015). For example the Health and Sustainability Guidelines for Federal Concessions and Vending Operations were developed in partnership with the U.S. Health and Human Services Department to translate the *Dietary Guidelines for Americans* into clear policy throughout federal workplaces. These guidelines attempt to include proper nutrition and sustainable practices of cafeterias and vending facilities offered to employees of a federal workplace (U.S. General Services Administration, n.d.).

Finally, workplace food services as part of a workplace health promotion nutrition priority program are often locally designed and implemented, building on workers' culture, ethnicity, and food interest as well as local community food products. One example of such a local food service design is the Dole Corporation corporate headquarters employee cafeteria (Figure 11.1). The cafeteria (café) food service menu is dominated by healthy food choices; discounts on healthy foods, such as the US$1.50 salad bar; a "smoothie" machine, which makes a thick drink by mixing fruits, vegetables, herbs, or teas often with yogurt; and healthy fat-free or low-fat desserts. The café offers breakfast, lunch, and take-away dinners, which are heavily subsidized, particularly considering the quality of the meals. Breakfasts cost around US$3.00, and lunches US$4.75 on average, which is about half the cost of restaurant meals of similar quality in the surrounding area (California). The "Daily Dole" is a lunch special costing US$4.25. There are no beef, pork, cream, whole milk, or sugary drinks. Protein sources are chicken, turkey, fish, and soya and other beans. Traditional beef dishes such as hamburgers are served with meat substitutes, such as soya or vegetable meal with the same consistency as beef. Chile con carne

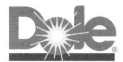

Dole Garden Court Cafe
Week of April 6

Breakfast News!!!
We are now offering
Pancakes with Wheat,
Gluten and Dairy Free
Better Tasting Fewer
Calories

Made to Order Sushi at
Dole Garden Court Cafe
every other Thursday

Fresh Smoothies or
Vegetable Juice Available at
Dole Garden Court Cafe
From 8:00 AM-10:00 AM
Smoothies made with your
favorite fruit and booster

Freshly Roasted Herbed
Rotisserie Chicken
Packed to Go

Hours
Monday-Friday
8:00am-2:00pm

Manager
Alma Medina x 6722

Chef
Emmanuel Prodet x 6722

Monday
Sun Creek Breakfast:	Buckwheat Waffles with Fresh Berries	$2.75
Copper Pot:	Gazpacho Blanco	$1.35/1.85
Chef Features:	Grilled Chicken breast with Olive Pesto Crust	$5.25
Daily Dole:	Poached Sole with Roasted Red Pepper Sauce	$5.25
Sage Deli:	Mediterranean Pita	$4.25
Sedona Grill:	Mushroom Turkey Burger with Grilled Onions	$4.25
Exhibition Salad:	Tropical Fruit Spinach Salad Tossed with Citrus Vinaigrette	$4.95

Tuesday
Sun Creek Breakfast:	Smoked Salmon Omlet with Chives	$3.25
Copper Pot:	Onion Soup	$1.35/1.85
Chef Features:	Mexican Grouper	$5.25
Daily Dole:	Poached Sole with Roasted Red Pepper Sauce	$5.25
Sage Deli:	Mediterranean Pita	$4.25
Sedona Grill:	Mushroom Turkey Burger with Grilled Onions	$4.25
Exhibition Salad:	Tropical Fruit Spinach Salad Tossed with Citrus Vinaigrette	$4.95

Wednesday
Sun Creek Breakfast:	Buckwheat Waffles with Fresh Berries	$2.75
Copper Pot:	Black Bean Soup	$1.35/1.85
Chef Features:	Grilled Halibut	$5.25
Daily Dole:	Turkey Cutlet Red Pepper Sauce	$5.25
Sage Deli:	Shrimp Po'boy	$4.25
Sedona Grill:	Mushroom Turkey Burger with Grilled Onions	$4.25
Exhibition Salad:	Tropical Fruit Spinach Salad Tossed with Citrus Vinaigrette	$4.95

Thursday
Sun Creek Breakfast:	Buckwheat Waffles with Fresh Berries	$2.75
Copper Pot:	Mushroom Barley	$1.35/1.85
Chef Features:	Grilled Blackened Talapia	$5.25
Daily Dole:	Poached Sole with Roasted Red Pepper Sauce	$5.25
Sage Deli:	Mediterranean Pita	$4.25
Sedona Grill:	Roasted Vegetable open face sandwich	$4.25
Exhibition Salad:	Almond Turkey Salad Tossed with Cranberry Vinaigrette	$4.95

Friday
Sun Creek Breakfast:	Buckwheat Waffles with Fresh Berries	$2.75
Copper Pot:	Potato Leek Soup	$1.35/1.85
Chef Features:	Grilled Chicken Fajita	$5.25
Daily Dole:	Fresh Wild Salmon	$5.25
Sage Deli:	Mediterranean Pita	$4.25
Sedona Grill:	Mushroom Turkey Burger with Grilled Onions	$4.25
Exhibition Salad:	Tropical Fruit Spinach Salad Tossed with Citrus Vinaigrette	$4.95

Figure 11.1   Dole Corporation Headquarters Cafe Menu
Source: Wanjek, 2005.

is served as "chile non carne." A typical daily lunch menu includes cilantro (coriander) black bean soup, grilled halibut with melon salsa, turkey cutlet pomodoro, vegetable curry with marinated tofu, shrimp focaccia sandwich with herb mayonnaise, tuna melt with organic potato chips and three-grain trio salad (Wanjek, 2005).

Vending Programs

Many workplaces are more frequently adopting the use of vending machines to provide healthy food and drink options for their employees. By having a healthy vending machine program, employees are able to have quick access to healthful foods when otherwise they may only have access to foods high in calories, fat, and sugar. A workplace may take several steps to adopt a healthy vending program. These steps include evaluation of the current vending program, discussion of available options with the companies' decision-making person and the machine vendor, implementation of the proposed program, and marketing of the new program to the employees. It is common, especially in the beginning stages of the new program, to offer both healthy and less-healthy options within the same machine. Many workplace health vending programs include stickers on the products denoting the level of healthfulness of the snack for quick reference. Table 11.1 provides examples and a comparison of healthy, acceptable, and excluded snack options and beverages (Centers for Disease Control and Prevention [CDC], 2012a).

Food Safety and Inspection Services

Food and drink offered within the workplace must be safely stored, handled, prepared, and served in accordance to industry standards. Regular food safety inspections ensure that the food services provided to employees are safe, keeping the employees healthy and free of food-borne illness. The Food Safety and Inspection Services (FSIS) is an agency within the USDA that ensures that all commercial meat, poultry, and eggs are safe, wholesome, and correctly labeled and packaged (USDA, FSIS, 2015).

Local public health departments regularly inspect businesses (e.g., workplace cafeterias and food outlets) serving food to ensure they are following safe food handling procedures. Local laws determine how frequently these inspections take place, and the specific items the inspectors look for. However, in general, environmental health inspectors check that safeguards are in place to protect food from contamination by food handlers, cross-contamination, and contamination from other sources in the restaurant. Some examples include ensuring that employees regularly wash their hands in a sink equipped with soap, hot water, and paper towels;

Table 11.1   Healthy Vending Machine Snack Option Comparison (Centers for Disease Control and Prevention, 2012a)

Snacks		
Healthy	**Acceptable**	**Excluded**
Animal Crackers, Graham Crackers	Granola bars, whole-grain fruit bars	Cookies (including low-fat)
Nuts, seeds	Nuts with sugar or honey coating	Candy or yogurt covered nuts
	Baked chips	Regular chips
Trail mix	Popcorn/nut mix	Trail mix with chocolate or candy
		Candy bars, chocolate bars, toaster pastries
Beverages		
Milk (nonfat or low-fat)	Flavored or vitamin enhanced water	Regular soft drinks
Juice (at least 50% juice)	Low-calorie/diet soda	
Water, pure		

that utensils and surfaces that contact raw meat are not used to prepare ready-to-eat foods; and that rodents and other pests are not present.

As part of the federal government workplace health promotion program, food safety inspections are provided to federal facilities that prepare and serve food. The Environment Health and Safety program goal is to reduce or eliminate risks regarding food safety. The program helps to identify and address environmental safety issues, including food safety, through assessments, abatement programs, regular monitoring, and employee and management training. It is designed to help food workplace food services to comply with state and local regulations by identifying food safety risks, examining storage methods, identifying cross-contamination risks, ensuring safe staff sanitation procedures, and reviewing facilities for possible risks in design, layout or equipment (Federal Occupational Health, n.d.).

Health Coaches

More health insurance policy products now feature health coaching services for employees, making the services part of nutrition priority health program implementation. Participation in a health coaching program is typically incentivized with employees getting some type of reward (e.g., reduced health premium cost) for talking with a coach about health risk assessment results and any current employee health promotion activities. Because of the concern with obesity among Americans, health coaches often focus on nutrition and diet. Health coaching sessions can be face-to-face, but most health insurance plans offer health coaching only as a set number of 1-hour telephone conversations (e.g., three to four sessions) between the insurance company health coach and the employee at a time convenient for the employee to talk outside of the work day.

Health coaching, also referred to as wellness coaching, is a process that facilitates healthy, sustainable behavior change by challenging clients to listen to their inner wisdom, identify their values, and transform their goals into action. Health coaching draws on the principles of positive psychology, motivational interviewing, and goal setting. The terms "health coaching" and "wellness coaching" are used interchangeably. Health coaches are supportive mentors who motivate individuals to cultivate positive health choices. They support clients to achieve health goals through lifestyle and behavior modification. The focus is on maintaining a supportive environment for behavior change with an emphasis on nutrition, mindfulness, and physical health (CDC, 2012b).

Workplace Farmers' Markets

Farmers' markets at the workplace are an innovative strategy to potentially increase healthy nutritional workplace environments. Workplace farmers' markets vary in structure and size, including average number of patrons and vendors. For example vendors can number from a few (less than 6) to large (30 plus). The variety of vendor products spans organic, meats, baked goods, prepared foods, and other items (such as flowers). Workplaces partner with farmers' market association or independent market operators to coordinate the operational logistics. Depending on the market management structure of the site, the day-to-day market operations and vendor communications are handled by a market manager from the market association, an independent operator, or a vendor. Most markets are held one time per week on a weekday for 4 hours, though some take place every other week. Many markets operate year round, while others are seasonal, open only during spring, summer, and early fall. An early leader in workplace farmers' markets is the Kaiser Permanente Health system. A recent study found that workplace farmers' markets appear to have an impact on what people are eating, with 74% of all patrons reported eating more fruits and vegetables as a result of coming to the market (Cromp et al., 2012).

Factory Floor- and Office-Level Evidence-Based Nutrition Interventions and Practices

Workplaces have factory floor- and office-level nutrition interventions and practices to address their particular workforce health needs. From small and midsized organizations to large national employers, these programs engage employees at the workplace (factory floor and office), and are low cost and practical, with fairly easy administration. Outside vendors both national and local compete for contracts to offer the interventions. Examples of widely implemented evidence-based interventions and practices are:

Weight Watchers Groups: Within the workplace, employees can have access to weight loss support groups such as Weight Watchers program groups. The use of a weight watchers group significantly increases weight loss when compared to the self-help approach (Johnston, Rost, Miller-Kovach, Moreno, & Foreyt, 2013). Weekly Weight Watchers group meetings include topics to help stay motivated, weigh-ins, and tools and strategies for overcoming personal and group obstacles. The group activities and materials can also be used in content for social media, websites, Twitter campaigns, blogs, e-mails, videos, and text messaging to extend the program reach beyond the workplace and workday (Cook, Billings, Hersch, Back, & Hendrickson, 2007).

Overeaters Anonymous: Overeaters Anonymous (OA) is a program that provides support for individuals who are recovering from compulsive eating using a 12-step and 12-tradition approach. The groups provide a community of like-minded people to discuss struggles, strategies, and tools for overcoming the problem of compulsive overeating. The meetings provide strength, hope, and fellowship while maintaining anonymity among meeting participants. While OA addresses diet, weight loss, and obesity, the meetings also focus on mental health and spiritual well-being. OA is a member-supported organization but does not charge participants for attending meetings. All financial support comes from member donations (Overeaters Anonymous, 2015).

The Biggest Loser at Work: The Biggest Loser at Work Program is a weight loss challenge program among employees of a workplace. Usually, teams are created among the employees. The participants are given a certain amount of time to lose as much weight as possible through exercise and diet. Incentive programs or motivational tools are often used throughout the contest to keep the participants motivated and focused. After the given time period and usually at given intervals throughout, the participants are weighed and the winners and losers are determined. Sometimes the participants will buy into the contest, and winners will receive all of the money at the end or some other prize determined by the organizer of the contest. This type of program has become increasingly popular since the increase in popularity of *The Biggest Loser* television show (WeightLossWars, n.d.).

Take-Away Meals: Fast-food establishments and supermarkets have responded to the demand for quick meals by providing family "take-home" or "take-away" meal options. As part of workplace food service cafeterias, a growing number of companies provide take-away meals for the family or individual. This type of workplace-based meal option offers two advantages: the food tends to be as healthy as the cafeteria lunch, which is usually nutritionally balanced; and the meal is ready for the employees when they leave. Employees purchasing a meal for home outside the company would otherwise need to pick it up from a shop, and this could easily add 30 minutes to the commute home. The approach is straightforward. Each day in the late afternoon 2 to 4 meal options are available from the cafeteria: fully cooked, hot, and packaged to take home. Meals include protein (meat, fish), starches (rice, potatoes, pasta) and vegetables. Vegetarian meal options may be available (Wanjek, 2005).

Seattle 5-a-Day Program: The Seattle 5-a-Day program is designed for workplaces to increase fruit and vegetable consumption (Beresford, Thompson, Bishop, Macintyre, McLerran, & Yasui, 2010). The program's intervention strategies are developed around the stages of change model, addressing the work environment and the individual-level behavior change. Seattle 5-a-Day's protocol defines a general structure for organizing the workplace, for implementing the individualized intervention activities, and for documenting the process. Employee buy-in of the program is enhanced through an employee advisory board. In addition to individually tailored activities, stage-specific messages (such as "Do something groundbreaking" or "5 ways to a 5-a-Day") are delivered to workers through posters, e-mails, flyers, food demonstrations, and a self-help manual.

Nutrition Implementation Challenges

Ideally the nutrition-focused programs in a workplace health promotion program are implemented in the context of employers and employees working together to improve the nutritional status of the workers. With obesity and related noncommunicable diseases at epidemic levels, the intention is for employers to offer and support employees' healthier eating and better access to healthier foods. Challenges to program implementation include employee food preferences, food marketing, weight bias, and ethical concerns about food production, consumption, and transport.

Addressing Ethnic and Cultural Food Preferences

Different food preferences across different ethnicities and cultural groups are important to consider when implementing a nutrition plan for employees (Marra, King, & Holmes, 2014). Many times, food choices are made available to employees based on a traditional American diet. This diet however, may not be preferred by people of different cultures. It is important to understand individual preference of the employees being served by the food service. One must consider different varieties of food that both meet the needs and requirements of a healthful diet but also are preferred food for all cultures or ethnicities being represented (O'Neil, Nicklas, Kease, & Fulgoni, 2014). Likewise, consider that ethnic and cultural groups may have different daily meal patterns (e.g., large midday meals), which will need to be addressed and accommodated (Dooren, Marinussen, Blink, Aiking, & Vellinga, 2014).

Adopt Marketing Techniques to Promote Healthy Dietary Choices

Any food-oriented program operates within the larger context of food being marketed and promoted with food industry budgets that are in the millions of dollars. No workplace program will have enough funding to counter food industry advertising. However, being strategic about how and what is communicated related to employees' dietary choices and health as part of a workplace program is important to program success. For small and midsized companies this is particularly critical. For example, if food is available at a workplace, place the nutritious products so that they are easy for employees to choose, such as featuring fruits and vegetables, low-fat and fat-free milk and other dairy products, and whole grains in prominent places in cafeteria lines. Encourage businesses to promote healthy eating through family outreach and education. And use e-mails, text messages, and social media to highlight healthy eating behaviors to influence dietary choices. Furthermore talk with program partners and vendors to take the same approach to program-related activities and communications so as to provide a consistent and supportive dialogue with employees (American Heart Association, 2015).

Weight Bias/Discrimination

It is clear that overweight and obese individuals face employment discrimination that potentially reduces earning potential, reduces hiring opportunities, reduces promotion opportunities, and has serious mental and physical consequences for the individual being discriminated against. Twelve percent of adults report being subject to discrimination due to their overweight or obese status. This discrimination against overweight and obese individuals is often referred to as weight bias (Grant & Mizzi, 2014). The bias exists because of two main contributing factors: first, the idea that the shame will motivate the person to lose weight, and second, that people are solely responsible for their own bodies and it is the individuals' fault that they are overweight due to their lack of self-discipline or willpower (Vanhove & Gordon, 2013). Oftentimes the weight bias contributes to unhealthful and binge eating, which only worsens the situation. Currently, there are no federal policies protecting people from weight discrimination in the workplace. However, there are a few state and local policies that address the issue.

Food Production Ethical Concerns

Ethical concerns impact upon food production, consumption, and transport. Ethical consumption of food centers on localism, as a means of promoting environmental sustainability and social justice through reducing "food miles" and the creation of alternate food networks (DuPuis & Goodman, 2005). It provides a venue for the construction of identity through food choice. That choice provides a mark of membership of cultural groups (Fischler, 1988). Soper (2007) associates ethical consumption with the acquisition of status. The purchasing of organic and local food may reflect a form of asceticism in which distinction is marked by restraint, not only in type of food consumed but also in the amount consumed (Guthman, 2002), leading Soper (2007) to suggest that ethical food consumers may be more "obedient to 'consumerist' rather than 'citizenly' urges."

The recent surge in popularity of foods that are produced naturally and locally has driven employers to reconsider their nutrition programs to match the demand. The focus of many people's diets recently has been on foods that they can feel a connection with, such as local grown food, chicken eggs from local coops, and so forth. These types of food are typically more expensive and in shorter supply, which makes it hard for companies to consistently use such products in employee nutrition plans. However, in reaction to this movement, many employers have gone to great lengths and reorganized the traditional model of food service to do just that. Examples of steps that are taken include purchasing from local farms, providing many fruits and vegetable food options, having onsite gardens, and onsite chicken coops (Bittman, 2015).

Advocacy and Resource Partnerships and Organizations

An increasing number of national and international organizations are working with employers to create workplace environments that support employees' healthy eating and diets. They provide ongoing research, materials, and advocacy for the best, evidence-based practices to promote employees, nutritional health. Among those groups are:

The California Worksite Program Fit Business Kit (www.cdph .ca.gov)

Tools and resources developed by the Network for a Healthy California—Workplace Program to help employers develop and implement a culture and environment at their workplaces that support healthy eating and physical activity among workers. The kit contains 10 individual components, all of which have been evaluated by a diverse mix of businesses from across California and have been designed for easy implementation at any workplace. The tools can be used individually or as part of a comprehensive workplace health promotion program. The tools assist employers and employees in combating declining employee health and increasing health care costs. The four nutrition components are:

1. Vending Machine Food and Beverage Standards

2. Healthy Dining Menu Guidelines

3. Simple Steps to Ordering Farm Fresh Produce for the Worksite

4. A Guide to Establishing a Worksite Farmers' Market

Vending Machine Toolkit (www.banpac.org)

The Bay Area Nutrition and Physical Activity Collaborative (BANPAC) is a collaboration of over 200 regional organizations that work to promote health of area residents through nutrition, physical activity and policy support. BANPAC along with Imperial Regional Nutrition Network developed a Vending Machine Toolkit for schools to help them assess, strategize, and implement a healthier vending program. This toolkit includes fact sheets, policy updates, informational brochures, assessment tools and more.

National Automatic Merchandising Association (NAMA) (http://www.vending.org/)

NAMA is the national trade association of the food and refreshment vending, coffee service, and food service management industries including onsite, commissary, catering, and mobile services. Its 1,800-plus company membership comprises companies, equipment manufacturers, and suppliers of products and services to operating service companies. The basic mission of the association is to collectively advance and promote the automatic merchandising and coffee service industries. NAMA supports, with administrative, logistical, and financial assistance, a network of 30-plus affiliated state councils encompassing 36 states, where the vending and coffee service industries focus on local issues and concerns as well as gather frequently for networking opportunities. In 2005, NAMA created FitPick (www.fitpick.org) a healthy vending and micromarket labeling program, to help vending operators, workplace food vending program users (i.e., employees), and consumers identify products that meet recognized nutrition guidelines with maximum limits on calories, fat, sugar, and sodium.

American Heart Association Healthy Workplace Food and Beverage Toolkit (http://www.heart.org)

These tools and resources designed by the American Heart Association are geared for anyone involved with workplace food and beverages, from the office vending machine to an offsite special event involving catering. The toolkit provides practical, actionable suggestions that are easy to understand and apply. While the toolkit was originally designed for workplaces and corporations, it is recognized for its applicability to many different organizational settings.

American Diabetes Association—My Food Advisor (http://www.diabetes.org/)

The American Diabetes Association (ADA) is an organization that leads the fight against the deadly consequences of diabetes and for persons with diabetes. The organization funds research, delivers services, provides information, and offers a forum for people with diabetes to talk. Included in these objectives and services, the ADA sponsors My Food Advisor. My Food Advisor is an online nutrition resource for people with diabetes. It provides vast nutritional information, recipes, a food tracker, and more. It is a great way for those with diabetes to achieve proper nutrition and health.

The Center for Food Safety (http://www.centerforfoodsafety.org/#)

The Center for Food Safety (CFS) is a nonprofit interest and advocacy organization working to protect human health and modify the impact of food production on the environment by promoting the use of organic and other forms of sustainable agriculture. The CFS also provides educational materials and motivational tools to promote sustainability in food production. Finally, the CFS archives a body of case law suits on the food and agriculture business.

Center for Science in the Public Interest (https://www.cspinet.org/)

The Center for Science in the Public Interest (CSPI) is an organization whose twin missions are "to conduct innovative research and advocacy programs in health and nutrition, and to provide consumers with current, useful information about their health and well-being." CSPI accomplishes this mission through education, policy support, research, and advocacy. Currently, CSPI is working to eliminate all "junk" food from public school cafeterias nationwide, rid the food supply of partially hydrogenated oils, reduce sodium in processed foods, and increase food safety policy.

Summary

The goal of nutrition priority–focused program implementation is to engage and support employees to eat well for good nutrition. It champions a properly fed and healthy workforce as an indispensable element of productive, high-quality employees. Furthermore such a program provides access to healthy, nutritional food at work to fight malnutrition, obesity, chronic diseases, and food safety among the poorest and lowest skilled workers. Critical to the implementation of nutrition priority–focused programs is recognition that workers' diets and eating reflect larger dynamics related to food and society. Implementation in workplace programs balances healthy dietetic practice and dietary habits within a supportive environment that is respectful of workers' family, ethnic, economic, and community influences. Programs increasingly are raising awareness to challenge employers and employees to think critically about issues and dilemmas involving food production, food consumption behaviors, and nutritional outcomes as controversies in contemporary society.

For Practice and Discussion

1. How do what we eat and the way we eat it express our social identities (as members of social classes, ethnic groups, religions, etc.)? How do preparing and consuming (or not consuming) food reproduce gender roles? How does the economic system for producing and marketing food affect what (and how much) we eat?

2. In 2014 the Sodexo Corporation (a large foodservice corporation) joined the Partnership for a Healthier America and announced new commitments to battle the nation's obesity epidemic. These initiatives included engaging and motivating consumers toward healthy choices by widely deploying a mindful healthy dining program, expanding healthier food choices in hospitals, offering more free breakfast meals in schools, and increasing the selection of healthier, more nutritious options in its vending and K–12 lunchroom programs. Research and review the strategies of Partnership for a Healthier America. Make recommendations to Sodexo and Partnership for Healthier America for future workplace initiatives as part of workplace health promotion programs.

3. The local Business Group on Health has invited you to speak with the executive leadership from 25 local small and midsized employers about implementing a nutrition priority–focused workplace health promotion program. The group wants to promote employee engagement in local food production, food to table (i.e., local grown food sourcing for markets and restaurants), summer farmers' markets, food pantries, and family food services (federal and local) for low-wage workers. Prepare a 60-minute talk on how the employers can implement their program ideas.

4. An eating disorder is an illness that causes serious disturbances to an individual's everyday diet, such as eating extremely small amounts of food or severely overeating. A person with an eating disorder may have started out just eating smaller or larger amounts of food, but at some point the urge to eat less or more spiraled out of control. Severe distress or concern about body weight or shape may also signal an eating disorder. Common eating disorders include anorexia

nervosa, bulimia nervosa, and binge-eating disorder (National Institute of Mental Health, n.d.). Investigate the impact of eating disorders on individuals. Discuss concerns about addressing eating disorders in workplace health promotion programs. Recommend an approach to raising awareness of eating disorders as part of a workplace wellness nutrition program.

5. Explore how food is an object of politics (e.g., a target for government regulation, as with the Department of Agriculture and the Food and Drug Administration), a subject of politics (e.g., agriculture, food industry lobby groups), and an economic force employing millions of workers (e.g., food service, agriculture and food production, full service restaurants and fast food, food marketing industries). What are the roles and influences on workplace health promotion implementation of a nutrition-priority program by the following: government departments lobbying interest groups, and food production and service corporations and businesses? How are they focused and not focused on the U.S. workers' diet, eating patterns, and nutrition?

Case Study: Nutrition Program Implementation—What Would You Do?

Zhang Li, a director of corporate health for a midsized manufacturing company, wants to offer employees a web-based nutrition program designed to help people improve their eating habits by reducing fat intake and increasing fruit and vegetable intake. He proposes an initial e-mail to all employees with screening questions on fat and fruit and vegetable intake. The employees who fill out the screening instrument will receive a dietary analysis comparing their fruit and vegetable intake with recommended levels, suggestions for improving their intake, and an opportunity to enroll to receive additional e-mails over the course of the 12-week program. Once enrolled, employees will receive weekly e-mails that may include dietary information, suggestions to improve diet, and weekly nutrition goals chosen by the employee.

Mr. Li can use the company health insurance provider or an outside vendor to offer the program. A third option is to offer the program internally through the human resource department. He needs to decide the selection criteria upon which to make his decision. If you were Mr. Li what would you do?

KEY TERMS

Dietary Guidelines

Nutrition

Nutrition education

Dietitian services

Screening disordered eating

Food services

Food service industry

Vending programs

Food safety and inspection services

Health coaching

Workplace farmers' markets

Ethnic and cultural food preferences

Food marketing

Weight bias discrimination

Food production ethical concerns

References

American Dietetic Association. (2011). *Desktop dining survey: 2011 results: Americans' food safety knowledge and practice at work.* Retrieved from http://www.homefoodsafety.org/vault/2499/web/files/Desktop%20Dining%20 Executive%20Summary%20FINAL.pdf

American Heart Association. (2015). *Healthy workplace food and beverage toolkit.* Retrieved from http://www.heart.org/idc/groups/heart-public/@wcm /@fc/documents/downloadable/ucm_465693.pdf

Beresford, S., Thompson, B., Bishop, S., Macintyre, J., McLerran, D., & Yasui, Y. (2010). Long-term fruit and vegetable change in worksites: Seattle 5 a Day follow-up. *American Journal of Health Behavior, 34*(6), 707–720.

Bittman, M. (2015). *A bone to pick.* New York, NY: Pam Kraus Books.

Centers for Disease Control and Prevention. (2012a). *Health and sustainability guidelines for federal concessions and vending operations.* Retrieved from http://www.cdc.gov/chronicdisease/pdf/Guidelines_for_Federal_Concessions _and_Vending_Operations.pdf

Centers for Disease Control and Prevention. (2012b). *Steps to wellness: A guide to implementing the 2008 physical activity guidelines for Americans in the workplace.* Retrieved from http://www.cdc.gov/nccdphp/dnpao/hwi /downloads/Steps2Wellness_BROCH14_508_Tag508.pdf

Cook, R. F., Billings, D. W., Hersch, R. K., Back, A. S., & Hendrickson, A. (2007). A field test of a web-based workplace health promotion program to improve dietary practices, reduce stress, and increase physical activity: Randomized controlled trial. *Journal of Medical Internet Research, 9*(2), e17.

Cromp, D., Cheadle, A., Solomon, L., Maring, P., Wong, E., & Reed, K. M. (2012). Kaiser Permanente's Farmers' Market Program: Description, impact, and lessons learned. *Journal of Agriculture, Food Systems, and Community Development,* *2*(2), 29–36. Retrieved from 10.5304/jafscd.2012.022.010

Dooren, C., Marinussen, M., Blonk, H., Aiking, H., & Vellinga, P. (2014). Exploring dietary guidelines based on ecological and nutritional values: A comparison of six dietary patterns. *Food Policy, 44,* 36–46.

DuPuis, E. M., & Goodman, D. (2005). Should we go "home" to eat? Toward a reflexive politics of localism. *Journal of Rural Studies, 21*(3), 359–371.

Federal Occupational Health. (n.d.). *Food safety services.* Retrieved May 3, 2015, from https://www.foh.hhs.gov/Productfocus/June2006/foodsafetyasp

Fischler, C. (1988). Food, self and identity. *Social Science Information, 27*(2), 275–292.

Grant, S., & Mizzi, T. (2014). Body weight bias in hiring decisions: Identifying explanatory mechanisms. *Social Behavior and Personality: An International Journal, 42*(3), 353–370.

Guthman, J. (2002). Commodified meanings, meaningful commodities: Rethinking production–consumption links through the organic system of provision. *Sociologia Ruralis, 42*(4), 295–311.

Harvard School of Public Health. (2015). *Worksite obesity prevention recommendations: Complete list.* Retrieved from http://www.hsph.harvard.edu/obesity-prevention-source/obesity-prevention/worksites/worksites-obesity-prevention-recommendations-complete-list/

Henderson, J., Coveney, J., & Ward, P. (2010). Who regulates food? Australians' perceptions of responsibility for food safety. *Australian Journal of Primary Health, 16*(4), 344–351.

Johnston, C. A., Rost, S., Miller-Kovach, K., Moreno, J. P., & Foreyt, J. P. (2013). A randomized controlled trial of a community-based behavioral counseling program. *The American Journal of Medicine, 126*(12), 1119–1143.

Kruger, D. J., Greenberg, E., Murphy, J. B., DiFazio, L. A., & Youra, K. R. (2014). Local concentration of fast-food outlets is associated with poor nutrition and obesity. *American Journal of Health Promotion, 28*(5), 340–343.

Marra, M., King, B. W., & Holmes, J. (2014). Trivial, mundane or reveling? Food as a lens on ethnic norms in workplace talk. *Language & Communication, 34*(1), 46–55.

National Institute of Mental Health. (n.d.). *Health education: Eating disorders.* Retrieved from http://www.nimh.nih.gov/health/topics/eating-disorders/index.shtml

O'Neil, C. E., Nicklas, T. A., Kease, D. R., & Fulgoni, V. L., III. (2014, November 18). Ethnic disparities among food sources of energy and nutrients of public health concern and nutrients to limit in adults in the United States: NHANES 2003-2006. *Food Nutrition Research, 58,* 15784.

Overeaters Anonymous. (2015). *Program of recovery.* Retrieved from http://www.oa.org

Sommer, W., Stürmer, B., Shmuilovich, O., Martin-Loeches, M., & Schacht, A. (2013). How about lunch? Consequences of the meal context on cognition and emotion. *Plos ONE, 8*(7), e70314.

Soper, K. (2007). Re-thinking the Good Life: The citizenship dimension of consumer disaffection with consumerism. *Journal of Consumer Culture, 7*(2), 205–229.

U.S. Department of Agriculture. (2015). *Scientific report of the 2015 Dietary Guidelines Advisory Committee.* Retrieved from http://www.health.gov /dietaryguidelines/2015-scientific-report/PDFs/Scientific-Report-of-the-2015-Dietary-Guidelines-Advisory-Committee.pdf

U.S. Department of Agriculture, Food Safety and Inspection Service. (2015, March 24). Retrieved from http://www.fsis.usda.gov/wps/portal/fsis/home

U.S. Department of Agriculture & U.S. Department of Health and Human Services. (2010). Dietary guidelines for Americans 2010. Retrieved from http://www.health.gov/dietaryguidelines/dga2010/DietaryGuidelines2010.pdf

U.S. General Services Administration. (n.d.). Concessions and cafeterias: Healthy food in the federal workplace. Retrieved May 23, 2015, from http://www.gsa.gov/portal/content/104429

Vanhove, A. & Gordon, R. A. (2013). Weight discrimination in the workplace: A meta-analytic examination of the relationship between weight and work-related outcomes. *Journal of Applied Social Psychology, 44*(1), 12–22.

Wanjek, C. (2005). *Food at work: Workplace solutions for malnutrition, obesity and chronic diseases.* Geneva, Switzerland: International Labour Organization.

WeightLossWars. (n.d.). *Start a Biggest Loser at Work right now!* Retrieved May 3, 2014, from http://www.thebiggestloseratwork.com

WORKPLACE HEALTH PROMOTION PROGRAM IMPLEMENTATION HEALTH PRIORITY: PHYSICALLY HEALTHY AND SAFE ENVIRONMENTS

Physically Healthy and Safe Workplace Environments Priority

The goal of program implementation focused on a physically healthy and safe workplace environment priority is to address recognizable workplace hazards generally categorized as physical, chemical, and biological. Physical hazards cause injury to workers when an object, piece of equipment, or material comes in contact with a worker. Physical hazards are often associated with an uncontrolled source of energy, such as kinetic, electrical, pneumatic, or hydraulic. Examples of physical hazards are:

- Exposure to unguarded or unprotected electrical equipment
- Working with high voltage equipment
- Exposure to electromagnetic fields
- Incorrect wiring
- Loose surface conditions
- Wet surface conditions
- Object(s) on the floor
- Blocked walkways
- Uneven surfaces
- Small or inadequate walkways
- Force of movement

LEARNING OBJECTIVES

- Discuss program implementation with physically healthy and safe workplace environment priority

- Identify evidence-based physically healthy and safe workplace environment policies, practices, interventions, and services

- Explain physically healthy and safe workplace environment program challenges

- Describe advocacy partnerships and organizations

- Repetition of movement
- Awkward postures
- Sustained/static postures
- Contract stress
- Vibration
- Poor work station design
- Fast moving equipment
- Flash arc
- Working at heights
- Restricted/confined spaces
- Working with powered equipment
- Working with unguarded equipment
- Unguarded machines or work areas
- Overhead hazards
- Sharp edges
- Poor design or layout of work area

Chemical hazards are substances that, because of their characteristics and effects, may cause harm to human health and safety. Chemical hazards can be broken down to include exposure to vapors, gasses, mists, dusts, fumes, and smoke. Examples of chemical hazards include exposure to:

- Chemical reactions
- Production of chemicals
- Chemical incompatibility
- Chemical storage
- Flammable Substances
- Combustible substances
- Carcinogenic substances
- Oxidizing substances
- Corrosive substances
- Pressurized container

Biological hazards are organisms (or substances produced by organisms) that may pose a threat to human health and safety. Biological hazards include exposure to:

- Blood or other body fluids or tissue

- Human waste

- Anthrax

- Fungi/molds

- Bacteria and viruses

- Poisonous plants

- Animal waste

- Threat of insect or animal bites

- Drugs/cytotoxic substances

Each one of these hazards potentially has serious negative effects and consequences on employees' health. Implementing a program with a focus on establishing a physically healthy and safe workplace environment—to prevent these negative consequences can not only safeguard employees health but also contribute to lowering health care costs for the employees and employer. The specific health care cost most linked with this implementation priority is workers' compensation as the result of workplace hazard accident, injury, disability, or illness. Workers, as a consequence of an accident, injury, disability, or illness, can qualify for workers' compensation to provide wage replacement benefits, medical treatment, vocational rehabilitation, and other benefits to certain workers or their dependents who experience work-related injury or occupational disease. Employers have an incentive to implement physically healthy and safe workplace environment programs as a means to control workers' compensation expenses (i.e., insurance premium rate increases) and costs (e.g., lost production, fines, and legal expenses related to unsafe conditions).

Evidence-Based Physically Healthy and Safe Workplace Environment Policies, Practices, Interventions, and Services

Physically healthy and safe workplace environment policies, practices, interventions, and services reflect the unique characteristic of any given workplace and its employees. They also reflect and are concerned with the health of employees' families and communities. Employers are increasingly motivated to implement programs to avoid negative publicity, punitive legislative restrictions, and legal actions as a result of an organization's action or lack of action to address a health hazard that might negatively impact families and communities as well as the employee.

Safety Standards

The Occupational Safety and Health Administration (OSHA) is the federal administrative agency in charge of regulating workplaces and taking action when safety violations occur. Many states also regulate workplace safety and are in charge of investigating workplace conditions related to safety hazards, occupational diseases, and other risks in the workplace. By law state standards must be as rigorous as OSHA's or more so (OSHA, 2015a). The federal and state standards protect workers from dangerous work conditions and place a burden on the employer to ensure the workplace is safe. OSHA has passed a huge variety of different laws and regulations on everything from work surfaces to ladder and scaffolding safety to noise in the workplace to the number and location of exits in work environments (OSHA, 2015a). Certain workplaces, exempted from OSHA inspections because they fall outside of the scope of the Occupational Safety and Health Act, are regulated by other agencies, or are exempted through Department of Labor appropriations bills. For example:

- Mine and quarry workers (regulated by the Mine Safety and Health Administration—Department of Labor)
- Independent contractors and other self-employed individuals are exempted
- Public (government) sector employees (covered only in jurisdictions with state plans; the United States Postal Service is covered under the Postal Employees Safety Enhancement Act)
- Domestic workers (those whose workplace is a household) are exempted
- Flight crews (covered by the Federal Aviation Administration)
- Long distance truck drivers (covered by the Department of Transportation and OSHA)
- Farms employing only family members and farms employing fewer than 10 employees with no migrant labor housing are exempted

Additionally, workplaces participating in OSHA's voluntary protection programs are exempted from programmatic inspections, though they can still be subject to accident-, complaint-, or referral-initiated inspections. It is incumbent upon workplace health promotion professionals implementing physically safe and healthy priority–focused programs to know the state and federal legislation impacting the workplace as well as the occupations found at the workplace.

Worker Safety Programs

Many different types of programs fall under the title of Worker Safety Programs. They are mandated by the OSHA General Duty Clause: "Each employer shall furnish to each of his employees employment and a place of employment which are free from recognized hazards that are causing or are likely to cause death or serious physical harm to his employees" (OSHA, 2015c). A safe work environment is integral to the success of a facility and the health of its employees. Worker safety programs contribute action toward the common goal of the safe workplace, which can show itself in many different ways. See the list of programs below that may be required by OSHA across all industries as well as specific industries.

Common Worker Safety Programs

- First aid training
- Hearing loss prevention programs
- Fall protection
- Back injury
- Bloodborne pathogen
- Drug free and safe workplaces
- Fire evacuation
- Hazard communication
- Fleet safety (transportation)
- Emergency response
- Accident investigation

Two examples of state programs include the Washington State Department of Labor and Industries and the Maine Department of Labor. Washington State's program is called the Health and Safety Core Rules. This program focuses on goal-oriented programming to accomplish the application of predetermined rules to follow to make a workplace safer and healthier (Washington State Department of Labor and Industries, 2015). The state of Maine provides the SafetyWorks program, which is an outreach program whose goal is to reduce work-related injuries, illnesses, and deaths. The constructs of the SafetyWorks program include the "Ask a SafetyWorks Expert" link as well as workplace safety training programs, safety and health consultations, and videos and publications (State of Maine Department of Labor, 2015).

Mine Safety Training

In 2012 there were a total of 36 deaths resulting from mining-related accidents as opposed to 242 in 1978. The Mine Safety and Health Administration (MSHA) works to develop safety programs to reduce injuries, illnesses, and deaths related to the mining industry by instituting education, inspections, training, outreach, and technical support for those within the mining industry. This program succeeded to spend an average of 61 hours per mine doing safety inspections while issuing almost 140,000 citations and orders for safety hazards (MSHA, 2015).

All miners are trained in mine maintenance, storage, location, and usage of all emergency equipment and systems. The training follows MSHA guidelines with emphasis placed upon the systems and equipment incorporated within the overall mining scheme at the particular operation. Selected management personnel are given specific emergency training detailing procedures utilized in certain emergency situations. This type of training enables foremen to make a quicker and more intelligent decision when faced with an emergency. The mine operator formulates and informs each employee of the Mine Emergency Plan. This plan is drawn from a mixture of ideas resulting from meetings between management and labor, as well as any consultants the operator may wish to invite for the formulation process. A chain of command (e.g., superintendent of operations, general mine foreman, safety director, or safety coordinator) is established in case of an emergency. Procedures are developed in the event of a fire, explosion or other dangerous situation, personal injury, and emergency transportation of injured persons.

OSHA Facility Safety Inspections and Reporting

OSHA is authorized to conduct workplace inspections and investigations to determine whether employers are complying with standards issued by the agency for safe and healthful workplaces. The inspections are conducted without notice by an inspections officer unless under special circumstances. Because there are 7 million OSHA sites around the country, priority is given to certain sites in determining which sites to inspect. The justification or reason for inspections is based on four priorities. These priorities are, in order of highest to lowest: imminent danger situations, catastrophes, or fatal accidents; complaints, referrals, and follow-up inspections; and planned inspections. The higher the risk, the more frequent the inspections. The OSHA inspections focus on compliance: sites are complying with all requirements (e.g., daily inspections of chemical leakage and dangerous worksites) rather than waiting and only occurring when the OSHA inspector is present to monitor the workplace.

The normal inspection process will consist of an initial verification of the compliance officer's credentials, followed by an opening conference, a walk around, and a closing conference. After the compliance officer reports the results of the inspection, citations issued or resulting penalties must be issued within 6 months of the inspection. Violations are categorized as other-than-serious, serious, willful, repeated, and failure to abate (OSHA, n.d.-a).

OSHA inspectors perform a hazard analysis process. It compares site practices with recognized expert practices, assesses recent changes in safety practices, as well as routine examinations of jobs, processes, and phases of work (e.g., different work stations). While an alert and competent workforce is the constant "real time" protection against accident and injury, inspections provide the final clear and concentrated focus on potential problems. OSHA encourages employee participation in the inspections and ongoing safety programs.

OSHA Encourages Employee Workplace Safety Participation

- Meet OSHA or other legal obligations
- Involve employees in safety
- Form a safety committee
- Identify areas of undue risk and high loss potential
- Provide safety education
- Check past training and skill development
- Identify and develop positive safety attitudes
- Suggest better job methods
- Reinforce the positive efforts of people in the workplace

Ergonomics

Musculoskeletal disorders (MSDs) affect the muscles, nerves, and tendons. Work-related MSDs (including those of the neck, upper extremities, and low back) are one of the leading causes of lost workday injury and illness. Workers in many different industries and occupations can be exposed to risk factors at work, such as lifting heavy items, bending, reaching overhead, pushing and pulling heavy loads, working in awkward body postures, and performing the same or similar tasks repetitively. Exposure to these known risk factors for MSDs increases a worker's risk of injury. But work-related MSDs can be prevented. Ergonomics—fitting a job to a person—helps lessen muscle fatigue, increases productivity, and reduces the number and severity of work-related MSDs (OSHA, 2015b).

Work-related musculoskeletal disorders (WMSDs) are among the most prevalent and costly health concerns within today's workplace. A basic ergonomics program is designed to educate and aid employees regarding the topic of ergonomics to reduce the health and financial impact on the employers. The National Institute of Occupational Safety and Health (NIOSH) recognizes seven steps to implementing an effective ergonomics program within the workplace. They are as follows (Cohen, Gjessing, Fine, Bernard, & McGlothlin, 1997):

1. Looking for signs of a potential musculoskeletal problem in the workplace (aches, pains, repetitive movements, etc.).

2. Showing administrative and management commitment and problem focus.

3. Offering training to expand management and employee ability to recognize potential musculoskeletal problems.

4. Collecting data to determine most problematic jobs or work conditions.

5. Identifying control populations within the workplace to later analyze improvements in program population.

6. Establishing health care management to promote early detections and treatment for musculoskeletal injuries or disorders.

7. Minimizing risk factors for musculoskeletal disorders when planning new work processes and operations.

Workers' Compensation Management

An evolving model for workers' compensation management couples case management, workers' compensation, and absence programs making the argument that the model improves tracking; ensures regulatory compliance; and enhances the company's productivity and bottom line. There is a growing need for employers to be consistent in their approach to absence management regardless of the cause. There is increasing employer compliance risk due to tighter regulations associated with the Family Medical Leave Act (FMLA), the Americans with Disabilities Act (ADA), and the ever-changing state workers' compensation systems. Employers must comply with FMLA and ADA regulations while employees are off work with occupational and nonoccupational illnesses and injuries. For companies that use separate outside vendors for case management, workers' compensation, and leave of absence benefits, the information is not easily shared or integrated between all parties. With multiple processes and vendors to oversee, managing the details of each benefit can become a challenging task for an employer's risk management, human resources, and legal teams, as well as the employee's direct supervisor. The coupled model using a team approach handles the clinical steps, such as evaluation and duration management, stay-at-work and return-to-work planning, job accommodation, and vocational rehabilitation. For long-term disability cases, integrated services include return-to-work planning, case management, and Social Security assistance (Sedgwick, 2014).

Factory Floor- and Office-Level Evidence-Based Physically Healthy and Safe Workplace Interventions and Practices

Workplaces have factory floor- and office-level physically healthy and safe workplace interventions and practices to address particular workforce health needs. From small and midsized organizations to large national employers, these engage employees at the workplace (factory floor and office) and are lower cost and practical, with fairly easy administration. Outside vendors both national and local compete for contracts to offer the interventions. Examples of widely implemented evidence-based interventions and practices are:

Hazardous Material Program: The U.S. Department of Transportation's Hazmat Intelligence Portal states that in 2012, 15,436 hazardous materials incidents occurred, resulting in 12 deaths, 184 injuries, and over $79 million in damages (U.S. Department of Transportation, Pipeline and Hazardous Materials Safety Administration, 2015). One program that has been set into place to counteract the possibility of these types of accident is the Hazardous Materials Registration Program. The program requires providers and transporters of hazardous materials and waste to file a registration with the U.S. Department of Transportation as well as to pay an annual fee to promote the safety and compliance among all transporters of hazardous materials.

Safe Driving Programs: Safe driving is an important aspect of everyday life within the workplace as well as outside the workplace. Many employees are required to drive as part of their jobs in addition to the daily commuting that most people do via automobile. Many programs exist to promote safe driving to the general population and the employee population. Private employers as well as public organizations support these programs. One example of a public safe driving program is I Drive Safely. This program provides online driving courses that include fleet driver training, mature driver improvement courses, teen driver's education, and more. One benefit of completing a safety course is the most obvious: safer driving, which reduces risk for injury and death from a car accident. The benefits also include possibly reducing or erasing the impact of a traffic ticket on your license, reduction of stress, increased use of responsible driving habits, and more (Drive Safely, 2015). A second example is the Share the Road Safely program sponsored by the Federal Motor Carrier Safety Administration (FMCSA). This program's goal is to increase knowledge of road sharing between cars, trucks, motorcycles, and bicycles to ultimately reduce the amount of accidents, injuries, and fatalities that are a result of crashes between different types of motor vehicle. It does this through print and online materials, partnerships, and various educators (Share the Road, 2015).

Emergency response: Businesses are required to be prepared for emergencies such as natural disasters, technological and accidental hazards, terrorist hazards, hurricanes, and winter storms. Being prepared for all of these things requires constant attention, regular practice, and recognition that every emergency situation is unique. The Federal Emergency Management Agency (FEMA) suggests a plan to stay in business during or after an emergency if possible. Good preparation strategies include: having a continuity plan, creating an emergency plan for employees, having emergency supplies, planning to stay or go in specific situations, having an evacuation plan, and making a shelter-in-place plan. Next it is recommended to communicate with your employees, coworkers, and customers before, during, and after an emergency about the businesses current plan and plan for the future. It is recommended to practice the plan with your coworkers, promote family and individual preparedness, write a crisis communication plan, and to support employee health after a disaster. Finally, the business needs to protect its prosperity by securing the physical assets in the case of an emergency. FEMA suggests that a business review its insurance coverage, prepare for utility disruptions, secure facilities, buildings and plants, and finally improve its cyber security.

Physically Healthy and Safe Workplace Environment Priority Implementation Challenges

Physically healthy and safe workplace environment priority implementation involves challenges, in particular for small employers. Employees have a number of rights and protections that, when coupled with employers' obligations and their abilities to comply with OSHA standards, result in compromises for all parties. Finally, OSHA as the leading but not the only government regulating safety and health agency (others include the Federal Aviation Administration, Department of Transportation, FEMA, and those in individual states) has faced increased procedural requirements, shifting political priorities, and a rigorous standard of judicial review that have contributed to lengthy time frames for developing and issuing OSHA standards.

Small Business

Small employers place a high value on the well-being of their employees. Often small businesses employ family members and personal acquaintances. And, if they don't know the employees before they are hired, then chances are that the very size of the workplace will promote the closeness and concern for one another that small businesses value. At the same time, small employers typically have few resources and even less time to attend to personnel issues such as complying with OSHA requirements. The OSHA requirements often are perceived as a burden, taking time and energy away from tasks that the small employers need to accomplish to maintain their operations. Taking this reality into consideration, OSHA tailors services to small employers. Table 12.1 shows a seven-step process recommended for small employers to comply with the OSHA standards. Table 12.2 shows the first step in the recommended process. OSHA has streamlined the process to highlight the importance of complying and the value added by doing so (OSHA, n.d.-b).

To further support small employers OSHA operates five programs that address the needs of the employers:

1. Alliance Program works with unions, consulates, trade or professional organizations, businesses, faith- and community-based organizations, and educational institutions to promote the prevention of workplace fatalities, injuries, and illnesses.

Table 12.1   Compliance Assistance Quick Start: General Industry

Follow the steps below to identify the major OSHA general industry requirements and guidance materials that may apply to your workplace. These steps will lead you to resources on OSHA's website that will help you comply with OSHA requirements and prevent workplace injuries and illnesses.

Step 1: OSHA Requirements That Apply to Most General Industry Employers

Step 2: OSHA Requirements That May Apply to Your Workplace

Step 3: Survey Your Workplace for Additional Hazards

Step 4: Develop a Comprehensive Jobsite Safety and Health Program

Step 5: Train Your Employees

Step 6: Recordkeeping, Reporting, and Posting

Step 7: Find Additional Compliance Assistance Information

Table 12.2   Step 1: OSHA Requirements That Apply to Most General Industry Employers

1. Hazard Communication Standard. This standard is designed to ensure that employers and employees know about hazardous chemicals in the workplace and how to protect themselves. Employers with employees who may be exposed to hazardous chemicals in the workplace must prepare and implement a written Hazard Communication Program and comply with other requirements of the standard.

2. Emergency Action Plan Standard. OSHA recommends that all employers have an Emergency Action Plan. A plan is mandatory when required by an OSHA standard. An Emergency Action Plan describes the actions employees should take to ensure their safety in a fire or other emergency situation.

3. Fire Safety. OSHA recommends that all employers have a Fire Prevention Plan. A plan is mandatory when required by an OSHA standard.

4. Exit Routes. All employers must comply with OSHA's requirements for exit routes in the workplace.

5. Walking/Working Surfaces. Floors, aisles, platforms, ladders, stairways, and other walking/working surfaces are present, to some extent, in all general industry workplaces. Slips, trips, and falls from these surfaces constitute the majority of general industry accidents. The OSHA standards for walking and working surfaces apply to all permanent places of employment, except where only domestic, mining, or agricultural work is performed.

6. Medical and First Aid. OSHA requires employers to provide medical and first-aid personnel and supplies commensurate with the hazards of the workplace. The details of a workplace medical and first-aid program are dependent on the circumstances of each workplace and employer.

2. OSHA Challenge is an incentive program that provides participating employers and workers an avenue to work with their designated Challenge Administrators to develop and/or improve their safety and health management program.

3. OSHA Strategic Partnership Program (OSPP) provides opportunities for OSHA to partner with employers, workers, professional or trade associations, labor organizations, and other interested stakeholders to enhance workplace safety and health.

4. Safety and Health Achievement Recognition Program (SHARP) works to recognize small businesses and employers who exemplify above-average injury and illness prevention programs.

5. Voluntary Protection Plan is a cooperative program to recognize employers and workers (both private and federal) who implement effective safety and health management systems and maintain injury and illness rates below national Bureau of Labor Statistics averages for their respective industries.

Employee Rights

OSHA provides employees with a number of important rights and protections. First and foremost, if an employer is violating safety rules in a way that presents an imminent threat to employee health and safety, he or she has the right to refuse work. Employees also have the right to be trained on health and safety standards; to get trained on dangerous chemicals in the workplace; to request correction of any hazardous conditions in violation of OSHA; and to request that an OSHA inspection take place. If an OSHA inspection does take place, employees have the right to the results of the inspection. Employee rights also include:

- Get clear training and information in layman's terms on the hazards of their workplace, ways to avoid harm, and applicable OSHA standards and laws.

- Obtain and review documentation on work-related illnesses and injuries at the job site.

- Confidentially make a complaint with OSHA to have an inspection of the workplace.

- If desired, accompany and take part in a requested OSHA inspection of the workplace.

- Get copies of any tests done to measure workplace hazards (e.g., chemical, air, and similar testing).

If an employee is injured at work, he or she can file a claim with the employer in order to obtain benefits through workers' compensation. The workers' compensation program will provide the employee with benefits regardless of whether a safety violation occurred at work or not. Workers' compensation is a strict liability system. Employee benefits do not hinge on whether the employer was negligent or broke the law. If an employee gets injured at work, he or she should let the employer know right away. This is true if the employee is injured in an accident, injured due to a repetitive stress condition, or becomes ill as a result of exposure to toxins or hazardous materials. The employer will then need to notify the workers' compensation insurer representing the employee to receive benefits.

OSHA's Whistleblower Protection Program for employees enforces the whistleblower provisions of more than 20 whistleblower statutes protecting employees who report violations of various workplace safety regulations in the areas of airline, commercial motor carrier, consumer product, environmental, financial reform, food safety, health insurance reform, motor vehicle safety, nuclear, pipeline, public transportation agency, railroad, maritime, and securities laws. Rights afforded by these whistleblower acts include, but are not limited to, worker participation in safety and health activities, reporting a work-related injury, illness or fatality, or reporting a violation of the statutes.

Tension Between Employers' Obligations and Ability to Comply

A tension exists between the employers' obligations and their abilities to comply. Employers do not have enough time, resources, and energy to address all possible workplace hazards. The obligations can be viewed as overwhelming. For example, employers are required but not limited to provide a safe workplace free of serious hazards; find health and safety hazards; if hazards exist, eliminate or minimize them; if workplace hazards cannot be eliminated, provide employees with adequate safeguards and protective gear at no cost to them; notify employees of any hazards and provide the training necessary to address them; post a list of OSHA injuries and citations, plus place an OSHA poster in a place where employees will see them; and maintain records of work-related injuries (OSHA, 2015a). In large and midsized organizations, dedicated safety departments are tasked with the responsibility for the OSHA compliance. Small organization owners have to find the time to comply.

The result of the tension between obligations and compliance is compromise and balance for employers. They take the approach of hazard risk assessment: determine and eliminate the most likely hazards and those with the most severe consequences. With this approach the employers will try first to engineer and use job design to eliminate the hazard. Next they will use administrative policy and procedures to limit access and contact. Finally they use protection (e.g., clothing) to negate the hazardous effects (Sedgwick, 2013).

OSHA Standard-Setting Concern

Concerns exist about how long it takes OSHA to issue its standards. For OSHA to develop and issue safety and health standards, it can take anywhere from 15 months to 19 years, and the process averages more than 7 years. Furthermore OSHA is the leading but not the only government agency regulating safety and health (others include the Federal Aviation Administration, Department of Transportation, FEMA, and those in individual states), which often leaves it mired in bureaucratic procedures and politics. Experts and OSHA officials cite increased procedural requirements, shifting political priorities, and a rigorous standard of judicial review as contributing to lengthy time frames for developing and issuing standards. For example, they said that a shift in OSHA's priorities toward one standard took attention away from several other standards that previously had been a priority. Furthermore OSHA can address urgent hazards by issuing emergency temporary standards, directing additional attention to enforcing relevant existing standards, and educating employers and workers about hazards. However, OSHA has not issued an emergency temporary standard since 1983 because it has found it difficult to compile the evidence necessary to meet the statutory requirements. The consequence of the lengthy time for new standards to be issued and inability for OSHA to issue temporary standards is that OSHA focuses on enforcement and education when workers face new and urgent hazards (Labaton, 2007; U.S. Government Accountability Office, 2012).

Working to create physically healthy and safe environments, employers are quick to note the shortcomings of the OSHA standard-setting process. On the one hand, OSHA might offer potential guidance that is based on OSHA expertise and its collaboration with the National Institute on Occupational Safety and Health (NIOSH). On the other hand, many employers view OSHA compliance as a burden both financially and timewise and encumbered by politics, so the fact that OSHA is slow means OSHA is not adding to the existing employer burden (Delp, Mojtahedi, Sheikh, & Lemus, 2014).

Advocacy and Resource Partnerships and Organizations

Many business and nonprofit groups provide ongoing research, materials, and advocacy for the best evidence-based practices that support and maintain physically healthy and safe workplaces. Among the groups are:

Commission on Health and Safety and Workers' Compensation (http://www.dir.ca.gov/chswc/chswc.html)

The Commission on Health and Safety and Workers' Compensation (CHSWC) is a joint labor-management body created by the workers' compensation reform legislation of 1993. CHSWC is charged with examining the health and safety and workers' compensation systems in California and recommending administrative or legislative modifications to improve their operation. The commission was established to conduct a continuing examination of the workers' compensation system and of the state's activities to prevent industrial injuries and occupational illnesses and to examine those programs in other states. CHSWC also administers the Worker Occupational Safety and Health Training and Education Program (WOSHTEP), which sponsors workplace health and safety training programs and distributes educational materials on job safety.

Workers' Compensation Institute (http://www.wci360.com/)

The Workers' Compensation Institute (WCI) is a nonprofit educational organization that serves as a comprehensive resource to all workers' compensation stakeholders. The WCI is an outgrowth of the long-established Florida Workers' Compensation Institute. FWCI remains in existence under the WCI umbrella and continues its Florida focus, while the national organization provides a broader outreach across all states. The WCI sponsors an annual Workers' Compensation Educational Conference (WCEC) in Orlando in August, familiar to many through the sponsorship of FWCI. The conference brings together workers' compensation professionals from across the country for networking and information sharing and provides an opportunity for vendors to display their products and services.

Occupational and Environmental Professional Organizations

There are many professional organizations that exist in the occupation and environmental fields. Some organizations deal with professional advancement, education, and promotion while others are industry specific. Table 12.3 provides several examples of these organizations.

Mine Safety and Health Administration (http://www.msha.gov/)

The Mine Safety and Health Administration (MSHA) is an agency of the United States Department of Labor that administers the provisions of the Federal Mine Safety and Health Act of 1977 (Mine Act) to enforce compliance with mandatory safety and health standards as a means to eliminate fatal accidents, to reduce the frequency and severity of nonfatal accidents, to minimize health hazards, and to promote improved safety and health conditions in the nation's mines.

Workplace Wellness American Lung Association (http://www.lung .org/stop-smoking/workplace-wellness/)

Many potential causes of lung disease can be found in the workplace, but with the proper measures, they can be easily controlled to create safer and healthier working conditions for all employees. The American Lung Association offers many resources to help employers adopt and implement workplace policies that support a healthy work environment while providing health education resources to support lung health. Making the decision to focus on improving air quality indoors and providing resources for employees who smoke or are living with a chronic lung disease

Table 12.3 Occupational and Environmental Professional Organizations

American College of Occupational and Environmental Medicine (ACOEM) Professional association of physicians and other health care professionals specializing in the field of occupational and environmental medicine (http://www.acoem.org). The ACOEM is a proponent of combining workplace health protection and health promotion.

American Association of Occupational Health Nurses (AAOHN) Professional association of licensed nurses engaged in the practice of occupation and environmental health nursing (http://www.aaohn.org). The AAOHN advocates for workplace health promotion with a number of strong policy statements including the prevention of workplace violence.

American Society of Safety Engineers (ASSE) Professional organization for occupational safety, health and environmental (SH&E) professional members who manage, supervise, research, and consult on safety, health, and the environment in all industries, government, and education (http://www.asse.org/).

American Biological Safety Association Professional organization for those working in biological safety professions. It works to provide a forum for the continuing exchange of biological safety information and as a representative of the interests and concerns of biological safety professionals (http://www.absa.org).

American Chemical Society (ACS) Largest professional organization for chemists, chemical engineers, and related professions. Within the ACS, a committee on chemical safety exists. The ACS promotes and facilitates safe practices in chemical activities by calling attention to potential hazards and stimulating education in safe chemical practices (http://www.acs.org).

National Fire Protection Association (NFPA) A group of over 70,000 members who work to reduce the burden of fire-related hazards by enforcing codes and standards, research, training, and education (http://www.nfpa.org).

Campus Safety Health and Environment Management Association (CSHEMA) The goal of CSHEMA is to educate and support campus-based environment, health, and safety professionals to improve the profession as a whole and the specific campus environments (http://www.cshema.org).

will curb rising health care costs, help employees adopt healthier lifestyles, and lower the risk of developing costly chronic diseases.

U.S. Chemical Safety and Hazard Investigation Board (http://www.csb.gov/)

Chemical Safety Board, or CSB, is an independent U.S. federal agency charged with investigating industrial chemical accidents. Formed as part of the Clean Air Act of 1990 amendments. Following the successful model of the National Transportation Safety Board and the Department of Transportation, Congress directed that the CSB's investigative function be completely independent of the rulemaking, inspection, and enforcement authorities of the Environmental Protection Agency and Occupational Safety and Health Administration. Congress recognized that CSB investigations would identify chemical hazards that were not addressed by those agencies.

Summary

The goal of implementing a physically healthy and safe workplace environment priority-focused program is to address recognizable workplace hazards generally categorized as physical, chemical, or biological. The specific health care cost most linked with this implementation priority is workers' compensation, as the result of workplace hazard accident, injury, disability, or illness. Employers have an incentive to implement physically healthy and safe workplace environment programs as a means to control workers' compensation expenses (i.e., insurance premium rate increases) and costs (e.g., lost production, fines, and legal expenses related to unsafe conditions). The Occupational Safety and Health Administration (OSHA) is the federal administrative agency that is in charge of regulating workplaces and taking action when safety violations occur. Many states also regulate workplace safety and are in charge of investigating workplace conditions related to safety hazards, occupational diseases, and other risks in the workplace. Program implementation includes worker safety programs, mine safety, OSHA facility safety inspections and reporting, ergonomics, and workers' compensation and absence management. Challenges to a physically healthy and safe workplace include small employers' ability to comply with OSHA standards, employees' rights, tension between employers' obligations, and ability to comply with OSHA standards, as well as concerns related to the OSHA standard-setting process.

For Practice and Discussion

1. Select a physically healthy and safe workplace program area (e.g., worker safety programs, mine safety, OSHA facility safety inspections and reporting, ergonomics, or workers' compensation and absence management). Research the program offerings for the area by industry type (e.g., manufacturing, health care, education, mining, transportation). Compare and contrast the scope of the programs and training currently offered at workplaces. How can the programs be improved?

2. How would large, midsized, and small employers respond to federal legislation proposals to limit the authority of OSHA to enforce the OSHA General Duty Clause? "Each employer shall furnish to each of his employees employment and a place of employment which are free from recognized hazards that are causing or are likely to cause death or serious physical harm to his employees." What are pros and cons that each group of employers might list in deciding whether or not to support the legislation?

3. You have been asked to prepare a 2-hour training session for a group of 25 small employers on the use of the OSHA Safety and Health Management Systems eTool (Figure 12.1) (https://www.osha.gov/SLTC /etools/safetyhealth/index.html). The employers work in the housing and construction trades. The employers are interested in learning how to use the eTool and its benefits. They are skeptical that it really saves them time and money as well as makes for safer conditions at workplaces.

4. OSHA's Whistleblower Protection Program (http://www .whistleblowers.gov/) enforces the whistleblower provisions of more than 20 whistleblower statutes protecting employees who report violations of various regulations in workplace safety, airline, commercial motor carrier, consumer product, environmental, financial

Safety and Health Management Systems eTool

Does a safety and health program really make a difference? Definitely!

The best safety and health programs involve every level of the organization, instilling a safety culture that reduces accidents for workers and improves the bottom line for managers.When safety and health are part of the organization and a way of life, everyone wins.

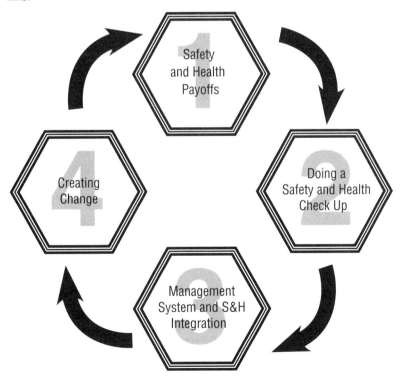

Figure 12.1 OSHA Safety and Health Management Systems eTool

reform, food safety, health insurance reform, motor vehicle safety, nuclear, pipeline, public transportation agency, railroad, maritime, and securities laws. Although workers have many rights and protections under the law, why do many individuals hesitate to report hazards in the workplace? For a safer and hazard-free workplace, what actions do you suggest that might reduce employee hesitation and reluctance to report hazards?

5. Midsized and small employers are expressing increased interest in total absence management programs to help them administer different types of occupational and nonoccupational disability leave (e.g., workers' compensation, FMLA) while using integrated data to create healthier workplaces. How can the integrated disability management programs developed for large employers many years ago be modified for midsized and small employers?

Case Study: Safety Inspector Career Guidance Unit—What Would You Do?

A safety inspector, sometimes called an occupational health and safety technician or specialist, examines and evaluates workplaces and practices to ensure compliance with state and federal regulations for a physically healthy and safe workplace environment. This career involves extensive travel to inspect a wide range of settings such as factories, offices, hospitals, and schools. Work as a safety inspector includes office hours, work in the field, and quite a bit of travel. Because most inspectors work for governments, job security is associated with this career. Inspectors may be exposed to a range of risks and must wear protective clothing and gear to ensure their personal safety while completing inspections. Inspectors primarily work full-time during the business day, although some nights and weekends may be required in an emergency.

Frances Albert is a high school guidance counselor preparing career and job exploration educational units for high school students as part of a regular social studies or history class period. For the upcoming school year one of the units Ms. Albert is asked to prepare is on a career and job working at OSHA as a safety inspector to ensure compliance with state and federal regulations for a physically healthy and safe workplace environment. If you were she, what would you include? Prepare your unit's content information, activities, and assignments. Typically units involve both small-group and individual activities that are completed, over the course of a month, as part of guidance curriculum delivered in the classroom.

KEY TERMS

Physical, chemical, and biological hazards	Workers' compensation
OSHA	Absence management
Worker safety programs	OSHA Small Business Program
General duty clause	Employee rights
Mine safety	Employer obligations
Facility safety inspections and reporting	OSHA standard setting
Ergonomics	

References

Cohen, A. L., Gjessing, C. C., Fine, L. J., Bernard, B. P., & McGlothlin, J. D. (1997). *Elements of ergonomics programs.* Retrieved from http://www.cdc.gov/niosh/docs/97-117/pdfs/97-117.pdf

Delp, L., Mojtahedi, Z., Sheikh, H., & Lemus, J. (2014). A legacy of struggle: The OSHA ergonomics standard and beyond, Part I. *NEW SOLUTIONS: A Journal of Environmental and Occupational Health Policy, 24*(3), 365–389.

Drive Safely (2015). *About I Drive Safely.* Retrieved May 24, 2015, from https://www.idrivesafely.com/about-us/

Labaton, S. (2007, April 25). OSHA leaves worker safety in hands of industry. *New York Times.* Retrieved from http://www.nytimes.com/2007/04/25/washington/25osha.html?pagewanted=all&_r=0

Mine Safety and Health Administration. (2015). *Protecting miners' safety and health since 1978.* Retrieved from http://www.msha.gov/

Occupational Safety and Health Administration. (2015a). *OSHA laws and regulations.* Retrieved from https://www.osha.gov/law-regs.html

Occupational Safety and Health Administration. (2015b). *Prevention of musculoskeletal disorders in the workplace.* Retrieved from https://www.osha.gov/SLTC/ergonomics/index.html

Occupational Safety and Health Administration. (2015c). *Workers' rights booklet.* Retrieved from https://www.osha.gov/workers/index.html

Occupational Health and Safety Administration. (n.d.-a). *OSHA inspections.* OSHA Fact Sheet. Retrieved May 23, 2014, from https://www.osha.gov/OshDoc/data_General_Facts/factsheet-inspections.pdf

Occupational Health and Safety Administration. (n.d.-b). *Small business.* Retrieved May 23, 2014, from https://www.osha.gov/dcsp/smallbusiness/index.html

Sedgwick. (2013). *OSHA compliance.* Retrieved from https://www.sedgwick.com/resources/Documents/Services/OSHACompliance.pdf

Sedgwick. (2014). *Integrated disability management.* Sedgwick White Paper. Retrieved from https://www.sedgwick.com/news/Documents/Studies /IntegratedDisabilityManagementWhitePaper.pdf

Share the Road. (2015). *Facts about the Share the Road specialty license plate.* Florida Bicycle Association. Retrieved from http://sharetheroad.org/about/

State of Maine Department of Labor. (2015). *Workplace safety and health.* Retrieved from http://www.maine.gov/labor/workplace_safety/

U.S. Government Accountability Office. (2012). *Workplace safety and health multiple challenges lengthen OSHA's standard setting.* Retrieved from http://www .gao.gov/assets/590/589825.pdf

U.S. Department of Transportation, Pipeline and Hazardous Materials Safety Administration. (2015). *PHMSA portal.* Retrieved from pdm.phmsa.dot.gov/

Washington State Department of Labor and Industries. (2015). *Get started in safety and health.* Retrieved from http://www.lni.wa.gov/SAFETY /GETTINGSTARTED/DEFAULT.ASP

WORKPLACE HEALTH PROMOTION PROGRAM IMPLEMENTATION HEALTH PRIORITY: PSYCHOLOGICALLY HEALTHY AND SAFE ENVIRONMENTS

Program Implementation: Psychologically Healthy and Safe Workplace Environments Priority

A psychologically healthy and safe workplace environment promotes employees' psychological well-being and does not harm employee mental health in negligent, reckless, or intentional ways. A psychologically healthy workplace is one where every reasonable effort is made to promote mental health through awareness, resources, and education. A psychologically safe workplace is where every reasonable precaution is taken to avert injury or danger to employee psychological health (Bureau de normalisation du Québec & Canadian Standards Association, 2013). Table 13.1 lists 12 psychosocial protective and risk factors known to impact workplace psychological health and safety.

Similar to implementing a program to promote physically healthy and safe environments, implementing a psychologically healthy and safe workplace environment contributes to lowering employer and employee health care costs. Likewise, high workers' compensation costs as the result of a psychologically unhealthy and unsafe workplace environment are a driving force and incentive for employers to implement programs in this priority area.

LEARNING OBJECTIVES

- Discuss program implementation with a psychologically healthy and safe workplace environment priority

- Identify evidence-based psychologically healthy and safe workplace environment policies, practices, interventions, and services

- Explain psychologically healthy and safe workplace environment program challenges

- Describe advocacy partnerships and organizations

Table 13.1   Psychosocial Protective and Risk Factors Known to Impact Workplace Psychological Health and Safety (University of Alberta Human Resources, 2012)

1. *Psychological support*: an environment where psychological and mental health concerns are supported and responded to appropriately.

2. *Organizational culture*: the environment is characterized by trust, honesty, and fairness.

3. *Leadership and expectations*: effective leadership exists that enables staff members to know what to do, how their work contributes, and if change is approaching.

4. *Civility and respect*: staff and faculty are respectful, considerate, and collegial with one another.

5. *Psychological job fit*: a good fit between interpersonal/emotional competencies, job skills, and the position.

6. *Growth and development:* staff members receive encouragement and support in the development of interpersonal, emotional, and job skills.

7. *Recognition and reward*: acknowledgment and appreciation of staff members' efforts in a fair and timely manner.

8. *Involvement and influence*: staff members are included in discussions about how work is done, how decisions are made, and their impact.

9. *Workload management:* tasks and responsibilities can be accomplished successfully within the time available.

10. *Engagement*: staff members enjoy and feel connected to their work and are motivated to do a good job.

11. *Balance:* recognition and support for balance between the demands of work, family, and personal life.

12. *Protection of physical safety*: appropriate action to protect employees' physical safety at work.

Different about psychologically unhealthy and unsafe work environments is their pervasive impact upon a workplace culture and climate with potentially serious negative impacts on workplace production, product quality, and consumer satisfaction and service. Workers can feel bad, concerned, and upset about a fellow employee's injury and accident, perhaps increasing their own physical safety efforts without their productivity being negatively impacted. However, the pervasive nature of a psychologically unhealthy and unsafe workplace permeates (and literally infects) workers' sense of well-being. The potential negative consequences can be quite high for employers.

Evidence-Based Psychologically Healthy and Safe Environment Policies, Practices, Interventions, and Services

The mandates, guidance, and oversight on what employers implement in this priority area have a number of sources. The Occupational Safety and Health Administration (OSHA) in 1989 published voluntary, generic safety and health program management guidelines for all employers to use as a foundation for their safety and health programs, which can include workplace violence prevention programs. OSHA's violence prevention guidelines build on these generic guidelines by identifying common risk factors and describing some feasible solutions. Although not exhaustive, the workplace violence guidelines include policy recommendations and practical corrective methods to help prevent and mitigate the effects of workplace violence. Likewise, OSHA recommends, as part of a program to promote psychologically healthy and safe work environments, to reduce worker stress with programs for employees, supervisors, crisis, and specific work environments (Centers for Disease Control and Prevention [CDC], n.d.). An executive order in 1987 put in place requirements for a drug-free workplace. The 1978 Civil Rights Act, Americans with Disability Act, and more recently the Mental Health Parity Act address the rights and treatment of individuals with a mental health concern and illness. Sexual harassment is a form of sex discrimination that violates Title VII of the Civil Rights Act of 1964, which states that employers with 15 or more employees as well as the federal, state, and local government are required to comply with the Act. Pritchard, Griffin, and O'Leary-Kelly (2004) and Zins, Elias, and Maher (2013) summarize psychologically healthy and safe environment program priorities in four categories. Programs to prevent harm to others: verbal and psychological (e.g., bullying), physical violence, and sexual harassment. Programs to prevent harm to the individual: substance use, tobacco use, and depression (these are addressed as part of the mental health priority area). Programs to prevent harm to the organization that have specific financial costs: absenteeism, theft of assets or property, destruction of assets or property, and violations of laws, codes or regulations. Programs to prevent harm that have nonspecific costs but can be toxic to the culture: destructive political behaviors, mismanagement, fraud, and breach of confidentiality.

Psychologically healthy and safe workplace environment priority program implementation mirrors other priority area implementations (Figure 13.1). However, the pervasive nature of the risks to harm the organization creates a different type of urgency to deal with risks that may not be specifically mandated by law.

Sexual Harassment Prevention Policies and Training

The U.S. Equal Employment Opportunity Commission (EEOC) defines harassment as "unwanted conduct of a sexual nature, or other conduct based on sex affecting the dignity of women and men at work which include physical, verbal, and non-verbal conduct" (EEOC, n.d.-b). The harasser or

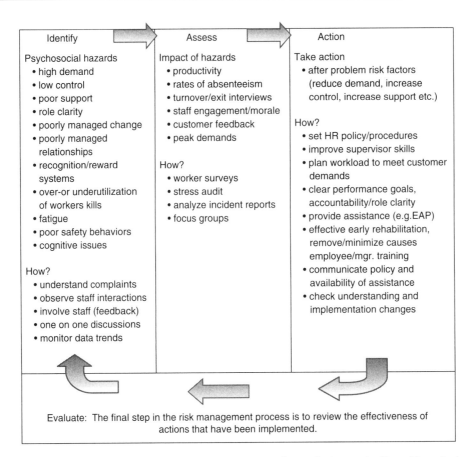

Figure 13.1   Psychologically Healthy and Safe Workplace Environment Priority Program Implementation (State of Queensland Department of Justice and Attorney-General, 2012)

victim can be of either sex and the two can be of the same sex. Recognizing and preventing sexual harassment in the workplace can be tough, although current policies, training, and other prevention strategies can be effective. Sexual harassment programs in the workplace commonly consist of three levels of intervention: primary, secondary, and tertiary. Primary interventions are programs and policies to prevent or reduce sexual harassment incidents. This level of intervention includes implementation of legislation and policies both within the workplace and at the governmental level. Furthermore it includes assessment of risk factors, regular training of employees, evaluation of training, and formal monitoring of prevalence rates. Secondary intervention deals with responding to incidents and complaints procedures. Secondary intervention commonly includes a network of advisers, formal responses, advocacy, active coping strategies, supportive environments, and eradication of negative psychological outcomes.

Tertiary intervention includes crisis intervention, legal advice, counseling, rehabilitation, and systematic monitoring (Hunt, Davidson, Fielden, & Hoel, 2010).

Recently, with gay marriage laws being passed allowing gay and lesbians to marry in all 50 states, there is a need for companies to be more accepting and tolerant. There are not always policies in place to protect lesbian, gay, bisexual, and transgender (LGBT) employees from harassment or termination. While there are currently 21 states and the District of Columbia that prohibit sexual orientation discrimination, not all do. The proposed federal legislation—the Employment Non-Discrimination Act—hopes to "provide basic protection against workplace discrimination on the basis of sexual orientation or gender identity" and end this type of discrimination throughout the country (Human Rights Campaign, 2015). Programs such as Straight Allies focus on helping end discrimination and increase LGBT employees' right to be out at work. By being able to come out to coworkers and bosses, LGBT employees feel more included in the workplace and are often more productive (Miles, 2011). A study on LGBT workplace programs shows how heterosexual employees underestimate the level of discrimination toward LGBT minorities in the workplace, and LGBT employees may not be able to fight back against discrimination for fear of termination or other job ramifications (Gates & Mitchell, 2013).

Drug-Free Workplace Programs

A drug-free workplace is an organization where the employer has specific policies and procedures to make sure employees are not using illegal drugs or other substances during working hours. Under the Drug-Free Workplace Act of 1988, all organizations that receive federal grants, and some federal contractors, are required to maintain a drug-free workplace. Even if an organization is not connected to a federal contract or grant, establishing a drug-free workplace will promote the well-being, safety, and productivity of employees, and will reduce employer absenteeism, medical, workers' compensation, and damaged product costs.

A comprehensive drug-free workplace program includes a clear policy, employee education, supervisor training, an employee assistance program (EAP), and possibly drug testing. If employers choose to conduct random drug tests, they must be sensitive about employees' invasion of privacy objections. The goal of a drug-free workplace program is to support and enable an employee with a substance abuse problem to receive treatment, recover, and return to work (Table 13.2).

An evolving change for employers related to a drug-free workplace program is there are now more options for legal drugs with the legalization

Table 13.2   Drug-Free Workplace Program Components and Strategies

Drug-Free Workplace Program Components	Implementation Strategies
Clear policy that specifies: • zero tolerance for prohibited substances • what consequences will be applied • what assistance is available • return to work procedures • all levels of the organization are subject to the same policy	• new hire orientation • seminars • web-based programs • brochures • posters
Employee education	• information about substance abuse and the effects of substance abuse on work performance • encourage employees to seek help • team building exercises to develop employee support networks and communication skills
Supervisor training	• know and understand the policy and program • be aware of legal issues • recognize drug-related work issues • maintain confidentiality • refer to appropriate services • reintegrate into the workforce
Employee assistance program	• easily accessible • includes family members • confidential • broad range of services (see above)
Drug testing	• if required by law or other customer, contract, insurance, nature of the work requirements • sends a clear message about workplace culture • must have employee consent • must be private and confidential • must be random; cannot single out particular individuals • can be background screening for all new hires

of marijuana in some states. Recently, the legalization for medical marijuana passed in 23 states, and four states—Colorado, Washington, Oregon, and Alaska—and DC passed recreational marijuana usuage laws. The legislation broadly defines marijuana or cannabis as not only the cannabis plant itself, but also any oils, ointments, tinctures, liquids, gels, pills, or similar substances made from the cannabis plant. And while there appears to be no immediate action as to whether employers will still drug test for marijuana, companies need to think about the social ramifications as well as ramifications for the company. One study suggests that guidelines be put into place to help companies decide whether someone is under the influence of marijuana and how to properly test for it. It is suggested that employers can provide literature to educate employees where marijuana is legal in order to help employees navigate the new laws and workplace policies (Phillips et al., 2015).

Workplace Violence Prevention

Workplace violence is a significant occupational health and safety issue that occurs when workers experience verbal abuse, bullying, horizontal violence, intimidation, physical threats, physical assault, sexual assault, and/or homicide. About 2 million workers report being victims of workplace violence every year (OSHA, 2015). Workplace violence contributes to increased stress, fear, anxiety, self-blame, carrying weapons for self-protection, decreased trust of management, decreased job satisfaction, and increased employee turnover. Employers are affected via increased health care costs, legal costs, worker turnover, absenteeism, and decreased productivity (American Association of Occupational Health Nurses, 2015).

Common workplace violence prevention programs include primary, secondary, and tertiary prevention. Primary prevention consists of prevention of workplace violence from occurring through risk assessments, workplace reporting and surveillance, prevention policies, sound hiring practices (background checks), visitor policies, walk-through surveys, employee and employer training, and increased awareness. Secondary prevention looks to address early detection of potentially violent behavior and situations by developing violent event procedures, reviewing company risk factors, and developing risk reduction strategies. Tertiary prevention strategies work to address workers and workplaces after a violent incident has occurred. Common strategies used in tertiary prevention are post–violent event investigation, monitoring of incident trends, provision of health care and employee assistance programs (EAPs) to victims, legal counseling, workers' compensation, and reporting to police (American Association of Occupational Nurses, 2015).

Dignity and Respect Programs

Civility, dignity, and respect programs in the workplace address issues of harassment, bullying, racism, and more among employees. The goal of these programs is to create or maintain a positive interpersonal environment for all employees. A program commonly will consist of a workplace consultation, awareness campaign, training, policy development, and evaluation. An example of this type of program is the Civility, Respect, and Engagement in the Workplace (CREW) program developed by the Veteran's Health Association (VHA) and utilized by the National Center for Organization Development at non-VA locations. This program focuses on improving the culture of respect and civility in the workplace through meetings, dialogue, and awareness (Department of Veterans Affairs, 2014).

Another aspect of dignity and respect programs for employers is to consider their workforce composition and assess to what degree it reflects its consumers and communities of its workplaces, especially if the business deals directly with the community. For example, when civil rights events or other protests occur in the community, employers need to be sensitive to employees' perception of these events. Through understanding dignity, that dignity is one's own perception of events, and that dignity revolves around an employee's expectations, employees can continue to feel heard and respected in the workplace, despite outside events (Lucas, 2015).

Workplace Bullying Prevention

Workplace bullying is when one or more individuals perceive themselves to be the target of repeated and systematic negative acts on at least a weekly basis over a period of 6 months or longer. Bullying is usually correlated with real or perceived imbalance of power among workers. Increasingly, workplace bullying is being carried out through uses of technology and the Internet on social media sites and e-mail (i.e., cyberbullying).

Differences in rates of bullying are reported by occupation. For example, some studies suggest that 44% of nurses have been bullied during the course of their working activities (Dellasega, 2009). Other occupations in which there is evidence of bullying include restaurant employees, school faculty and staff, business professionals, transportation workers, and police officers (Mathisen, Einarsen, & Mykletun, 2008; McKay, Arnold, Fratzl, & Thomas, 2008; Niedhammer, David, & Degioanni, 2007).

Increasingly workplace programs focus specifically on reducing bullying and bullying awareness within the workplace (Privitera & Campbell, 2009). Often they will utilize strategies to limit job demands (lower stress and susceptibility to being the target of bullying) and increase job resources to reduce workplace bullying (e.g., hot lines and supervisor training). One group identified as high risk for experiencing bullying are young women who feel dissatisfied with their working conditions (Ariza-Montes, Muniz, Montero-Simó, & Araque-Padilla, 2013).

Factory Floor- and Office-Level Evidenced-Based Psychologically Healthy and Safe Workplace Interventions and Practices

Workplaces have factory floor- and office-level psychologically healthy and safe workplace interventions and practices to address their particular workforce health needs. From small and midsized organizations to large national employers, these practices engage employees at the workplace (factory floor and office), and are lower cost and practical, with fairly easy administration. Outside vendors both national and local compete for contracts to offer the interventions. Examples of widely implemented evidence-based interventions and practices are:

Criminal behavior and fraud protection: Crime within the workplace is not an uncommon occurrence. Possible offenses include steeling, robbery, vandalism, fraud, and more. The National Crime Prevention Council developed the Workplace Safety program to address criminal behavior within the workplace. This program works to promote employer and employee awareness of possible criminal problems within the workplace. Employer education includes safe and knowledgeable hiring practices, the use of background checks, and creation or implementation practice of emergency action plans. Employee education programs include recognition of unidentified patrons, angry patrons, as well as other angry employees (National Crime Prevention Council, n.d.).

Workplace fraud can be common and be financially devastating to an employer or employee. Some common types of fraud include workers' compensation fraud, health care provider fraud, employer fraud, and injured worker fraud. The Washington State Department of Labor and Industries has established a program to educate employers and employees about fraud to reduce fraud within the workplace and prevent the financial repercussions felt by the employees and employers alike. This program includes online educational resources, fraud reporting systems, policy and legislature support, and fraud detection tips/information (Washington State Department of Labor & Industries, n.d.).

Microaggressions prevention: The notion of microaggressions has garnered national attention in recent years as individuals (employees) have begun to use social media to express their frustration of having to endure examples of this behavior on a daily basis. Microaggressions—defined as brief and commonplace daily, verbal, behavioral, or environmental indignities, whether intentional or unintentional, that communicate hostile, derogatory, or negative slights and insults directed toward an individual due to their group membership—often automatically and unconsciously have been found to be a significant barrier to performance (Sue, 2010). Examples of microaggressions include joking that you cannot give a female office worker constructive feedback or she'll cry, using derogatory names, saying to an employee *it's not your fault so don't take it personally* or *but that's just the way long-term employees are*, and denying participation in a homophobic behavior. As part of creating a psychologically safe environment, efforts to prevent microaggressions focus on interrupting and stopping the behavior among employers and employees.

Privacy safeguards: With the increase in the use of technology, information sharing, and workplace health promotion, information confidentiality and privacy becomes an important issue to consider. While certain personal and health information about employees is made available to their employers, other information is not needed or should not be made available to the employer. Many employers pursue background checks, health screenings, references, and new employee screenings for their new and existing employees. The use of the information gained through these interactions is sensitive material that must be protected to various degrees.

Emergency Communication Systems/Alert lines: OSHA recommends that "employers should establish effective safety and health management systems and prepare their workers to handle emergencies before they arise" (OSHA, 2014). A successful emergency action plan, especially in large companies and universities, includes an alert line or emergency communication system. An emergency communication system is a method or methods to notify a large group of people, such as employees, students, or workers, with the details of an occurring or pending emergency situation. An emergency communication system in the workplace often includes automated phone calls, text messages, and/or e-mails to notify employees, workers, students, or affiliated persons of a site-specific emergency or the business's reaction to a current large-scale emergency.

Psychologically Healthy and Safe Workplace Environment Priority Implementation Challenges

Workplaces are social organizations. The value of individual and social processes in organizations are recognized to be positive. They enhance and improve a workplace in one or more ways—to boost productivity, improve morale, or make the workplace more effective From a positive perspective they motivate and engage employees to excel. They contribute to a psychologically healthy and safe work environment. These same processes also have a dark side (Furnham & Taylor, 2004; Pritchard, 2004; Zins et al., 2013). The processes can have negative outcomes. They manifest themselves at the individual, group, and organizational levels. They reflect intentional choices by individuals, groups, and organizations. Implementation of the psychologically health and safe workplace program priority requires an awareness of the individual and social processes outcomes that are barriers and deterrents to psychologically healthy and safe workplace environments.

Subtle (and Not-So-Subtle) Discrimination in Organizations

At one time unfair and unhealthy behavior and discrimination in the workplace were open, tolerated, and even encouraged. Blatant discrimination against women and minorities, the disabled, and older workers only began to diminish to a substantial degree in the United States after the civil rights legislation of the 1960s. Subsequently the workplace has become more open and tolerant. Nevertheless, a variety of groups and individuals continue to suffer from unfair treatment in the workplace despite laws, court decisions, and social pressure (Dipboye & Halverson, 2004). Differential treatment is not necessarily unfair but becomes unfair when it is based on "attributes irrelevant to judgment of a person's competence or worth" (Piper, 1993) and is "selectively unjustified" (Gaertner & Dovidio, 1986).

Employers by law are prohibited from using neutral employment policies and practices that have a disproportionately negative effect (i.e., discriminate) on applicants or employees of a particular race, color, religion, sex (including pregnancy), or national origin, or on an individual with a disability or class of individuals with disabilities, if the policies or practices at issue are not job-related and necessary to the operation of the business. Employers are also prohibited from using neutral employment policies and practices that have a disproportionately negative impact on applicants or employees age 40 or older, if the policies or practices at issue are not based on a reasonable factor other than age (EEOC, n.d.-a). Blatant varieties of discrimination include racism (EEOC, 2014b), sexism (EEOC, 2014c, and ageism (EEOC, 2014a).

Subtle-variety discrimination is harder to report but is as damaging, if not more damaging, to the workplace environment. Box 13.1 illustrates a subtle-variety discrimination that most likely would not be reportable or a successful basis for a lawsuit. Social exclusion, marginalization, private

BOX 13.1   NOT-SO-SUBTLE WORKPLACE DISCRIMINATION (ADAPTED FROM DIPBOYE & HALVERSON, 2014)

A recently transitioning female-to-male worker for a large corporation in a professional position is afraid he may lose his job and feels isolated from his cisgender male coworkers. An invitation to lunch is seldom extended. At meetings he often feels as though his male coworkers interrupt him and fail to give his contributions the serious consideration they deserve. He feels that when he asserts himself in meetings he is seen as overly aggressive, but when he is quiet he is considered to be "too emotional." The coworkers, on the other hand, generally feel he is qualified in several respects and would admit that he has done well in the technical aspects of his job. In private they say that he lacks some of the business savvy and social skills needed for the job. They assume he will not be promoted anytime soon and may even be fired due to his appearance and inability to currently pass as completely male.

misgivings of colleagues, and interruptions in meetings create an unhealthy workplace environment. People hold stereotypical beliefs in check out of concern with violating personal and public standards of conducts. Things go unspoken, creating an environment of ambiguity and ambivalence among all parties.

Person-Specific Arrangements

In person-specific arrangements individual workers seek special treatment or working conditions differing from what their coworkers receive. Despite the advantages for an employee, supervisor, and employer, these deals skirt the dark side of an organization. They can be collusive, causing bad feelings, injustices, and resentments. Rousseau (2004) identifies three workplace categories of special arrangements. The first category, *preferential*, is favored treatment to workers by a supervisor or manager to strengthen their relationship, as in the case of holding lower standards for a friend of the boss or extending special privileges (e.g., extended lunch breaks, leaving work early). The second, *unauthorized*, applies to illicit appropriation of workplace resources by workers, as in the case of theft or misrepresentation (e.g., taking home office supplies and tools, setting aside products until on sale and purchasing at lower price). The third category, *idiosyncratic*, involves negotiations between employer and employee based on the perceived employee value to the workplace, as in the case of getting special training and distinct job titles. The boundaries among the three person-specific arrangements can be ambiguous (Figure 13.2). The first

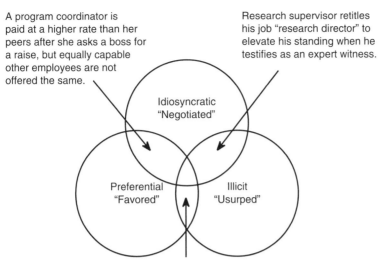

A program coordinator is paid at a higher rate than her peers after she asks a boss for a raise, but equally capable other employees are not offered the same.

Research supervisor retitles his job "research director" to elevate his standing when he testifies as an expert witness.

Idiosyncratic "Negotiated"

Preferential "Favored"

Illicit "Usurped"

Boss tells worker it is okay to help himself to the store's food when working nights.

Figure 13.2   Blurry Boundaries Among Person-Specific Employment Practices
Source: Rousseau, 2004.

two categories (preferential and unauthorized) are particularly problematic, and in some cases illegal, but they are common in the workplace and pose a threat to a psychologically safe and healthy workplace environment. The third category, idiosyncratic, serves the interest of both worker and the organization and is common. The potential for these relationships to be positive, not negative and destructive, lies in creating arrangements so that third parties—particularly immediate coworkers, supervisors, and managers—view them as fair.

Engaging workers to create a psychologically health and safe workplace environment involves frank discussion and knowledge of the person-specific arrangements that occur in the workplace. Supervisors and managers are key to program implementation that assumes everyone is being treated equally. It is therefore important to be honest about the person-specific arrangements to avoid being perceived as dishonest, uninformed, or naïve about how an organization really works.

Employee Family and Intimate Partner Needs and Concerns

Creation of a psychologically healthy and safe workplace environment opens up that workplace to the employee family and intimate partner needs and concerns. Part of the workplace health promotion program implementation recognizes and perhaps will rely on employee families and loved ones to influence and support healthy employee behaviors. A family/work-life program as part of mental health workplace priority program implementation is a vehicle to recognize the importance of families and partners. Likewise, employers through the FMLA address the needs and rights of employees to attend to family member needs.

Creating a psychologically healthy and safe workplace environment brings with it the knowledge that family problems and struggles, and in particular intimate-partner violence (i.e., domestic violence), are behaviors that the employer is willing and ready to address. Intimate-partner violence can affect workplace in at least four ways: (1) when a perpetrator harasses, stalks, is physically violent, or otherwise present at the workplace, (2) when employee workplace performance is diminished due to abusive behavior occurring outside the workplace, (3) when a perpetrator is less productive because of past, present, or planning abusive behaviors, and (4) when coworkers of perpetrators or victims are fearful for their own safety or less productive because of the abuse being experienced or perpetrated by their coworker (Reeves, 2004). A challenge of creating healthy and safe workplaces includes dealing with difficult employee issues and concerns such as initiate-partner violence.

Root Causes Beyond the Workplace

Three root cause issues flow from the larger environment surrounding the organization into the workplace. First, high-quality, affordable, stable housing located close to the workplace and resources leads to reduced exposure to toxins and stress, stronger relationships and willingness to act collectively among neighbors, greater economic security for families, and increased access to services (including health care) and resources (such as parks and supermarkets) that influence health. Second, improve transit options by providing incentives for use of mass transit and nonmotorized vehicle transportation. Advocate for streets that are safe and accessible for all users to encourage walking and bicycling (Smart Growth for America's Complete Streets, 2015). Enhancing the safety, accessibility, and afford-ability of mass transit is also essential. Increased use of these types of transit will decrease air pollution and increase physical activity, which will lead to healthier individuals and communities. Third, work with schools to increase high school graduation rates of poor and minority students. These students are the future workforce for the organization. In general the students do not receive equitable resources at the schools that they attend. The proportion of minority students attending high-poverty, high-minority schools is 60%, while less than 20% of Whites attend high-poverty, high-minority schools (Orfield & Lee, 2005). High-poverty schools often have inadequate, run-down facilities (Acevedo-Garcia, Osypuk, McArdle, & Williams, 2008) or receive lower per-pupil spending allocations from federal, state, and local districts. Long-term, a psychologically healthy and safe workplace environment requires that organizations address issues external to the workplace that potentially are harmful and destructive to the workplace.

Advocacy and Resource Partnerships and Organizations

An increasing number of organizations are working with employers to create psychologically healthy and safe workplace environments. They provide ongoing research, materials, and advocacy for the best, evidence-based practices that support and maintain psychologically healthy and safe workplace environments. Among those groups are:

American Psychological Association Center for Organization Excellence—Psychologically Healthy Workplace Program (http://www.apaexcellence.org/resources/)

An online employer resource center to support employees' psychological health and well-being and enhance organizational performance and productivity. Resources are in five categories: employee involvement, work-life balance, employee growth and development, health and safety, and employee recognition.

Work Safe Victoria—Workplace bullying: prevention and response (https://www.worksafe.vic.gov.au/)

A guide on how employers can implement measures to eliminate or reduce workplace bullying, so far as is reasonably practicable. It also provides practical information for employers on what to do when an issue is raised.

The Canadian Centre for Occupational Health and Safety Mental Health in the Workplace (http://www.ccohs.ca/)

The Canadian Centre for Occupational Health and Safety (CCOHS) fulfills its mandate to promote workplace health and safety, and encourage attitudes and methods that will lead to improved worker physical and mental health, through a wide range of products and services. Mental health claims are the fastest growing category of disability costs in Canada, and represent a significant health problem in Canadian workplaces across all sectors. Mental Health Works helps workplaces better address the issues of mental health and mental illness at work by raising awareness of the effects of unaddressed mental health issues at work, training managers in effective communication and accommodation approaches, and educating employers and employees about creating mentally healthy workplaces.

Society for Industrial and Organizational Psychology (http://www .siop.org/default.aspx)

Industrial-organizational (I-O) psychology is the scientific study of the workplace. Rigor and methods of psychology are applied to issues of critical relevance to business, including talent management, coaching, assessment, selection, training, organizational development, performance, and work-life balance. The Society for Industrial and Organizational Psychology is a division of the American Psychological Association.

American Association of Critical-Care Nurses—Healthy Workplace Standards (http://www.aacn.org)

The American Association of Critical-Care Nurses recognizes the inextricable links among quality of the work environment, excellent nursing practice, and patient care outcomes. AACCN created model standards for a psychologically healthy workplace environment to produces high staff performance and good patient outcomes.

Mental Health Commission of Canada—Psychological Health & Safety: An Action Guide for Employers (http://www.mental healthcommission.ca)

The guide is mainly intended for employers and human resource personnel who are considering programs and policies to improve psychological health in their organizations. This material is also relevant to union leaders, occupational health care providers, frontline managers, legal and regulatory professionals, and others with a stake in maintaining the psychological health and safety of workers. To make it easier for employers to foster an integrated process of change, the Mental Health Commission created a six-step implementation process—Policy, Planning, Promotion, Prevention, Process and Persistence—to create and sustain a psychologically healthy and safe workplace environment.

National Standard of Canada for Psychological Health and Safety in the Workplace (http://www.mentalhealthcommission.ca/English /node/5346)

The National Standard of Canada for Psychological Health and Safety in the Workplace, the first of its kind in the world, was launched in January 2013. The Standard is a voluntary set of guidelines, tools, and resources focused on promoting employees' psychological health and preventing psychological harm due to workplace factors. The Standard focuses on prevention, promotion, and guidance to staged implementation.

Summary

A psychologically healthy and safe workplace environment promotes employees' psychological well-being and does not harm employee mental health in negligent, reckless, or intentional ways. Implementing a program to promote psychologically healthy and safe workplace environments is similar to programming to promote physically healthy and safe environments and thereby contributes to lowering employer and employee health care costs. Different about psychologically unhealthy and unsafe work environments is their pervasive impact upon a workplace culture and climate with potentially serious negative impacts on workplace production, product quality, and consumer satisfaction and service. The pervasive nature of a psychologically unhealthy and unsafe workplace permeates (and literally infects) workers' sense of well-being. Program implementation includes sexual harassment prevention; drug-free workplace programs; violence prevention; dignity and respect (civility) programs; bullying (including cyberbullying); criminal behavior and fraud protection; and privacy safeguards. Challenges to a psychologically healthy and safe workplace result from an organizations' social process, which both creates positive outcomes (e.g., motivated, engaged, productive employees) and negative, dark-side outcomes (e.g., discrimination, person-specific arrangements, human resource practices concerns). Finally, creating healthy and safe workplaces includes dealing with difficult employee issues and concerns such as initiate-partner violence and root causes of mental health problems beyond the workplace.

For Practice and Discussion

1. Any workplace that has money exchange and transfer on its premise (e.g., retail stores, banks, movie theaters, supermarkets) prepares an Accident Prevention Program, which includes evaluating the hazards for violence in the workplace (e.g., robbery). Select a local workplace with money exchange and transfer on its premise. Prepare an Accident

Prevention Program with a plan that outlines measures to reduce this risk, such as training workers on de-escalation techniques, installing adequate lighting in parking lots, and providing drop safes. Some workplaces may also consider if personal protective equipment is needed (e.g., body armor for some law enforcement personnel), and address this as well. What is your emotional reaction to preparing the Accident Prevention Program?

2. Select a psychologically healthy and safety workplace program area (e.g., sexual harassment prevention, drug free workplace, violence prevention, dignity and respect/civility programs, bullying and cyber-bullying, criminal behavior and fraud protection, privacy safeguards). Research the program offerings for the area by industry type (e.g., manufacturing, health care, education, mining, transportation). Compare and contrast the scope of the programs and training currently offered at workplaces. How can the programs be improved?

3. Social processes in organizations create positive outcomes (e.g., motivated, engaged, productive employees) and negative, dark-side outcomes (e.g., discrimination, person-specific arrangements, human resource practices concerns). Identify and describe a social process that you have witnessed and/or knowingly or unknowingly participated in. Describe the outcomes (positive and negative).

4. A large percentage of workplace problems such as absenteeism, lower productivity, turnover, and excessive use of medical benefits are due to family violence. Battered women arrive an hour late for work and are harassed by their partner while they are at work. How best can workplaces address initiate partner violence? Research and brainstorm strategies.

Case Study: Sexual Images and Videos on Employee Computer—What Would You Do?

While working on a colleague's computer, Renee Brown, a university human resource office manager, found sexual images and videos. The images ranged from photographs of nude women to graphic videos of sexual acts. According to the university's human resource policies and union agreements, the images and videos are not permitted. The images create an unsafe psychological workplace environment. Ms. Brown feels very negatively about the images. She wants to confront the colleague. If you were Ms. Brown, what would you do?

KEY TERMS

Psychological healthy and safe workplace environments

Negative consequences

Sexual harassment prevention

Drug free workplace

Violence prevention

Dignity and respect (civility)

Bullying (including cyberbullying)

Criminal behavior and fraud protection

Microaggressions

Privacy safeguards

Discrimination

Person-specific arrangements

Human resource practices

Intimate-partner violence

Root causes

References

Acevedo-Garcia, D., Osypuk, T. L., McArdle, N., & Williams, D. R. (2008). Toward a policy-relevant analysis of geographic and racial/ethnic disparities in child health. *Health Affairs, 27*(2), 321–333.

American Association of Occupational Health Nurses. (2015). *Preventing workplace violence.* Retrieved May 22, 2015 from http://www.aaohn.org/practice/position-statements.html/

Ariza-Montes, A., Muniz, N. M., Montero-Simó, M. J., & Araque-Padilla, R. A. (2013). Workplace bullying among healthcare workers. *International Journal of Environmental Research and Public Health, 10*(8), 3121–3139.

Bureau de normalisation du Québec, & Canadian Standards Association. (2013). *Psychological health and safety in the workplace.* Retrieved from http://www.csagroup.org/documents/codes-and-standards/publications/CAN_CSA-Z1003-13_BNQ_9700-803_2013_EN.pdf

Centers for Disease Control and Prevention. (n.d.). *Stress . . . at work.* NIOSH Pub. No. 99-101. Retrieved from http://www.cdc.gov/niosh/docs/99-101/

Dellasega, C. A. (2009). Bullying among nurses. *The American Journal of Nursing, 109*(1), 52–58.

Department of Veterans Affairs, National Center for Organization Development. (2014, July 17). *Civility, respect, and engagement in the workplace (CREW).* Retrieved from http://www.va.gov/ncod/crew.asp

Dipboye, R. L., & Halverson, S. K. (2004). Subtle (and not so subtle) discrimination in organizations. In R. W. Griffin & A. M. O'Leary-Kelly (Eds.), *The dark side of organizational behavior* (pp. 131–158) San Francisco, CA: Jossey-Bass.

Furnham, A., & Taylor, J. (2004). *The darker side of behaviour at work: Understanding and avoiding employees leaving, thieving and deceiving.* London, England: Palgrave Macmillan.

Gaertner, S. L., & Dovidio, J. F. (1986). *The aversive form of racism.* San Diego, CA: Academic Press.

Gates, T. G., & Mitchell, C.G. (2013). Workplace stigma-related experiences among lesbian, gay, and bisexual workers: Implications for social policy and practice. *Journal of Workplace Behavioral Health, 28*(3), 159–171.

Human Rights Campaign. (2015, March 9). *Employment Non-Discrimination Act.* Retrieved from http://www.hrc.org/resources/entry/employment-non-discrimination-act

Hunt, C., Davidson, M., Fielden, S., & Hoel, H. (2010). Reviewing sexual harassment in the workplace—An intervention model. *Personnel Review, 39*(5), 655–673.

Lucas, K. (2015). Workplace dignity: Communicating inherent, earned, and remediated dignity. *Journal of Management Studies, 52*(5), 630–643.

Mathisen, G. E., Einarsen, S., & Mykletun, R. (2008). The occurrences and correlates of bullying and harassment in the restaurant sector. *Scandinavian Journal of Psychology, 49*(1), 59–68.

McKay, R., Arnold, D. H., Fratzl, J., & Thomas, R. (2008). Workplace bullying in academia: A Canadian study. *Employee Responsibilities and Rights Journal, 20*(2), 77–100.

Miles, N. (2011). *Straight allies: How they help create gay-friendly workplaces.* Stonewall. Retrieved from http://www.stonewall.org.uk/documents/straight_allies_2.pdf

National Crime Prevention Council (n.d.). *Workplace safety.* Retrieved from http://www.ncpc.org/topics/workplace-safety

Niedhammer, I., David, S., & Degioanni, S. (2007). Economic activities and occupations at high risk for workplace bullying: Results from a large-scale cross-sectional survey in the general working population in France. *International Archives of Occupational and Environmental Health, 80*(4), 346–353.

Occupational Safety and Health Administration. (2015). *Help.* Retrieved from https://www.osha.gov/SLTC/workplaceviolence/

Orfield, G., & Lee, C. (2005, January). *Why segregation matters: Poverty and educational inequality.* The Civil Rights Project at Harvard University. Retrieved from http://civilrightsproject.ucla.edu/research/k-12-education/integration-and-diversity/why-segregation-matters-poverty-and-educational-inequality/orfield-why-segregation-matters-2005.pdf

Phillips, J., Holland, M., Baldwin, D., Meuleveld, L., Mueller, K., Perkinson, B., . . . Dreger, M. (2015). Marijuana in the workplace: Guidance for occupational health professionals and employers: Joint guidance statement of the American Association of Occupational Health Nurses and the American College of Occupational and Environmental Medicine. *Journal of Occupational and Environmental Medicine, 57*(4), 459–475.

Piper, A. M. S. (1993). Higher order discrimination. In O. Flanagan & A. O. Rorty (Eds.), *Identity, character, and morality: Essays in moral psychology* (3rd ed., pp. 285–309). Cambridge, MA: MIT Press.

Pritchard, R. D. (2004). Foreword. In R. W. Griffin & A. O'Leary-Kelly, A. *The dark side of organizational behavior* (p. xv.): San Francisco, CA: Jossey-Bass.

Privitera, C., & Campbell, M. A. (2009). Cyberbullying: The new face of workplace bullying? *CyberPsychology & Behavior, 12*(4), 395–400.

Reeves, C. A. (2004). When the dark side of families enters the workplace: The case of intimate partner violence. In R. W. Griffin & A. O'Leary-Kelly (Eds.), *The dark side of organizational behavior* (pp. 103–127). San Francisco, CA: Jossey-Bass.

Rousseau, D. M. (2004). Under the table deals: Preferential, unauthorized or idiosyncratic. In R. W. Griffin & A. O'Leary-Kelly (Eds.), *The dark side of organizational behavior* (pp. 262–290). San Francisco, CA: Jossey-Bass.

Smart Growth for America's Complete Streets. (2015). *National Complete Streets Coalition.* Retrieved May 15, 2015, from http://www.smartgrowthamerica.org/complete-streets

State of Queensland Department of Justice and Attorney-General. (2012). *Psychological health for small business.* Retrieved from http://www.deir.qld.gov.au/workplace/resources/pdfs/psychhealth-smallbusiness.pdf

Sue, D. W. (2010). *Microaggressions in everyday life: Race, gender, and sexual orientation.* Hoboken, NJ: Wiley.

U.S. Equal Employment Opportunity Commission (n.d.-a). *Prohibited employment policies/practices.* Retrieved from http://www.eeoc.gov/laws/practices/index.cfm

U.S. Equal Employment Opportunity Commission. (n.d.-b). *Sexual harassment.* Retrieved from http://www.eeoc.gov/laws/types/sexual_harassment.cfm

U.S. Equal Employment Opportunity Commission. (2014a). *EEOC sues Memphis Light, Gas & Water for age discrimination* [Press release]. Retrieved from http://www.eeoc.gov/eeoc/newsroom/release/2-28-14.cfm

U.S. Equal Employment Opportunity Commission. (2014b). *Sparks restaurant to pay $56,000 and provide injunctive relief in EEOC retaliation lawsuit* [Press release]. Retrieved from http://www.eeoc.gov/eeoc/newsroom/release/2-5-14a.cfm

U.S. Equal Employment Opportunity Commission. (2014c). *Wal-Mart to pay $87,500 to settle EEOC suit for unlawful retaliation* [Press release]. Retrieved from http://www.eeoc.gov/eeoc/newsroom/release/1-27-14a.cfm

University of Alberta Human Resources. (2012). *Framework for a psychologically healthy & safe workplace.* Retrieved from http://www.hrs.ualberta.ca/HealthandWellness/~/media/hrs/HealthWellness/WorkplaceHealth/Leaders_Package_PHSW-1.pdf

Washington State Department of Labor & Industries. (n.d.). *Fraud & complaints.* Retrieved May 3, 2015, from http://www.lni.wa.gov/ClaimsIns/FraudComp/default.asp

Zins, J. E., Elias, M. J., & Maher, C. A. (2013). Prevention and intervention. In J. E. Zins, M. J. Elias, & C. A. Maher (Eds.), *Bullying, victimization, and peer harassment: A handbook of prevention and intervention* (pp. 3–8). New York, NY: Routledge.

WORKPLACE HEALTH PROMOTION PROGRAM IMPLEMENTATION HEALTH PRIORITY: HEALTH EDUCATION IN AN eHEALTH ENVIRONMENT

Program Implementation: Health Education Priority in an eHealth Environment

The goal in implementing the health education priority–focused workplace health program is to promote a variety of workers' learning experiences to facilitate voluntary action that is conducive to health (Green, Kreuter, Deeds, & Partridge, 1980). These educational experiences facilitate gaining new knowledge, adjusting attitudes, and acquiring and practicing new skills and behaviors that could change health status. The educational strategies are delivered through individual (one-to-one) or group instruction or interactive electronic media in order to promote changes in individuals, groups of individuals, or the general population. Mass communication strategies that might be used include public service announcements, webinars, social marketing techniques, and other new strategies from text messaging to blogging. Social media (media for social interaction, using highly accessible and scalable publishing techniques and web-based platforms) is now viewed as a tool to promote health with the options to communicate health and safety information in the workplace as it changes with each new technological advance.

Health education in the workplace now relies on health communications, which is defined as the art and technique of informing, influencing, and motivating individual,

LEARNING OBJECTIVES

- Discuss program implementation with a health education priority in an eHealth environment

- Identify evidence-based health education policies, practices, interventions, and services

- Explain health education workplace program challenges

- Describe advocacy partnerships and organizations

institutional, and public audiences about important health (and health care) issues (U.S. Department of Health and Human Services, 2000). It has been described further as "a multifaceted and multidisciplinary approach to reach different audiences and share health-related information with the goal of influencing, engaging, and supporting individuals, workplaces, communities, health professionals, special groups, policy makers, and the public to champion, introduce, adopt, or sustain a behavior, practice, or policy that will ultimately improve health outcomes" (Schiavo, 2007).

eHealth (e-Health) is a relatively recent term connected with health promotion and health care practice supported by electronic processes and communication (Table 14.1). Usage of the term varies: some would argue it is interchangeable with health informatics with a broad definition covering electronic/digital processes in health, while others use it in the narrower sense of health care practice using the Internet. It can also include health applications and links on mobile phones, referred to as m-Health. Since about 2011, the increasing recognition of the need for better cybersecurity and regulation may result in the need for these specialized resources to develop safer eHealth solutions that can withstand these growing threats. The term "eHealth" can encompass a range of services or systems that are at the edge of health, medicine, health care, and information technology.

The health education priority–focused program implementation is the union of health education, health communication, and eHealth with the potential to be transformative for workers' health. The priority represents

Table 14.1   What Is e-Health? (U.S. Department of Health and Human Services, 2014)

What is e-Health? e-Health is the use of digital information and communication technologies to improve people's health and health care. The increasing use of technologies, especially the Internet and mobile devices, to manage health highlights the potential of e-Health tools to improve population health. There are numerous tools and resources that fall under "e-Health" including:

- Online communities and support groups
- Online health information
- Online health self-management tools
- Online communication with health care providers
- Online access to personal health records

Why is e-Health important? e-Health tools and resources enable health care consumers and their caregivers to improve health in a number of ways including:

- Real-time monitoring of health vital signs and indicators
- Managing chronic conditions
- Gathering information to make informed medical decisions
- Communicating with health care providers

a merging of health and medicine. No longer is health education in the workplace about health and safety but rather involves supporting employees' engagement and full participation in promoting their health as well as being decision makers in their health care. eHealth is not limited to the workplace, and therefore workplace health education is not limited to the workplace. It can now span employees' workplaces, communities, and homes, thereby involving family and friends.

Evidence-Based Health Education Policies, Practices, Interventions, and Services in an eHealth Environment

Health education in an eHealth environment can be a time and money saver for workplace health promotion programs. It has the potential to improve individuals' health status, life quality, and health care quality while lowering health care costs and expenses for the employer and employee. It provides a vehicle to deliver current workplace health and safety information that complies with OSHA regulations, monitors worker compliance, and provides individual employees feedback and support to improve productivity and health.

Health education in an eHealth environment creates awareness of an issue, changes attitudes toward a health behavior, and encourages and motivates individuals to follow recommended health behaviors. However, it is important to recognize that health education alone cannot change behavior. It can increase awareness and knowledge, prompt action, and reinforce attitudes, but it cannot compensate for inadequate health care services or for behaviors that are complex in nature and require more than just education (National Institutes of Health & National Cancer Institute, 2001). Health education in an eHealth environment impacts each of the other implementation priorities; it is the vehicle by which we communicate and interact with employees as we implement all of the workplace health promotion priority areas. It spans all of the potential employee populations, educating them about health promotion as well as current treatments and options when confronting a medical treatment decision. The health education in an eHealth environment implementation priority is dedicated to keeping employees up to date and supported in their quest for good health.

eHealth Technologies

eHealth technologies merge health and medicine to both promote employee health and engage and support employees to be decision makers in their health care. Some of the technologies are clearly for health promotion such as the personal health devices (e.g., pedometers and activity trackers, interactive daily food logs), while others are part of medical treatment including the medical devices (e.g., pacemakers, hearing aids). The majority of the eHealth technologies use technology to enhance and streamline health care, combining aspects of health promotion and medicine to improve individuals' life quality (e.g., e-Prescribing, telemedicine, virtual health teams). They increase service access and support for the individual who otherwise might not be able to access services in a timely matter. These eHealth technologies now exist, although maybe not in all locations. However, increasingly it can be expected that individuals (employers and employees) will question what might be potential benefits of the technologies for a particular organization and how to access and use the technologies. Therefore awareness and education of the technologies is considered as part of workplace health education. Prominent eHealth technologies include:

- ePrescribing: access to prescribing options, printing prescriptions to patients, and sometimes electronic transmission of prescriptions from doctors to pharmacists.

- Telemedicine: physical and psychological treatments at a distance, including telemonitoring of individual functions.

- Personal health devices: wearable fitness and medical devices that monitor activities, vital signs, and symptoms that interface individuals and health care providers via cloud, cell phones, apps, and GPS platforms.

- Health knowledge management: for instance, in an overview of latest medical journals, best-practices guidelines or epidemiological tracking (e.g., physician resources such as Medscape and MDLinx).

- Virtual health care teams: consisting of health care professionals who collaborate and share information on individuals through digital equipment (for transmural care).

- mHealth (or m-Health): includes the use of mobile devices in collecting aggregate and individual level health data; providing health care information to practitioners, researchers, and individuals; real-time monitoring of individual vitals; and direct provision of care (via mobile telemedicine).

- Medical research using grids: powerful computing and data management capabilities to handle large amounts of heterogeneous data.

- Health care information systems: also often refer to software solutions for appointment scheduling, individual data management, work schedule management, and other administrative tasks surrounding health.

- Medical devices: range from blood glucose test strips and stethoscopes to more complex products, such as hearing aids, pacemakers, and joint replacements. These technologies are used in hospitals, doctors' offices, and in patients' homes to diagnose, treat, or prevent illness. Many people have benefited from such recent advances, and Americans increasingly rely on medical devices.

Consumer Health Education and Informatics

Consumer health education and informatics refer to employees' use of electronic resources to investigate health and medical topics. Increasingly individuals use the Internet to determine a diagnosis or identify a medical condition (Fox & Duggan, 2013). Individuals can search for health information anytime and anywhere using computers and mobile devices (e.g., tablet and cell phones). A 2012 Pew survey of the Internet users revealed that 72% had looked online for health information in the past year (Pew Research Center, 2012). When the Pew survey started in the early 2000s, individuals were searching for information on:

- Specific diseases or medical problems
- Specific medical treatments or procedures
- Doctors or health-related professionals
- Hospital or medical facilities
- Health insurance, including private, health exchanges, Medicare, or Medicaid
- Environmental health hazards (Fox, 2011)

Over time, what consumers search for has expanded to include the following:

- Food safety or recalls
- Drug safety or recalls
- Pregnancy and child birth
- Memory loss and dementia or Alzheimer's
- Medical test results
- Management of chronic pain

- Long term care for elderly or disabled persons
- End of life decisions (Fox, 2011)

These topics suggest individuals (employees) are seeking online health information about time-sensitive topic (such as recalls) as well as for complex or chronic health conditions. Time-sensitive information requires the availability of dynamically updated online factual content. In contrast, complex or chronic health conditions do not require minute-to-minute updates but incremental changes as new information becomes available. In designing workplace health promotion programs it is therefore important to understand what employees are asking for when searching for health information and to design program consumer health education and informatics content to answer the questions. Likewise it is also essential to know the reasonable life span of the information that is posted and to update or retract it in a responsible fashion (Brixey, 2014).

Electronic Medical Records and Electronic Health Records

Electronic medical records (EMRs) and electric health records (EHRs) are two eHealth technologies that, while not directly part of a workplace health promotion program, can and do impact programs due to being sources of program information as well as being an indicator of the level of sophistication of the health care delivery that employees receive within health care systems.

EMRs are digital versions of the paper charts in clinicians' offices, clinics, and hospitals. EMRs contain notes and information collected by and for the clinicians in that office, clinic, or hospital and are mostly used by providers for diagnosis and treatment. EMRs are more valuable than paper records because they enable providers to track data over time, identify patients for preventive visits and screenings, and monitor patients. An EMR is more beneficial than a paper record because it allows providers to:

- Track data over time
- Identify individuals who are due for preventive visits and screenings
- Monitor how individuals measure up to certain parameters, such as vaccinations and blood pressure readings
- Improve overall quality of care in a practice

An EMR contains the standard medical and clinical data gathered in one provider's office. EHRs go beyond the data collected in the provider's office and include a more comprehensive individual history. EHRs are designed to contain and share information from all providers involved in an individual's care. EHR data can be created, managed, and consulted by authorized providers and staff from across more than one health care organization. Unlike EMRs, EHRs also allow an individual's health record to move with them—to other health care providers, specialists, hospitals, nursing homes, and even across states. An EHR can:

* Give quicker access to individual's health information

* Help to protect medical privacy

* Give a summary of each visit

* Help to prevent drug errors

* Make health information available to share with medical providers, according to individual's preferences, in order to coordinate care

Personal Health Records

A personal health record (PHR) is an electronic or paper health record maintained and updated by an individual for himself or herself; a tool that individuals can use to collect, track, and share past and current information about their health or the health of someone in their care (American Health Information Management Association, 2012). PHRs are one method to improve health for individuals and reduce the cost of health care (Hillestad et al., 2005). There is growing interest among employers for employee PHRs as part of a strategy to encourage employees to engage in their own health care and to empower personal responsibility for health. Unlike electronic medical records, PHRs allow employees to control the information and access to data within their PHR. Conceptually, the PHR is not linked to a single provider or health plan, spans an employee's lifetime, and can contain data entered by employees that might not normally be part of a medical record (e.g., nonprescription medications and supplements, alternative and complementary modalities of care). However, there are some concerns about employees' willingness to use a PHR if offered one by their employer. Trust and concern about confidentiality and security appear to be the major factors that contribute to this reluctance. Nevertheless, employers are looking carefully at PHRs as yet another eHealth tool to convey to their employees the importance of personal responsibility for health.

Concerns about PHRs include limited in functionality especially for individuals with health in emergencies. Additionally, most records are stored in an electronic, interoperable format, which limits the transfer of data from that source to an individual's PHR. Nevertheless, results from the Personal Health Working Group work in the early 2000s, part of the Markle Foundation's Connecting for Health initiative, indicated that more than 70% of respondents would use one or more features of a PHR to e-mail their doctor, track immunizations, note mistakes in the record, transfer information to new providers, and get and track test results (Markle Connecting for Health, 2003). A coalition of large employers, including Walmart and Pitney Bowes, has formed to develop and implement a PHR for their employees (Ahern, Buckel, Aberger, & Follick, 2009). Microsoft (2015) created a secure PHR called *Health Vault* that is available free to the public with partnerships with health care providers and institutions to enable interoperability of information flow between the PHR and the EMR.

Blue Button Initiative—Personal Health (Patient) Portal

A personal health (patient) portal is a secure online website that gives individuals convenient 24-hour access to personal health information from anywhere with an Internet connection. Using a secure username and password, patients can view health information such as:

- Recent doctor visits
- Discharge summaries
- Medications
- Immunizations
- Allergies
- Lab results

Some personal health portals allow individuals to exchange secure e-mail with their health care teams, request prescription refills, schedule nonurgent appointments, check benefits and coverage, update contact information, make payments, download and complete forms, and view educational materials. For workplace health promotion programs the portals can enhance employee health care provider communication, empower employees, support care between visits, and, improve health outcomes (Office of the National Coordinator for Health Information Technology, n.d.).

The Blue Button initiative, a public-private partnership between the health care industry and the federal government that aims to empower all Americans with secure access to their own health information, is a model personal health portal. In 2010, the U.S. Department of Veterans Affairs (VA) launched the Blue Button Initiative to give veterans the ability to access and download their medical records from their MyHealtheVet online portal. Blue Button has expanded to other federal agencies and the private sector. Private-sector companies and organizations have pledged their support to increase individual (employee) access to (and use of) their own health data as a way to empower individuals to better manage their health and coordinate their health care. In 2013 Blue Button was expanded to include a standardized, machine-readable data format and additional functionality for the trusted, automated exchange of health care data and a release of the Blue Button implementation guide (Department of Veterans Affairs, n.d.).

Personal health portals are widely used by health care systems and are part of workplace health promotion programs to engage employees in the program. For example, myMedicationAdvisor is designed to promote the safe and proper use of medications. It also offers ways to save money on medications and helps employees get the most out of their pharmacy benefit (Abacus Group, n.d.). The information and tools on the website can help employees and their families to save money on medications, take medications correctly and safely, and better communicate with their doctor and pharmacist. It is where employees obtain medication list(s), forms, and instructions they need for any special medication buying program(s) offered by their employer or health plan.

Factory Floor- and Office-Level Evidence-Based Health Education Interventions and Practices

eHealth environments for health education operate at all levels of the workplace. They are present at the factory floor and office level as well as the executive suite. The eHealth technologies are available from the small and midsized employers to large national employers that engage employees at the workplace (factory floor and office), and are lower cost and practical, with fairly easy administration. Examples of widely implemented evidence-based interventions and practices are:

> **E-mails, tweeting, texting:** The use of e-mail, Twitter, and text messages in workplace health promotion is a common strategy that includes private health care provider communications, tailored health feedback (e.g., physical activity, nutritional intake, appointment reminders), weekly health promotion e-mail messages, and health care consumer satisfaction questionnaires. Employees' e-mailing, tweeting, and texting and their willingness to receive health promotion e-mails, tweets, and texts may not depend on employees' health status and health behavior, making the technologies a vehicle for reaching a wide variety of employees in

the workplace and encouraging active participation in health care (Nundy et al., 2013).

Regular e-mail and tweeting are not secure, so tailoring personal messages is limited. Likewise employers are concerned with the amount of e-mails and Twitter messages employees receive, which may limit access and use. Texting is more personal and does allow messages to be tailored to the person, such as with the following examples: texting a daily medication reminder message ("Time to take your medications."), dietary message ("Remember to avoid salt. Items high in salt include canned soups, deli meats, and fried foods."), appointment support ("Please remember to go to your appointment and take all of your medicines with you."), health management if experiencing symptoms ("Have you noticed that your legs are swollen or you are having trouble fitting into your shoes? If yes, call your physician."), and health care navigation ("If you're having trouble paying for your medicines, please make sure your doctor knows."). With texting and tweeting there may be a need to provide tutorials on receiving, reading, and sending text messages and how to use Twitter (Nundy et al., 2013).

Smartphone applications (apps): As the digital technologies proliferate, persuasive health communications are delivered with consideration to individuals' preferences, personalities, health literacy levels, and medical histories. Apps on telephones and tablets offer a unique opportunity for tailoring health promotion messages. With decision making algorithms and personal data, health promotion can be integrated into people's lives with the right message at the right time through the right communication channel. Data compiled by personal devices like the Fitbit Surge, Mio Fuse, Garmin, Jawbone and UP24 lets people see how their diets, how much they exercise, and how well they sleep compare with others. Some newer services tackle more-specific health issues, such as infertility, neighbor safety and cleanliness, and asthma. Apps put health promotion at people's fingertips.

The iPhone's Health App permits individuals to put health data from all kinds of apps in one place. However, the iPhone app is designed to handle much more than simply recording data. It can help individuals get a grip on areas of wellness, such as vitamin intake (for managing deficiencies, for example), blood glucose tracking, sleep, and even vitals like heart rate and blood pressure. Apple designed its app for users to be able to make sense of their data. And, perhaps one day, share that data with their health care providers. This can lead to more-effective workouts and help people meet fitness goals (Dennison, Morrison, Conway, & Yardley, 2013).

Health education and promotion apps

Kindara Fertility Tracker (http://www.kindara.com) asks women to chart various details about their cycles, body temperature, fitness activity, vitamins, moods, and more. It analyzes the information and identifies peak fertility days. It can tell women whether their results are typical or unusual within their demographic.

Neighborland (http://www.neighborland.com) aims to help community groups and government offices work well together. The app combines photos, data, and APIs from sources including Twitter, Google Maps and Instagram, agencies that report on real-estate parcels, transit systems, and "311" complaints about nuisances like noise, broken lights, and garbage. In 2012, the New Orleans Food Truck Coalition used Neighborland to collect community ideas and map "food deserts," which are areas lacking easy access to groceries and healthy food.

Ginger.io (http://www.ginger.io) offers a mobile application in which individuals with select conditions agree, in conjunction with their providers, to be tracked through their mobile phones and assisted with behavioral-health therapies. The app records data about calls, texts, geographic location, and even physical movements.

Humetrix's iBlueButton® (http://www.humetrix.com/ibb.html) is a mobile health information exchange app system to access and exchange medical records. It combines the convenience of mobile phones with medical information and tracks sleep, manages diabetes, heart disease, and asthma. The app helps the user to understand behavior patterns and provides motivation for health promotion action.

Propeller Health (http://www.propellerhealth.com) collects data from patients and provides them with feedback, which helps them better manage their asthma. A mobile GPS-enabled tracking device attaches to asthma inhalers to monitor the time and location of events.

Online HRAs: Online health risk assessments are becoming increasingly popular related to their ease of administration, reduced respondent burden, reliability of responses, immediacy of results, and rapid availability of aggregated information in a database. Providing an online, interactive HRA allows employees to complete the HRA regardless of geographic location and at a convenient time (Ahern et al., 2009). Online HRAs have the flexibility to be customized to an employer and industry type. Employee Internet access and skills are two factors to consider in the decision to use an online HRA (Framer & Chikamoto, 2009).

Health Education Priority Implementation Challenges in an eHealth Environment

Employees work, live, play, and pray in a technology-savvy world where information is shared instantly across the globe. With e-mail, video chat, texting, cell phones, apps, tablets, social media, and other forms of communication, it is hard to go even a few minutes without being contacted or updated in some way. Having so much information available is great for being able to keep in touch with friends and relatives and for finding out information about current events, personal health, or really any possible topic of interest. However, it also is a stressor that people have to deal with, it is out of control, and it is ever-present. At any one moment, information and anxiety can show up at employees' doorsteps. At the same time, all of the information and all of the technology keeps individuals up to date and in contact with friends and family can also be a source of help, support, and resources when they need it. Given the reality of the eHealth environment, workplace health promotion programs have to be equally savvy with the additional burden of making sure the connections are respectful and supportive of individuals health and health decisions.

Health Literacy and eHealth Literacy

Health literacy skills are a major factor in determining individuals' (employees') health outcomes. Although experts are still debating the single definition of health literacy, the most commonly accepted definition is the degree to which individuals have the capacity to obtain, process, and understand basic health information and services needed to make appropriate health decisions (Selden, Zorn, Ratzan, & Parker, 2000).

Because the word "literacy" is included in the phrase, people often misinterpret health literacy to be an issue of concern only for those who cannot read or write. However, health literacy expands beyond reading and writing skills to include the ability to comprehend and assess health information in order to make informed decisions about mentally healthy behaviors, emotional, and social functioning, and stress management (Nielsen-Bohlman, Panzer, & Kindig, 2004). Given the reliance on the Internet and technologies for health information and knowledge, eHealth literacy is critical for individuals (employees) gaining access to needed information, resources, and support. eHealth literacy is the ability to seek, find, understand, and appraise health information from electronic sources and apply the knowledge gained to address or solve a health problem (Norman & Skinner, 2006). In an eHealth environment health visual literacy (ability to understand graphs and other visual information), numeric or computational literacy (ability to calculate or reason numerically), computer literacy (ability to use a computer), and technology literacy (having some basic knowledge about technology and to think critically about technological issues and act accordingly) all can influence health outcomes (Brixey, 2014; Committee on Assessing Technological Literacy, 2006).

Plain Language Strategies to Improve Health Literacy

Presenting information in plain language (or plain English) is an integral component of improving health literacy and eHealth literacy. The term "plain language" has many definitions, but is fundamentally defined as communication your audience can understand the first time they read or hear it (Plain Language Action and Information Network, n.d.). Material is in plain language if your audience can:

* Find what they need

* Understand what they find

* Use what they find to meet their needs

Although definitions vary, the essence of "plain language" focuses on the audience, clarity, and comprehension. Using clear and concrete words in a straightforward manner is the best way to organize information, particularly with health content. Using graphs and charts is recommended to clearly convey data and statistics.

Using plain language is especially important when communicating with individuals with low health literacy and eHealth literacy, but all people can benefit from information in plain language. Something to note, though, is that plain language refers not only to the specific words that are used, but also *how* information is presented.

Health Communication and Social Media Plan

Health communication and social media plans guide and develop the information exchange between and among the workplace health promotion program staff, employers, and employees. Plans can be formal or informal, but the important element is that there is a consistent strategy for what information is communicated and how that communication will occur (Table 14.2). The most effective workplace health promotion programs have consensus among staff, employer, and employees on what message(s) are being communicated to the employees and their families (and sometimes to the larger community and customers). The communication plan is about details. It can provide guides for communications with workers, supervisors, managers, leadership, and family members. It can provide standardized formats for letters and e-mails. Even press releases and crisis management communications might be included in a communication plan. The most effective plans are a team effort. Time has been spent thinking about and discussing what to communicate and how. Likewise the issues of health literacy and use of plain language are addressed in the plan.

Education and Skills That Support eHealth Deployment and Implementation

Health professionals are not embracing eHealth technologies and social media as rapidly as the public for health services or information dissemination. How could advocates for eHealth incentivize health professionals to embrace eHealth and social media, track their evolution, and work with

Table 14.2   Health Communication and Social Media Plan (National Institutes of Health & National Cancer Institute, 2001)

Intended audiences: Whom do you want to reach with your communications? Be specific.

Objectives: What do you want your intended audiences to do after they hear, watch, or experience this communication?

Obstacles: What beliefs, cultural practices, peer pressure, misinformation, etc., stand between your audience and the desired objective?

Key Promise: Select one single promise/benefit that the audience will experience upon hearing, seeing, or reading the objectives you've set.

Support Statements/Reasons Why: Include the reasons the key promise/benefit outweighs the obstacles and the reasons what you're promising or promoting is beneficial. These often become the messages.

Tone: What *feeling* or *personality* should your communication have? Should it be authoritative, light, emotional. . . ? Choose a tone.

Media: What channels will the communication use, or what form will the communication take? Television? Radio? Social media? Texts? E-mails? Alert line? Newspaper? Webpage? Poster? Point-of-purchase? Flyer? All of the above?

Opportunities: What opportunities (times and places) exist for reaching your audience?

Creative Considerations: Anything else we should know? Will it be in more than one language?

the public to fully unleash the power of these mediums to support workplace health and wellness? Meanwhile, is there a professional obligation for health professionals on social media to respond to inquiries or address misinformation if they choose to participate in social media (Ho & Peter Wall Workshop Participants, 2014)?

The successful utilization of eHealth is critically dependent on the eHealth skills and competencies of staff involved in the workplace health promotion program as well as colleagues throughout the health care fields. Workplace health promotion programs staff action is needed to identify the skills and knowledge deficiencies within health care systems and services and then advocate for eHealth skills development of programs for health care professionals and service providers. Organizations as part of their health communication and social media plan can examine the requirement for their organization to define and agree on common standards of competence and professionalism that they feel are needed to best deliver their services.

Finally, mobile health technologies fit well with the current emphasis on personalized health initiatives and hold great promise. Although there has been rapid growth in the use of these technologies in health care (e.g., various health apps), little evaluation has been conducted on usability of those health programs. Workplace health promotion professionals are well positioned to lead this endeavor as they have a great deal of experience with workers and family members and many opportunities to communicate with workers to assess their competencies in using these technologies (Nahm, 2013).

Harnessing Technology for Health and Wellness

At play in the eHealth environment are many social interactions and dynamics that can contribute to success or failure of workplace health promotion programs as well impact employees' health outcomes. Health education in an eHealth environment touches on how information is managed, employees' social support, health decision making, and action in support of employee and employer health goals. Although there is a common notion that eHealth can be very helpful to support health and wellness, it is not always clear how best to quantify these benefits. Furthermore how can eHealth optimally and effectively support workers' active pursuit of health and help them become experts of their own wellness? What more does eHealth need to accomplish to improve the health of the workforce? This is not limited by age, language and technological literacy, and types of social media used (e.g., Twitter, Facebook). It is about accessing the information and knowledge captured in the various dimensions of the eHealth environment (Ho & Peter Wall Workshop Participants, 2014).

Advocacy and Resource Partnerships and Organizations

Increasing numbers of organizations are working on implementing a focus on health education in the workplace in an eHealth environment. They provide ongoing research, materials, and advocacy for the best, evidence-based practices that create and support workplace health promotion and education in an eHealth environment. Among those groups are:

Compendium of Innovative Health Technologies for Low-Resource Settings (http://www.who.int/ehealth/resources/compendium/en/index.html)

All innovative solutions in the compendium are presented in one page summarizing the health problem addressed, the proposed solution, and the product specifications, based on data, information, and images provided by the developers of the technologies concerned. Note that for the selected technology, the inclusion in the compendium does not constitute a warranty for fitness of the technology for a particular purpose.

The Centers for Medicare & Medicaid Services (CMS) eHealth Initiative (http://www.cms.gov/eHealth/about.html)

The Centers for Medicare & Medicaid Services (CMS) eHealth initiative aligns health information technology (Health IT) and electronic standards programs. Together these eHealth initiatives will help the health care industry deliver higher quality care and reduce costs.

eHealth Tools You Can Use (http://www.healthit.gov/patients-families/ehealth)

This website offers a starting point to finding tools that meet some of the most common needs faced by employees and family members. Nearly everything you do to affect your health and the health of your loved ones happens outside of the doctor's office. Individuals (employees) and family members have access to more resources and tools than ever before to enhance personal health and become more involved with their health care.

National Network of Libraries of Medicine (http://nnlm.gov/)

The mission of the National Network of Libraries of Medicine (NN/LM) is to advance the progress of medicine and improve the public health by providing all U.S. health professionals with equal access to biomedical information and improving the public's access to information to enable them to make informed decisions about their health. The program is coordinated by the National Library of Medicine and carried out through a nationwide network of health science libraries and information centers.

Society for Public Health Education (SOPHE) (http://www .sophe.org/)

SOPHE is a professional organization to provide global leadership to the profession of health education and health promotion and to promote the health of all people by: stimulating research on the theory and practice of health education (including eHealth); supporting high-quality performance standards for the practice of health education and health promotion; advocating policy and legislation affecting health education and health promotion; and developing and promoting standards for professional preparation of health education professionals.

Summary

Health education in an eHealth environment has the potential to improve individuals' health status, life quality, and health care quality while lowering health care costs and expenses for the employer and employee. It spans all of the potential employee populations, educating them about health promotion as well as current treatments and options when confronting a medical treatment decision. The health education priority–focused program implementation is the union of health education, health communication, and eHealth with the potential to be transformative for workers' health. The priority represents a merging of health and medicine. No longer is health education in the workplace about health and safety but rather about supporting employees' engagement and full participation in promoting their health as well as being decision makers in their health care. eHealth is not limited to the workplace, and therefore workplace health education is not limited to the workplace. The eHealth environment spans employees' workplaces, communities, and homes, thereby involving family and friends.

For Practice and Discussion

1. Reflect on your own (and family members' and friends') eHealth engagement. Listed in the chapter are just some of the eHealth technologies that engage individuals in their own health and wellness (e.g., electronic health records, ePrescribing, telemedicine, personal health devices, consumer health informatics, health knowledge management, virtual health care teams, and mHealth, or m-Health, health care

information systems). Compare and contrast your personal eHealth experiences with those of your family members and friends.

2. Compare and contrast the privacy and security concerns of electronic medical records (EMRs), electronic health records (EHRs), personal health records (PHRs), and personal health portals. What are the benefits of employers supporting and encouraging employees to be fully engaged in the use of these eHealth innovations? Realistically, how much can employers encourage and support employees to fully participate in the eHealth environment?

3. Is the depth of the information or knowledge shared in an eHealth environment appropriate for pursuit of health? How could the inter-activity of the eHealth environment be best used to support health and health promotion? How can workplace health promotion program staff members build trust and credibility to nurture the relationships between themselves and employees?

4. eHealth has a disruptive nature, altering the way people (employees) get, create, and share information about their health. The disruptive nature of eHealth is creating positive tension to stimulate changes. How to harness this momentum of change toward empowering employees and health professionals alike in health information exchange and dissemination? What types of eHealth tools will continue to emerge in the future? How can individuals (e.g., staff, employees, employers) keep abreast of these changes and continue to adopt them for health and wellness?

Case Study: Union and Employee eHealth Concerns—What Would You Do?

Roy Creek works as a program director for health education in the Department of Knowledge Management and Sharing at a big health system. Mr. Creek knows that workplace health education has changed. Technology has transformed health education. His organization already uses brochures, posters, workshops, lunchtime speakers, and classes to promote employees' health and safety. The web, cloud, and mobile devices show real potential for eHealth tools to improve employees' health. His organization partners with business, community, state, and national groups to promote and strengthen workplace health education using communication technologies from applications on the factory floor to the administrative offices. They are involved with employees' health care, educating them about electronic health records, ePrescribing, telemedicine, consumer health information, health knowledge management (e.g., using WebMD), virtual health care teams, health apps, and personal devices. It is a lot.

Mr. Creek has a problem. The union and employees are concerned that it is too much. They are concerned about their personal information security. Recently, employees have begun to stop using the available technology to access their personal information as well as the organization's health education and promotion offerings. Mr. Creek's supervisor wants a plan to deal with the employees' anxiety and to get the employees engaged in using the eHealth system that the organization spent money to create. The executive leadership is wondering if they have done too much, if they have wasted their time, resources, and money. If you were Mr. Creek, what would you do?

KEY TERMS

eHealth	Personal health (patient) portal
Health education	E-mails, tweeting, and texting
Health communication+	Health information exchange (HIE)
eHealth technologies	Online HRAs
Consumer health education and informatics	Health literacy
Personal health record (PHR)	Plain Language Strategies
Electronic medical records (EMRs)	Communication and social media plan/strategy
Electric health records (EHRs)	Privacy
Blue Button Initiative	Security

References

Abacus Group. (n.d.). *My Medication Advisor.* Retrieved from https://www.mymedicationadvisor.com/Home/Login.aspx?ReturnUrl=%2fDefault.aspx

Ahern, D., Buckel, L., Aberger, E., & Follick, M. (2009). eHealth for employee health and wellness: Optimizing plan design and incentive management. *ACSM's worksite health handbook: A guide to building healthy and productive companies* (2nd ed., pp. 248–258). Champaign, IL: Human Kinetics.

American Health Information Management Association. (2012). *Pocket glossary for health information management and technology* (3rd ed.). Chicago, IL: Author.

Brixey, J. (2014). Consumer health informatics. In S. Fenton & S. Biedermann (Eds.), *Introduction to healthcare informatics* (pp. 321–346). Chicago, IL: American Health Information Management Association.

Committee on Assessing Technological Literacy. (2006). *Tech tally: Approaches to assessing technological literacy.* Washington, DC: National Academies Press.

Dennison, L., Morrison, L., Conway, G., & Yardley, L. (2013). Opportunities and challenges for smartphone applications in supporting health behavior change: Qualitative study. *Journal of Medical Internet Research, 15*(4), e86.

Department of Veterans Affairs. (n.d.). *Blue Button.* Retrieved from http://www.va.gov/BLUEBUTTON/index.asp

Fox, S. (2011). The social life of health information, 2011. *Pew Internet & American Life Project.* Retrieved from http://www.pewinternet.org/2011/05/12/the-social-life-of-health-information-2011/

Fox, S. & Duggan, M. (2013). The diagnosis difference. Retrieved from http://www.pewinternet.org/2013/11/26/the-diagnosis-difference/

Framer, E., & Chikamoto, Y. (2009). The assessment of health and risk: Tools, specific uses, and implementation processes. *ACSM's worksite health: A guide to building healthy and productive companies* (2nd ed., pp. 140–150). Champaign, IL: Human Kinetics.

Green, L., Kreuter, M., Deeds, S., & Partridge, K. (1980). *Health promotion planning: A diagnostic approach.* Mountain View, CA: Mayfield.

Hillestad, R., Bigelow, J., Bower, A., Girosi, F., Meili, R., Scoville, R., & Taylor, R. (2005). Can electronic medical record systems transform health care? Potential health benefits, savings, and costs. *Health Affairs, 24*(5), 1103–1117.

Ho, K., & Peter Wall Workshop Participants. (2014). Harnessing the social web for health and wellness: Issues for research and knowledge translation. *Journal of Medical Internet Research, 16*(2), e13.

Markle Connecting for Health. (2003). *Americans want benefits of personal health records.* Retrieved from http://www.markle.org/publications/950-americans-want-benefits-personal-health-records

Microsoft. (2015). *HealthVault.* Retrieved May 10, 2015, from https://www.healthvault.com/us/en

Nahm, E.-S. (2013). Mobile technologies for health education: What do we need to consider? *Online Journal of Nursing Informatics, 17*(2). Retrieved from http://ojni.org/issues/?p=2655

National Institutes of Health & National Cancer Institute. (2001). *Making health communications programs work.* Retrieved from http://www.cancer.gov/publications/health-communication/pink-book.pdf

Nielsen-Bohlman, L., Panzer, A. M., & Kindig, D. A. (2004). *Health literacy: A prescription to end confusion.* Washington, DC: National Academies Press.

Norman, C. D., & Skinner, H. A. (2006). eHealth literacy: Essential skills for consumer health in a networked world. *Journal of Medical Internet Research, 8*(2), e9. doi:10.2196/jmir.8.2.e9

Nundy, S., Razi, R. R., Dick, J. J., Smith, B., Mayo, A., O'Connor, A., & Meltzer, D. O. (2013). A text messaging intervention to improve heart failure self-management after hospital discharge in a largely African-American population: Before-after study. *Journal of Medical Internet Research, 15*(3), e53. doi:10.2196/jmir.2317

Office of the National Coordinator for Health Information Technology. (n.d.). *What is a patient portal?* Retrieved from http://www.healthit.gov/providers-professionals/faqs/what-patient-portal

Pew Research Center (2012). *Fact sheet.* Retrieved May 12, 2015 from http://www.pewinternet.org/fact-sheets/health-fact-sheet/

Plain Language Action and Information Network (n.d.). *Plain language.* Retrieved May 10, 2015, from http://www.plainlanguage.gov/

Schiavo, R. (2007). *Health communication: From theory to practice.* Hoboken, NJ: Wiley.

Selden, C., Zorn, M., Ratzan, S., & Parker, R. (2000). *National Library of Medicine current bibliographies in medicine: Health literacy* (NLM Pub. No. CBM 2000-1). Bethesda, MD: National Institutes of Health, U.S. Department of Health and Human Services.

U.S. Department of Health and Human Services, Office of Disease Prevention and Health Promotion. (2000). *Healthy People 2010: With understanding and improving health and objectives for improving health.* Retrieved May 3, 2014, from http://www.healthypeople.gov/2020/default.aspx

U.S. Department of Health and Human Services, Office of Disease Prevention and Health Promotion. (2014). *What is e-Health?* Retrieved May 15, 2015, from http://www.health.gov/communication/ehealth/

PART FOUR

EVALUATION

CHAPTER 15

BEST PRACTICES IN WORKPLACE HEALTH PROMOTION PROGRAM EVALUATION

Population Health Management Evaluation Framework

Population health has been defined as the health outcomes of a group of individuals, including the distribution of such outcomes within the group. A population health management program (e.g., workplace health promotion program) strives to address health needs at all points along the continuum of health and well-being through participation of, engagement with, and interventions for the population (employees). Its goal is to maintain or improve the health and well-being of individuals through cost-effective and tailored program policies, practices, interventions, and services (Population Health Alliance, 2014). Population health management for workplace health promotion is a coordinated effort across all of the program implementation priority health areas that addresses employees' health (Shortell et al., 2002; Terry, 2012).

The population health management evaluation framework (Figure 15.1) identifies the general components and stakeholders of population health (employees). It depicts the health assessment and stratification of employees as the starting point to understand the health of the employees and flows to the core of the framework that includes the program priority health areas (e.g., physical, mental, nutrition). The interaction of policies representing the organizational culture and environment; the evidence-based practices, interventions, and services; along with teams, partnerships, and collaborations—all produce a continuum to address employee health (at the center of the

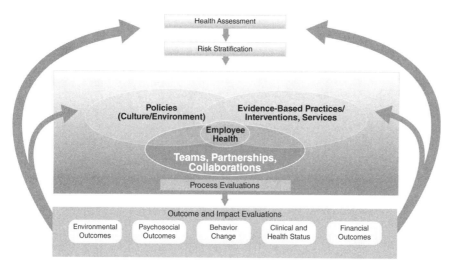

Figure 15.1   Population Health Evaluation Framework
Source: Adapted from Population Health Alliance, 2014.

framework). Process, outcome, and impact evaluations yield information that is part of the information loop depicted by the large curved arrows.

The population health evaluation framework provides information to the stakeholder groups of the workplace health promotion programs: employers, program staff, employees, and program providers (i.e., vendors). Individual employees are not evaluated as part of the program evaluation. Employees benefit from the evaluation but the evaluation is not about employees, rather the evaluation's focus is the program's ability to address employees' health needs. The information and data as part of the evaluation process support decisions for program improvement (employee health improvement) and accountability (costs). Program improvement involves identifying sources of employee health risk and addressing those through the policies, practices, intervention, and services in the program's implementation of health priority areas. Accountability identifies opportunities for program delivery process improvement to impact employees' health.

The population health management evaluation framework provides a continuous feedback cycle for ongoing program decision making by employers, program staff, employees, and program providers. Figure 15.2 shows the feedback loop with its data collection, analytics, stratification, and many decision-making points. The continuous feedback supports the program decision-making process that provides employers, program staff, and program providers with information to ensure the highest quality service. It links to the organization's strategic human resource management.

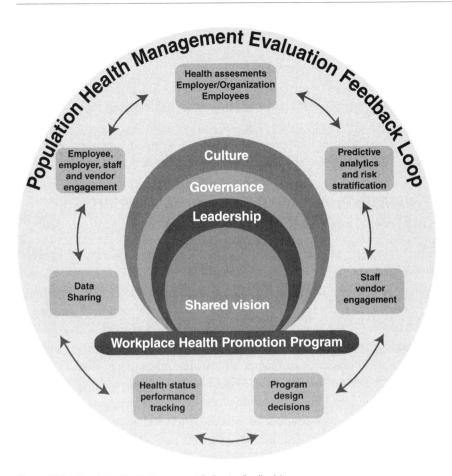

Figure 15.2   Population Health Management Evaluation Feedback Loop
Source: Adapted from Cassidy, 2013.

It keeps employee health as part of the organization's shared vision, leadership, governance, and culture.

Evaluations of the specific policies, practices, interventions, and services in the program of implementation health priority areas are completed within the population health evaluation framework. Employers, employees, program staff, and program providers raise questions as part of creating, operating, and sustaining a program, which are answered through the evaluation process. Evaluation in the most effective programs starts when a program is being planned and continues in tandem as the program is implemented and sustained in order to provide continual feedback to the stakeholders (Figure 15.2).

Finally, the 2010 Patient Protection and Affordable Care Act (ACA) raised the expectation for workplace health promotion programs to evaluate and report their quality, appropriateness, and efficiency, as well their program outcomes. The expectations are now for workplace health promotion programs as well as all health care providers and services to use evidence-based interventions and practices, reduce variability in strategies, methods, and resource use that cannot be clinically justified, increase coordination of programs through the use of information technology and team-based initiatives, while emphasizing prevention and disease management, and giving individuals (employees) a stronger voice in their own health and health care and in defining what matters.

Two Main Purposes of Program Evaluation: Improvement and Accountability

Combining the population health management framework and expectations of the ACA, the two main purposes of workplace health promotion program evaluations are program improvement and accountability. Approaches to measurement differ for each. In measurement for improvement, the general strategy is to measure just enough to learn. This approach is characterized by limited data and small, sequential samples. Hypotheses are flexible and are apt to change as learning takes place. Trend data are typically analyzed, and the data are used by those doing the improvement.

Measurement for accountability focuses on reporting, oversight, comparison, choice, reassurance, or motivation for change. It is not about hypothesis testing, but evaluation of current performance. It is important to make adjustments to reduce bias in comparisons, and important to collect all available, relevant data.

Because the purpose of measurement should determine the methods, mismatching purposes and methods can have adverse consequences (Table 15.1). For example, applying accountability methods in an improvement setting can slow down the learning process, and more importantly set the bar for statistical significance too high to detect potentially useful changes. Alternatively, applying improvement methods to accountability questions can lead to inappropriate generalization of findings.

Evaluation for Improvement

Evaluation for improvement has its roots in methods dating back to the early 1900s, led by the work in the science of improvement by W. Edwards Deming, Walter Shewhart, and Joseph M. Juran. The Model for Improvement, developed by Associates in Process Improvement (Institute for Healthcare Improvement, 2014) is a widely used tool focused on improvement. The Model for Improvement consists of two parts. The first part focuses on basic questions to frame and understand the improvement process.

Table 15.1   Two Purposes of Workplace Health Promotion Program Evaluation (Provost & Murray, 2007; Solberg, Mosser, & McDonald, 1997a, 1997b)

Aspect	Improvement	Accountability
Aim	Improvement of policies, practices, interventions, and services	Comparison, choice, reassurance, spur of change
Methods		
Test observability	Test observable	No test, evaluate current performance
Bias	Accept consistent bias	Measure and adjust to reduce bias
Sample size	"Just enough" data, small sequential samples	Obtain 100% of available, relevant data
Flexibility of hypothesis	Hypothesis flexible, changes as learning takes place	No hypothesis
Testing strategy	Sequential tests	No tests
Determining if a change is an improvement	Displays data over time (i.e., Run or Shewhart charts)	No change focus
Confidentiality of the data	Data used only by those involved with the improvement	Data available for public consumption and review

- What are we trying to accomplish?
- How do we know that a change is an improvement?
- What change can we make that will result in an improvement?

A clear goal statement is essential to answer the first question concerning what we are trying to accomplish. A useful technique for developing goal statements is to make them "SMART": specific, measurable, attainable, realistic, and time-bound. Data is collected and charted at various points (Figure 15.2) to observe change. From the goal statement, the data collection and observations occur that lead to understanding the change process as well as to learning changes that lead to the desired improvements (Provost & Murray, 2007). The Model for Improvement repeats itself. It is a feedback loop that consists of continuous cycles of Plan-Do-Study-Act to test and implement changes in real-world settings (Institute for Healthcare Improvement, 2014).

The ACA expectations also influenced the evaluation for improvement of workplace health promotion programs. Programs are now expected to use evidence-based interventions and practices, reduce variability in strategies, methods, and resource use that cannot be clinically justified, and increase coordination of programs through the use of information technology and team-based initiatives. As a result evaluation for improvement now asks additional questions (Saul & Gasser, 2014):

- Did the program advance the outcome that stakeholders care about?

- How far did the program move the needle on the outcome (how big is the change)?

- How does this program compare to others?

These questions reflect a time of diminishing resources and increasing need to implement high performance and quality programs that can meet the goal of improved health at lower cost. It is not enough anymore to just implement a program well. You need to show that the program is impacting employee behavior and adding value.

Predictive modeling is another tool used in workplace health promotion program evaluation for improvement. It relies on mathematical modeling to predict the probability of an outcome. It is used in many industries other than health care, including archeology and geology (e.g., to predict the likelihood of archeological sites or mineral deposits), insurance (e.g., to predict cost), and marketing (e.g., to predict what consumers will buy). Within the context of health promotion, predictive modeling is typically used to predict such outcomes as cost, resource utilization, or mortality by population segments. The ultimate goal of using a predictive model is the delivery of tailored interventions and resources to a specific population segment based on their specific needs. Predictive models in health promotion are used for a variety of purposes, including identification of individuals at risk for adverse health outcomes, high resource utilization, hospital stays/days/readmissions, expensive or risky procedures, large health care-related costs, or disenrollment from a health plan (Stiefel & Nolan, 2012).

Evaluation for Accountability

Evaluation for accountability is linked to the Institute for Healthcare Improvement's Triple AIM, which focuses on care (experience), health (improving population health), and costs (Berwick, Nolan, & Whittington, 2008). The methods for accountability focus on value of the health promotion program for the employer. For the employer the question is the health promotion program's worth, utility, or importance in comparison with other actions (i.e., programs) that an employer (organization) might decide to pursue (e.g., increasing salaries, hiring more staff, taking more profits).

Accountability is concerned with trying to understand the drivers or determinants of health and health costs (Figure 15.3). Workplace health promotion programs can impact different health drivers depending on

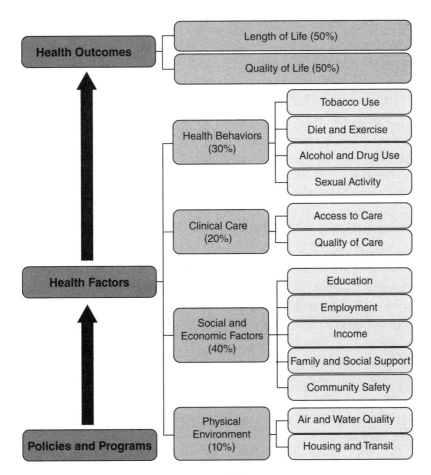

Figure 15.3   Drivers or Determinants of Health and Health Costs

Source: University of Wisconsin Population Health Institute, 2015.

the priority areas selected to be implemented. For example, workplace health promotion program investment to address health behaviors and clinical care (i.e., access to care and quality of care) can impact up to 50% of employers and employees' health costs. And since employers and employees are increasingly sharing the cost of health care the priority is to maximize program efforts that impact costs. Evaluation for accountability of workplace health promotion programs for that reason focuses on economic evaluation, one of which is return on investment (ROI).

Economic Evaluations Including Return on Investment

The Centers for Disease Control and Prevention (CDC) argues that decision makers in public health are faced with the need to consider the costs and effectiveness of these choices when it comes to offering preventive services to Americans (CDC, 1995). The decision makers need to consider not only what preventive programs work but also the additional costs associated with the use of these interventions. Businesses are also charged with finding affordable ways of keeping their workforce healthy and productive. The expense of providing health insurance to their workers is a good investment only if the workers remain healthy and productive.

It is argued that that improvements in the health of the population can be achieved through better use of evidence-based decisions concerning the use of finite resources in order to do the right thing at the right time. What is needed is faster and better use of scientific information that increases the return on investment (ROI) by having the desired effect on the health of the public (Brent, 2014; Fielding & Briss, 2006).

Furthermore the cost associated with poor health can also be part of an economic evaluation. For example, workplace programs typically have an objective to avert or reduce the occurrence of a specific health outcome. The economic analysis therefore might consider including all health outcomes (positive and adverse) that are caused or prevented during the lifetime of the participant as a result of the health promotion program. Fielding and Briss (2006) explain the fact that many improvements in health result from evidence-informed programs that affect the likelihood of acquiring a disease, the severity of the disease, and the receipt of appropriate and timely medical care.

The CDC (1995) offered a basic assessment scheme for the evaluation of costs and consequences of a workplace health promotion program (Table 15.2). The scheme offers a rationale for seeking and understanding the economics of a program.

Table 15.2   Economic Analysis of Workplace Health Promotion Programs (Centers for Disease Control and Prevention, 1995)

- A complete description of the program, the units in which the service(s) are provided, and the time frame of the program

- Health outcome(s) averted by the prevention program and the estimated time between its implementation and when the health outcome is averted

- The rates and societal burden of the health outcome

- The preventable fraction for the health outcome, with the program in place and used in a realistic manner (i.e., the proportion of the health outcome averted through the program)

- Intervention costs per unit of intervention, including the cost of any intervention side effects

- Direct medical treatment cost of the health outcome prevented

Economic Evaluations, ROI Is O

Economic evaluations attempt to disco
individuals healthy at a reasonable cos
evidence of improvement in health as a re~u.. ..i ..~uui...~ ..eing allocated for
policies, practices, interventions and services. There are several economic
evaluation tools available to measure these improvements and to rank
them in some logical order of success. Major methods used in economic
evaluations include cost analysis, cost-effectiveness analyses, cost-utility
analysis, cost-benefit analysis, and return on investment.

Cost analysis (CA) includes the cost of total illness estimates, including
direct and indirect costs of the problem. It represents an economic evaluation technique that involves the systematic collection, categorization, and
analysis of program costs. The results are actually a measure of the burden
of disease for some period of time.

Cost-effectiveness analysis (CEA) compares the costs of intervention
with the resulting improvement in health. It is an analysis used to compare
the costs of alternative interventions that produce a common health effect.
Table 15.3 shows the value of various health interventions to offer to
the population that are cost effective. The most cost-effective preventive
health services that can be offered for physical health in a workplace
health promotion program practice, according to the list, are smoking
cessation, aspirin therapy, and pneumococcal immunization. The list is a

Table 15.3   Comparison of Cost-Based Analysis and Return on Investment (adapted from Schottmuller, 2014)

	Cost-Based Analysis (CBA)	**Return on Investment (ROI)**
Formula	Benefits – Costs	(Benefits – Costs)/Costs
Example	$12,000 B – $1,000 C = $11,000 CBA	($12,000 B – $1,000 C /$1,000 C = 11 or 1100% ROI
Format	Dollar Value	Percentage or Ratio
Purpose	Analyze estimated cost impact (i.e., make a profit, break even, take a loss)	Analyze investment effectiveness for generating a profit
Focus	Profit	Investment Return
Common Use	Compare options using a common currency and justify bottom-line feasibility of spending	Assess profitability as a basis for continuing and prioritizing future investments
Answers. . .	Will we come out ahead?	How effective were we at coming out ahead? What kind of payback did we get for the investment?

good example of using economics to assist in making decisions about the utilization of health resources.

Nas (1996) argues that because of the difficulty in identifying and quantifying outcomes, health care services research usually uses CEA or cost-utility analysis (CUA) when determining value in the use of health resources. CEA provides a good measurement tool for determining the efficiency of a particular procedure or program in meeting its goal. The outcome in CEA is usually represented by a single health outcome, such as years of life saved or improvement in health status.

Cost-Effective Interventions (Johnson, 2006)

- Aspirin therapy
- Childhood immunizations
- Tobacco use screening, intervention
- Colorectal cancer screening
- Measuring blood pressure in adults
- Influenza immunizations
- Pneumococcal immunization
- Alcohol screening and counseling
- Vision screenings for adults
- Cervical cancer screening
- Cholesterol screening
- Breast cancer screening

- Chlamydia screening
- Calcium supplement counseling
- Vision screening in children
- Folic acid counseling
- Obesity screening
- Depression screening
- Hearing screening
- Injury prevention counseling
- Osteoporosis screening
- Cholesterol screening for high-risk patients
- Diabetes screening
- Diet counseling
- Tetanus-diphtheria boosters

Cost-utility analysis (CUA) is a type of cost-effectiveness analysis that uses years of life saved combined with quality of life during those years as a health outcome measure. These measures allow direct comparison.

Cost-benefit analysis (CBA) compares both costs and benefits in dollar terms. They are adjusted to their present value through a process called discounting. If a program demonstrates a net benefit after computations, the program is considered to provide a good economic value and should be continued or, perhaps, expanded.

Return on investment (ROI) measures the costs of a program (i.e., the investment) versus the financial return realized by the program. ROI is usually calculated from the perspective of the organization implementing the program, rather than from the perspective of government or society. ROI analysis is the most common form of investment analysis used by private companies and is useful when communicating the financial ramifications of a given program to a business audience. ROI analysis can be performed to evaluate the impact of an existing program, but it is more often used to determine whether a program should be implemented.

Table 15.3 shows a comparison of a CBA and ROI. The two analyses are used to answer different questions. CBA is asking about profits. Will the employer come out ahead using the program? ROI asks how effective were we at coming out ahead? What kind of payback did we get for the investment? Note that an ROI of 1% or 100% implies you'd get back what you put into it, while CBA has a $0 "break-even" point. Furthermore the CBA for two different workplace program interventions with very different costs could be the same. The respective ROI would shed light on the investment effectiveness of the interventions.

Consumers continually use economic techniques every day. Whenever they shop for a product or service, they usually compare price with value before making a purchase decision. The free-market economy usually allocates resources based on information that becomes available through the price system. This market efficiency operates under conditions first described by an Italian economist named Vilfredo Pareto. Nas (1996) defines "Pareto optimality" as an efficiency norm where no one can be made better off without first making someone worse off.

Nas (1996) argues that the impact of CBA grew significantly in the 1960s because the federal Office of Management and Budget made cost benefit a principal tool of evaluation of government programs. Using economic theory to evaluate performance in the Flood Control Act of 1936, the government developed a standard guide for water resources. In the 1960s the Planning Programming and Budgeting System (PPBS) adopted a system of analysis in the Department of Defense using economic evaluative methods.

The CDC has been pursuing CBA for years to justify the costs and potential benefits of prevention programs. These justifications can be easily applied to illness and injury programs in the workplace. The CDC (1995) pointed out that prevention effectiveness analysis methods, a form of CBA, could be used to measure the effects of public health programs. In order to compare different prevention strategies, there is a need for reliable and consistent cost and effectiveness data. This information is necessary to document which programs and activities provide the greatest benefit for the funds expended. Table 15.4 shows how each of these analysis methods can be applied to document economic effectiveness of programs.

Table 15.4   Economic Evaluation of Health Promotion Programs (Centers for Disease Control and Prevention, 1995)

Economic Evaluation Method	Comparison	Measurements of Health Effects	Economic Summary Measure
Cost Analysis	Compares net costs of different programs for planning and assessments	Dollars	Net costs Cost of illness
Cost-effectiveness analysis	Compares interventions that produce a common health effect	Health effect, measured in natural units	Cost-effectiveness ratio Cost per case averted Cost per life-year saved
Cost-utility analysis	Compares interventions that have morbidity and mortality outcomes	Health effects, measured as year of life, adjusted for quality of life	Cost per quality-adjusted life year
Cost-benefit analysis	Compares different programs with different units of outcomes (health and nonhealth)	Dollars	Net benefit or cost Benefit-to-cost ratio
Return of investment (ROI)	Compares costs of a program (i.e., the investment) versus the financial return realized by the program	Percentage or ratio	Benefits minus costs as percentage or ration of costs

It Is Just Not About Wellness or Disease Management ROI

Recent evaluations of workplace health promotion programs have focused on the ROI of workplace wellness and disease management programs (Baicker, Cutler, & Song, 2010; Caloyeras, Liu, Exum, Broderick, & Mattke, 2014; Mattke et al., 2013). One consequence of the reports is to narrow the view of what is a workplace health promotion program and how to evaluate programs. Furthermore they completely sidestep the opportunity for workplaces in adopting strategies expected by the ACA to demonstrate how their workplace programs are emphasizing prevention and disease management and giving employees a stronger voice in their own health and health care and in defining what matters.

ROI analysis (as well as other economic analyses) is a powerful tool for measuring the net financial benefits of an investment and is commonly used by business-oriented organizations when evaluating where to spend their resources. It is therefore important that workplace health promotion professionals and program staff understand ROI analysis, and all of the economic analyses, as well as limitations of the analyses. However, we do not want to limit the view of the workplace health promotion program to simply ROI and focus solely on programs of wellness and disease management. This is particularly important when considering that properly measuring ROI can be difficult. And that many companies simply avoid the challenge altogether: A 2012 ADP study, titled "Why You Should Care About Wellness Programs," showed that "while 79 percent of large and 44 percent of midsized companies offer wellness programs, over 60 percent of these companies do not measure their return on investment" (ADP, 2012).

Health promotion professionals and workplace health promotion program staff need to be prepared to discuss program benefits that are not so easily measured in financial terms. In addition to measurable financial benefits to the company's bottom line, there are other benefits from health improvements (e.g., lives saved, improved quality of life) that are difficult to value in dollar (economic) terms. Three actions that help broaden the evaluation focus are (Lavizzo-Mourey, 2014):

1. Define why an employer wants a program. Clearly decreasing overall health cost is important. Everyone wants to save money. What about increasing worker productivity? The ADP (2012) study of employers with workplace health promotion programs reported workers returned to work up to 9 days sooner from workers' compensation–related absences and 17 days sooner from short-term disability absences. Also important to employers were the company culture, attracting and retaining employees, and improving organizational performance and competitiveness.

2. Define what makes a "good" program (e.g., evidence-based interventions and practices, increase coordination of programs through the use of information technology and team-based initiatives). Many health promotion programs rely on activity measures (e.g., miles walked) and unreliable self-reported data (e.g., survey responses). Once a year employees log in to a site, promise to eat better, exercise more, and smoke less, and—presto—their health premiums are reduced. Instead, champion the use of clinical data measurement to prove health goals are met. Effective health promotion programs regularly track actual cholesterol levels, blood pressure, glucose, and more.

3. Keep employees engaged. Communicate a corporate vision with health and program participation a priority. Make it more than just wellness and disease prevention. The health education program priority area implementation is key to employer and employees holding the broad view of the workplace health promotion program.

Lavizzo-Mourey (2014) concludes that the broader program view requires not being limited to ROI calculations for wellness or disease programs. Clearly ROI matters for health promotion professionals and program staff, but they need to help their organizations establish ROI and other economic measures as part of an evaluation process and not be the sole measure of a program.

Feasible, Scalable, Sustainable, and Scientific Workplace Evaluations

Workplace health promotion program evaluations need to be feasible, scalable, sustainable, and scientific. Feasible means the evaluations can be carried out and completed, and the results used to make decisions. Scalable means that they encompass the gestalt of a program and engage all program levels and participants. Sustainable evaluations are ongoing, providing a feedback loop to participants and decision makers. Scientific evaluations are grounded in rigorous and agreed-upon methods and standards. The results are trusted and answer the questions people have asked.

The number of peer-reviewed, published articles evaluating workplace health promotion program research is growing. However, making the leap from the published articles to the factory floor is formidable. Workplace health promotion is an applied field. When a pharmaceutical company studies the effects of nicotine replacement on smoking use, they are able to use a small number of participants and randomize volunteers into a treatment group and a comparison or control group.

When professionals design an evaluation study of workplace health promotion programs, they typically are not able to perform this type of randomization process. The ability to randomly select participating and nonparticipating employees is often viewed as denying the opportunity to participate for many who may benefit. In some instances, it may be possible to use lotteries or randomization to tailor the timing when people can gain access to health promotion programs (thus enabling similar comparison groups to be used for evaluation purposes), but this is not always possible either. A solution to this dilemma may be to use rigorous statistical processes in the evaluation to assure that the demographic, health status, and other differences between participating and nonparticipating employees are accounted for before making inferences about the impact of the programs they use (Smeltzer, Ozminkowski, & Musich, 2014).

Ozminkowski and Goetzel (2001) argued that competent evaluation of a workplace health promotion program can address such issues, and many others. For example, they developed a checklist of items to consider when evaluating workplace programs. Included in the list are:

- Decide both financial and nonfinancial questions to address and which hypotheses to test in the impact study.

- Choose an evaluation design that is well suited to testing that addresses these questions and hypotheses.

- Before conducting any analyses of dollar metrics, adjust for inflation.

- Before generating the final ROI a
  estimate and discount costs for eacl
  consideration (for multiyear evaluat

- Similarly, estimate and discount monetary and nonmonetary benefits.

- Perform sensitivity analyses to deal with uncertainties and test assumptions that had to be made in order for the evaluation research to be conducted.

- Present results to aid effective decision making by senior leaders.

- Recognize and describe the consequences of any limitations in the analysis.

Money Isn't Everything, Though. . .

When designing workplace health promotion programs to be feasible, scalable, sustainable, and scientific, recognize that a hallmark of successful workplace programs is their contribution to multiple business objectives. And the varying goals of the health promotion program need to be established a priori. A common observation in program evaluation is the assumed main goal of medical benefit cost reductions. However, talking with corporate leaders substantiates that medical benefit cost reductions are not the primary goal in as many as 50% of all programs. If program goals such as lower employee turnover, improved morale, or other desired outcomes are important, the program evaluation must be tailored to gauge progress in reaching these goals. This is not to suggest that the financial evaluations should be minimized, but that a total picture of business objectives must be identified in order to establish the evaluation plan (Bartholomew & Smith, 2006; Musich, Adams, & Edington, 2000; O'Donnell, 1984).

Understand the Organizational Evaluation Culture

Evaluators may not be aware that attitudes within an organization about health, employees, and evaluation may influence the conduct of quality evaluation. The leaders of an organization may believe that the program is worthwhile solely because the employees "feel" better. Consequently, appropriate monies may not be budgeted for evaluation because of the perceived intrinsic value of a program. Clearly, evaluation is needed to justify the value of a program in demanding economic times and during corporate restructuring.

As we design program evaluations, the human factors that influence attitudes toward evaluation in the workplace must not be overlooked. Data, if misused, can be a powerfully influencing factor. Knowledge of high-risk employee health behaviors must be confidential in order to maintain worker support for programs. Compliance with appropriate experimental design and methodologies may be seen as factors that will compromise the employee-relation benefits of the program. The evaluation must balance the need for evaluative rigor with the need for good employee relations. Good evaluation is expensive. Program directors working with finite budgets may not believe that the benefits of evaluation will outweigh the cost. When money is tight, resources tend to be allocated in areas of personal expertise. Therefore, evaluation efforts are sacrificed to maintain program continuity and integrity.

Strategic Alignment, Innovation, and Business Intelligence and Knowledge Management

Workplace employee health promotion program evaluations are built on a foundation supported by a strategic organizational commitment and shared vision for innovation, strong and active leadership, a well-developed governance structure, and a culture continually striving for improvement. Cassell, Kontor, and Shah (2012) argue that feasible, scalable, sustainable, and scientific workplace health promotion program evaluations occur when three elements are present: strategic alignment, innovation, and business intelligence and knowledge management.

Strategic alignment: Achieving strategic alignment is critical to a workplace health promotion program being linked to the organization's strategic human resource management. In other words, the health promotion program evaluations need to be visible or aligned with the organizational vision and throughout the human resource department and wider organization (Figure 15.2). The evaluations provide continuous feedback to support the program decision-making to ensure the highest quality program. It keeps employee health as part of the organization's shared vision, leadership, governance, and culture. It creates a culture of accountability that fosters transparent approaches aligning incentives and engaging employees and employers. The four essential components of the organization's alignment strategy include:

1. **Shared vision:** A shared vision has been described by Peter Senge as "a force in people's hearts, a force of impressive power. At its simplest level, a shared vision is the answer to the question, 'What do we want to create?'" (Senge, 1990).

2. **Leadership:** Clarity and communication of purpose, progress, and challenges are integral to achieving strategic alignment. Program leaders will be required to empower and engage stakeholders within and outside the organization to successfully execute a vision in order to achieve measurable results.

3. **Governance:** An organization whose leadership has created a common vision requires a governance structure supporting the strategic mission. Governance should incorporate service coordination, data analytics and reporting, and drive shared decision making and accountability among key stakeholders.

4. **Culture:** An organization's culture promotes its values and the behaviors required to achieve its shared strategic vision. A culture of change can be extremely challenging to instill within an organization, especially in the midst of such significant ongoing modifications to the practice and health care delivery. However, investments in infrastructure, resources, and relationships with the greater community are not likely to succeed without engaging all stakeholders. Creating a health promoting workplace culture requires leadership and governance to effectively communicate and disseminate the organization's strategic mission, values, and vision while building the trust required to share risk.

    Innovation: Given the complexity of change, it is essential for an organization to have a foundation entrenched in a culture of innovation and change. Through this creative and improvement-driven culture, an organization will successfully engage employers, employees, providers, and other health promoting and health care stakeholders in leveraging the program's inherent capabilities and strengths.

    Business intelligence and knowledge management: An organization's business intelligence and relevant strategies to govern and manage data and information are essential components for successful evaluations. Knowledge management is an organizational asset that may be leveraged by employees and employers through informed decision making and data-driven improvement. This includes understanding how to take data and transform it into both information and knowledge to improve programs.

Summary

The population health evaluation framework provides information to the workplace health promotion program stakeholders. Individual employees are not evaluated as part of the program evaluation. The population health management evaluation framework provides a continuous feedback cycle for ongoing program decision making by employers, employees, program staff, and program providers (vendors). The information and data as part of the evaluation process support decisions for program improvement (employee health improvement) and accountability (costs). The ACA emphasis on the use of evidence-based interventions and practices; reduced variability in strategies, methods, and resource use that cannot be clinically justified; and increased coordination of programs through the use of information technology and team-based initiatives has influenced programs evaluation. Evaluation for accountability of workplace health promotion programs includes economic evaluation, one of which is return on investment (ROI). The major methods used in economic evaluations are cost analysis, cost-effectiveness analyses, cost-utility analysis, cost-benefit analysis, and return on investment. ROI (as well as other economic analyses) matters for health promotion professionals and program staff, but they need to help their organizations establish ROI and other economic measures as part of an evaluation process and not allow ROI to be the sole measure of a program. Finally workplace health promotion program evaluations need to be feasible, scalable, sustainable, and scientific, and built on a foundation supported by a strategic organizational commitment and shared vision for innovation, strong and active leadership, a well-developed governance structure, and a culture continually striving for improvement.

For Practice and Discussion

1. Workplace population health management is concerned with all of an organization's employees (and families). Propose a strategy for employers to use when deciding how to balance between program evaluation to improve programming and employee health status and to demonstrate accountability to meet program and fiscal goals.

2. How do the employer, program staff, and vendor's perspective of evaluation differ? How do the differences impact the evaluation feedback loop (Figure 15.2)?

3. As part of workplace program evaluations, what are you predicting? Why are you predicting it? How accurate are your predictions? What actions are taken based on the predictions?

4. Recommend why and when as part of a workplace health promotion program evaluation you would use a cost analyses, cost-effectiveness

analyses, cost-utility analysis, cost-benefit analysis, and return on investment. What question does each analysis answer?

5. Many benefits that can be measured, although not always easily, are employee productivity, short- and long-term disability, workers' compensation, absenteeism, pensions, and life insurance. Propose economic measures to evaluate the benefits.

6. Prepare a workshop for midsized employers (i.e., 200 to 500 employees) on a workplace health promotion program evaluation that used a population health management evaluation framework. Focus the workshop on teaching the employers about feasible, scalable, sustainable, and scientific workplace evaluations. What can you do to help the employers establish ROI and other economic measures as part of an evaluation process but not see it as the sole measure or view of their programs?

Case Study: Patient Protection and Affordable Care Act Program Evaluation Influence—What Would You Do?

The reality for workplace health promotion program directors is that the program evaluation questions being asked have changed. In the past, Christine Iocco, the director of employee health promotion at an aerospace and defense corporation, would answer questions such as, *did the programs fit the guidelines, did the programs do what they said they were going to do,* and *were the program approaches evaluated?* But now with the Patient Protection and Affordable Care Act 2010, workplace health promotion program evaluations have changed. The corporation's programs are now expected to use evidence-based interventions and practices, reduce variability in strategies, methods, and resource use that cannot be clinically justified, and increase coordination of programs through the use of information technology and team-based initiatives. Ms. Iocco now is being asked, *do the programs advance the outcome stakeholders care about, how far do the programs move the needle on the outcomes (how big is the change),* and *how do the programs compare to others?* What can Ms. Iocco do to prepare her staff and program vendors to answer these new questions? It is not enough anymore to just implement the program well. You need to show that the programs are impacting employee behavior and adding value. What would you do?

KEY TERMS

Population health management	Triple AIM
Population health management evaluation framework	Cost analyses
	Cost-effectiveness analyses
Population health management evaluation feedback loop	Cost-utility analysis
	Cost-benefit analysis
Program improvement	Return on investment
Model for Improvement	Feasible
Plan-Do-Study-Act	Scalable
Predictive modeling	Sustainable
Accountability	Scientific

References

ADP. (2012). *Why you should care about wellness programs.* Retrieved from http://www.adp.com/tools-and-resources/adp-research-institute/insights/~/media/RI/whitepapers/Why-You-Should-Care-About-Wellness-Programs.ashx

Baicker, K., Cutler, D., & Song, Z. (2010). Workplace wellness programs can generate savings. *Health Affairs, 29*(2), 304–311.

Bartholomew, S., & Smith, A. D. (2006). Improving survey response rates from chief executive officers in small firms: The importance of social networks. *Entrepreneurship Theory and Practice, 30*(1), 83–96.

Berwick, D. M., Nolan, T. W., & Whittington, J. (2008). The triple aim: Care, health, and cost. *Health Affairs, 27*(3), 759–769.

Brent, R. J. (2014). *Cost-benefit analysis and health care evaluations* (2nd ed.). Northampton, MA: Edward Elgar.

Caloyeras, J., Liu, H., Exum, E., Broderick, M., & Mattke, S. (2014). Managing manifest diseases, but not health risks, saved PepsiCo money over seven years. *Health Affairs, 33*(1), 124–131.

Cassell, C., Kontor, J., & Shah, L. (2012). *Population health management: Leveraging aging data and analytics to achieve value.* Retrieved from http://www.reliancecg.com/uploads/2_2012_Clinovations_PopulationHealthManagement_BriefingPaper.pdf

Cassidy, B. (2013). *Population health information management presents a new opportunity for HIM.* Retrieved May 3, 2014, from http://library.ahima.org/xpedio/groups/public/documents/ahima/bok1_050281.hcsp?dDocName=bok1_050281

Centers for Disease Control and Prevention. (1995). Assessing the effectiveness of disease and injury prevention programs: Costs and consequences. *Morbidity and Mortality Weekly Report, 44*(RR-10), 1–11.

Fielding, J. E., & Briss, P. A. (2006). Promoting evidence-based public health policy: Can we have better evidence and more action? *Health Affairs, 25*(4), 969–978.

Institute for Healthcare Improvement. (2014). How to improve. Retrieved from http://www.ihi.org/resources/Pages/HowtoImprove/default.aspx

Johnson T. (2006). Preventive services a good investment for health. *The Nation's Health, 36*(6).

Lavizzo-Mourey, R. (2014). *Workplace wellness: Not just about the dollars.* Retrieved from https://www.linkedin.com/today/post/article/20140117184103-43742182-workplace-wellness-not-just-about-the-dollars?goback=%2Egde_2007987_member_5830081233035485185

Mattke, S., Liu, H., Caloyeras, J., Huang, C., Van Busum, K., Khodyakov, D., & Shier, V. (2013). *Workplace wellness program study: Final report.* Santa Monica, CA: RAND Corporation. Retrieved from rand.org/t/RR254

Musich, S. A., Adams, L., & Edington, D. W. (2000). Effectiveness of health promotion programs in moderating medical costs in the USA. *Health Promotion International, 15*(1), 5–15.

Nas, T. F. (1996). *Cost-benefit analysis: Theory and application.* Thousand Oaks, CA: Sage.

O'Donnell, M. P. (1984). Health promotion in the workplace. *The Journal of Ambulatory Care Management, 7*(3), 79.

Ozminkowski, R. J., & Goetzel, R. Z. (2001). Getting closer to the truth: Overcoming research challenges when estimating the financial impact of worksite health promotion programs. *American Journal of Health Promotion, 15*(5), 289–295.

Population Health Alliance. (2014). Retrieved from http://www.populationhealthalliance.org/

Provost, L., & Murray, S. (2007). *The data guide* (pp. 3–15). Austin, TX: Associates in Process Improvement and Corporate Transformation Concepts.

Saul, J., & Gasser, N. (2014). Using big data to predict social impact. *Stanford Social Innovation Review.* Retrieved from https://event.webcasts.com/starthere.jsp?ei=1043480

Schottmuller, A. (2014). *Social media ROI: 14 formulas to measure social media benefits.* Retrieved from http://searchenginewatch.com/article/2249515/Social-Media-ROI-14-Formulas-to-Measure-Social-Media-Benefits

Senge, P. (1990). *The fifth discipline: The art and practice of the learning organization.* New York, NY: Random House.

Shortell, S. M., Zukoski, A. P., Alexander, J. A., Bazzoli, G. J., Conrad, D. A., Hasnain-Wynia, R.,. . . Margolin, F. S. (2002). Evaluating partnerships for community health improvement: tracking the footprints. *Journal of Health Politics, Policy, and Law, 27*(1), 49–92.

Smeltzer, P. A., Ozminkowski, R., & Musich, S. A. (2014). *Evaluating health promotion programs applying best practices to evaluate and study the impact of health promotion programs benefit costs, health and productivity.* Retrieved from http://www.corporatewellnessmagazine.com/issue-20/economics-issue-20/impact-of-health-promotion/

Solberg, L., Mosser, G., & McDonald, S. (1997a). The three faces of performance measurement: improvement, accountability, and research. *Joint Commission Journal on Quality and Patient Safety, 23*(3): 13–147.

Solberg, L., Mosser, G., & McDonald, S. (1997b). Why are you measuring? *Journal on Quality Improvement, 23*(3), 135–147.

Stiefel, M., & Nolan, K. (2012). *A guide to measuring the triple aim: Population health, experience of care, and per capita cost.* IHI Innovation Series white paper. Cambridge, MA: Institute for Healthcare Improvement. Retrieved from http://www.ihi.org/resources/Pages/IHIWhitePapers/AGuidetoMeasuringTripleAim.aspx

Terry, K. (2012). Construction of countywide EHR part of larger national IT program. *Fierce Health IT.* Retrieved from http://www.fiercehealthit.com/story/hennepin-health-project-looks-build-countywide-ehr-program-national-implica/2012-01-10

University of Wisconsin Population Health Institute (2015). *County health rankings & roadmaps.* Retrieved from www.countyhealthrankings.org

BIG DATA, HEALTH INFORMATION MANAGEMENT, HEALTH INFORMATICS, AND WORKPLACE HEALTH PROMOTION

Big Data for Workplace Health Promotion

Big data, which is increasingly used in the evaluation of workplace health promotion programs, refers to a set of information and data so large and complex that it becomes difficult to process using conventional database management tools (TechAmerica Foundation, 2012). Big data describes large and ever-increasing volumes of data that adhere to the following attributes (Zikopoulos, Eaton, DeRoos, Deutsch, & Lapis, 2012):

- Volume—ever-increasing amounts
- Velocity—quickly generated
- Variety—many different types
- Veracity—from trustable sources

The trend to larger data sets (big data) is due to the creation of related data sets, as compared to separate smaller sets with the same total amount of data, allowing correlations to be found to identify trends in the health of workers at workplaces, prevent diseases, organize health promotion activities, and determine and improve program outcomes.

Big data for workplace health promotion programs is the combination of all of the varied data sources that are now available to access (Figure 16.1). Together they

LEARNING OBJECTIVES

- **Explain big data for workplace health promotion**

- **Discuss health information management and health informatics professionals**

- **Describe how big data can enhance the impact and sustainability of workplace health promotion programs**

- **Present workplace health promotion big data evaluation challenges**

- **Describe big data platforms and frameworks for workplace health promotion**

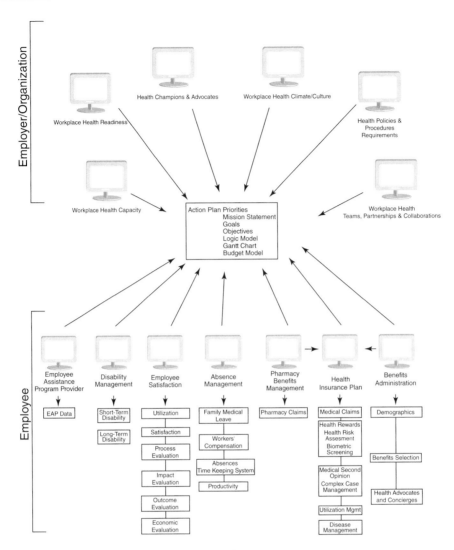

Figure 16.1   Big Data for Workplace Health Promotion Program Evaluation

create big data that can be analyzed as part of workplace health promotion program planning as well as program evaluation.

A series of changes and trends have created the opportunity to use big data in workplace health promotion programs (Figure 16.2). The U.S. federal government and other public stakeholders have been opening their vast stores of health care knowledge, including data from clinical trials and information on individuals covered under public insurance programs. A dramatic increase is due to incentives for electronic health record (EHR) adoption in the United States funded by the Health Information Technology for Economic and Clinical Health (HITECH) Act. Recent

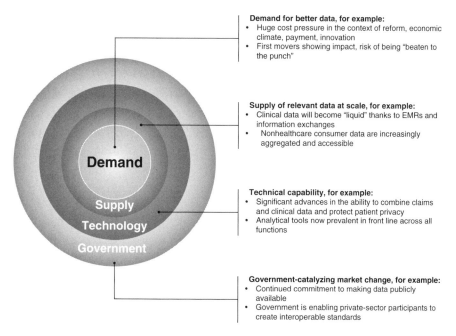

Demand for better data, for example:
- Huge cost pressure in the context of reform, economic climate, payment, innovation
- First movers showing impact, risk of being "beaten to the punch"

Supply of relevant data at scale, for example:
- Clinical data will become "liquid" thanks to EMRs and information exchanges
- Nonhealthcare consumer data are increasingly aggregated and accessible

Technical capability, for example:
- Significant advances in the ability to combine claims and clinical data and protect patient privacy
- Analytical tools now prevalent in front line across all functions

Government-catalyzing market change, for example:
- Continued commitment to making data publicly available
- Government is enabling private-sector participants to create interoperable standards

Figure 16.2   Recent Changes and Trends Have Created the Opportunity to Use Big Data in Workplace Health Promotion Programs
Source: Kayyali, Knott, and Van Kuiken, 2013.

technical advances have made it easier to collect and analyze information from multiple sources—a major benefit for health care and employers, since data for a single individual (worker) come from various hospitals, laboratories, pharmacies, and medical offices as well as the employer's human resource files (e.g., benefit usage, attendance, worker compensation, health promotion program satisfaction and interest, health risk appraisal). The supply of data has increased. For example, health care systems and insurance companies have digitized records and pharmaceutical companies have been aggregating years of research and development data into medical databases. Finally the demand for the data is high. Fiscal concerns, perhaps more than any other factor, are driving the demand for big data applications. Analyzing and using the data is seen as a means to maximize resources and improve worker health outcomes by designing health promotion programs and benefits matched to the needs of employees.

While health care costs may be paramount in big data's rise, health promotion program and clinical trends also play a role. Health professionals have traditionally used their judgment when making health program and treatment decisions, but in the past few years there has been a move toward evidence-based medicine and health programs, which involves system- atically reviewing clinical data, health program evaluations, and research literature, and making programmatic and treatment decisions based on the best available evidence. Aggregating individual (worker) data sets into big data algorithms often provides the most robust evidence, since nuances in subpopulations (such as the presence of workers with gluten allergies) may be rare enough that they are not readily apparent in small samples.

Although the health care industry has lagged behind sectors like retail and banking in the use of big data—partly because of concerns about individual confidentiality—it is catching up. Many large employers are achieving positive results that are prompting other large employers, as well as midsized and small employers, to take action lest they be left behind. These developments are encouraging, but they also raise an important question: Is the health care industry prepared to capture big data's full potential, or are there roadblocks that will hamper its use? At issue is how to access, distribute, and utilize this vast amount of "unstructured" data.

What Is Data Mining?

Data mining is the processing and modeling of large amounts of data to discover previously unknown patterns or relationships (Bellazzi & Zupan, 2008). Using data mining it is possible to examine all of the data sets available for a workplace health promotion program (Figure 16.1). For example, medical data management companies collect this information from health insurers, third-party administrators, health maintenance organizations, and pharmacy benefit managers and organize it into highly useful program outcomes, clinical utilization, and financial data sets. Sophisticated software allows analysts to sort, combine, and contrast key data elements to help decision makers and program managers take effective actions. Tools such as the National Committee for Quality Assurance's (NCQA) Healthcare Effectiveness Data and Information Set (HEDIS) are used in the mining process. HEDIS consists of 75 measures across eight domains of care. Using the HEDIS it is now possible to mine the various data sets available to workplace health promotion programs to help employers uncover problems and focus on areas for improvement. Kirby, Kersting, and Flick (2010) identified seven examples of how data mining can be used to evaluate workplace health promotion programs:

1. **Determine what diseases and conditions are driving trends.** This entails reviewing an organization's medical and prescription drug claims data to verify which health issues are most prevalent among employees and their families. Using this information, the employer can then tailor the health promotion program to help employees adopt healthier behaviors and reduce costs.

2. **Target intervention to high-risk segments of the workers and those who need the most care.** Reviewing the severity of employees' diseases and conditions will identify those who have complex needs and require significant care management. The goals of targeted intervention include reducing the rate of hospital readmission and directing care to high-quality, low-cost network providers.

3. **Identify gaps in medical treatment and direct employees to the proper care.** Gaps can be discovered by comparing employees' data to Healthcare Effectiveness Data and Information Set (HEDIS) benchmarks. Where possible, employees and their primary-care physicians should be encouraged to reduce or eliminate those gaps.

4. **Identify the best, most cost-effective network providers and guide employees to use them.** Data mining can, for example, pinpoint high-performance, high-quality providers and services. It can also identify providers that offer access to appropriate care and interventions that follow evidence-based guidelines. Workplace health promotion programs can then promote the use of these providers and services by employees who need care.

5. **Improve health habits through wellness, health promotion, education, and care-management programs that increase awareness and engage employees in their own care.** Using data mining, a health promotion program plan can determine if its benefit design is effective in promoting wellness and prevention. The result might be the design of a multifaceted, incentive-based plan that includes design, vendor performance, communications, and incentives that help manage costs.

6. **Measure the performance of vendors and administrators and hold them accountable for quality, cost-effective treatment by comparing their results to national benchmarks.** Health promotion programs can implement performance guarantees for the plan's financial, clinical, operational and utilization components. For example, utilization performance guarantees can help manage emergency room visits for chronic conditions, such as asthma.

7. **Determine what level of cost-sharing improves employee health and cuts costs.** One organization that had an upfront deductible and a copayment for office visits decided to try eliminating both. The next year virtually every employee visited his or her primary care physician and specialists, which doubled the plan's physician and specialist visit rates per 1,000 employees. This improved employee health and reduced long-term costs. The key is to be sure that cost-sharing encourages appropriate usage. For example, in a recent study

of individuals (employees) who self-referred, 61% visited the wrong specialist. If cost-sharing is structured to encourage individuals to visit a primary care physician first, he or she will select an appropriate specialist, which will cut costs and improve results.

Health Information Management and Health Informatics Professionals: Big Data Professional Fields

In the evaluation of workplace health promotion programs the professionals who work with big data are individuals trained in the fields of health information management and health informatics. Both terms are often used interchangeably even though they are quite different. *Health information management* is the accumulation, storage, and accuracy of health data. It is the management of personal health information in hospitals, health care organizations, health insurance providers, and public health programs enabling the delivery of quality services to the public. There is no implication of use of the data beyond viewing individual data records in a digital-based manner. It is simply the access of information. *Health informatics* is a much newer term in the public health and health care industries, and grounded in the history of business intelligence. Health informatics is the utilization of information technologies and information management tactics to enhance process efficiency and reduce costs. Health informatics applies the data gathered and stored through health information management systems and creates knowledge. Health informatics is concerned with the manipulation of organization-wide data to generate reports on outcomes, utilization, and cost to improve program (health promotion) quality and achieve better health care and health outcomes for the employee and employers. It leverages computer systems to help analyze and manage individuals' data.

Health Information Management and Health Informatics

Health Information Management is the management of personal health information in hospitals or other health care organizations enabling the delivery of quality health care to the public. Health information management deals largely with patient or individual-related data. It is responsible for the accumulation, storage, and accuracy of patient data (medical record); it operates the domain of medical records, billing, and data regulatory compliance; and it focuses on records management, terminology, coding, transcription, and the business of health care related to medical records management.

Health Informatics is the rapidly developing scientific field that utilizes computer technology in the advancement of medicine. It applies information technology in health care for knowledge creation and management. It is responsible for the design, development, analysis and utilization of individual and organization data systems. Health informatics has a foundation and background in information infrastructure and architecture, with a focus on database design and programming, information systems design, standards and analysis—health systems organization plus the business of health care systems computer information systems.

Increasingly, health information management professionals have been playing a role in workplace health through their focus on the collection, maintenance, and use of quality data to support the information-intensive and information-reliant health care system. They work with clinical, epidemiological, demographic, financial, reference, and coded health care data. Health information administrators plan information systems, develop health policy, and identify current and future information needs. In addition, they apply the science of informatics to the collection, storage, use, and transmission of information. Greater access to data has had a positive impact on workplace health promotion programs. Employers can look for trends in employees' health status, disease management, and service utilization. The data helps put preventive plans in place, watch for changes in a certain geography or demographic, as well as report information of interest or concern to the overall populace.

Health information management and health informatics have changed with the changing health care industry, but their main goal is still to analyze, manage, and utilize the information that is essential to individuals' health and ensure that providers can access the information when necessary. Some of the main subdisciplines of health informatics include: biomedical informatics, medical informatics, clinical informatics, nursing informatics, pharmacy informatics, public health informatics, business informatics, and health information management. As the fields have developed, a number of professional groups organized to support health information management and health informatics professionals.

Health Information Management and Health Informatics Professional Organizations

- American Society of Health Informatics Managers (ASHIM)

- American Health Information Management Association (AHIMA)

- Commission on Accreditation of Health Informatics and Information Management Education (CAHIIM)

- Healthcare Information Management and Systems Society (HIMMS)

Key Health Information Management and Health Informatics Terms

Algorithm. The process for carrying out a complex task, which is broken down into simple decision and action steps. Often assists the *requirements analysis* process carried out before programming.

Clinical data system. Any information system concerned with the capture, processing, or communication of individual (employee) data.

Clinical decision tool. Any mechanical, paper, or electronic aid that collects or processes data from an individual patient to generate output that aids clinical decisions during the doctor-patient encounter. Examples include *decision support systems*, paper or computer *reminders* and *checklists*, which are potentially useful tools in *public health informatics*, as well as other branches of medical informatics.

Consumer health informatics. The use of *medical informatics* methods to facilitate the study and development of paper or electronic systems that support public access to and use of health and lifestyle information.

Decision support system (computer decision aid). A type of *clinical decision tool*: a computer system that uses two or more items of *patient data* to generate case specific or encounter specific advice. An example is a computer risk assessor to estimate cardiovascular disease risk. Evidence-adaptive decision support systems are a type of decision aid with a knowledge base that is constructed from and continually adapts to new research based and practice based evidence.

Decision tree. A way to model a complex decision process as a tree with branches representing all possible intermediate states or final outcomes of an event. The probabilities of each intermediate state or final outcome and the perceived utilities of each are combined to attach expected utilities to each outcome.

Individual health record. The primary legal record documenting the health care services provided to a person in any aspect of the health care system. The term includes routine clinical or office records, records of care in any health-related setting, preventive care, lifestyle evaluation, research protocols, and various clinical databases. This repository of information about a single patient is generated by health care professionals as a direct result of interaction with a patient or with individuals who have personal knowledge of the patient.

Primary record. The record that is used by health care professionals while providing care services to review individuals' data or document their own observations, actions, or instructions.

Secondary record. A record that is derived from the primary record and contains selected data elements to aid nonclinical persons in supporting, evaluating, and advancing individual care. Individual care support refers to administration, regulation, and payment functions.

How Big Data Can Enhance the Impact and Sustainability of Workplace Health Promotion Programs

Big data enhances the impact and sustainability of workplace health promotion programs by integrating a growing quantity of varied data sources, along with methods to analyze and put the data to use, which can lead to improved personal health, health care delivery, and effective workplace health promotion programs. Adams and Klein (2011) suggested three levels of analytics to use for workplace health promotion program evaluations, each with increasing functionality and value:

- Descriptive: Standard types of reporting that describe current situations and problems

- Predictive: Simulation and modeling techniques that identify trends and portend outcomes of actions taken

- Prescriptive: Prescribing actions to optimize programmatic, financial, and other outcomes

In particular, workplace health promotion program evaluations use big data predictive and prescriptive analytics as a way to maximize resources and outcomes. To help employers think about the power of big data in the evaluation of workplace health promotion programs, Kayyali et al. (2013) created five evaluation objectives (pathways) to guide predictive and prescriptive analyses. Their goal is to produce practical data that can be used by employers to make decisions about their employee health promotion program that support employees' right living, right care, right provider, right value, and right innovation.

Five Pathways of Evaluations (Kayyali et al., 2013)

1. **Right living.** Employees must be encouraged to play an active role in their own health by making the right choices about diet, exercise, preventive care, and other lifestyle factors.

2. **Right care.** Employees must receive the most timely, appropriate health promotion programs and treatment available. In addition to relying heavily on protocols, right care requires a coordinated approach, with all health providers having access to the same information and working toward the same goal to avoid duplication of effort and suboptimal health promotion programs and treatment strategies.

3. **Right provider.** Any health professionals who serve workers must have strong performance records and be capable of achieving the best outcomes. They need to be selected based on their skill sets and abilities rather than their job titles. For instance, nurses or physicians' assistants may perform many tasks that do not require a doctor.

4. **Right value.** Employers, health professionals, and health insurance companies need to continually look for ways to improve value while preserving or improving health care quality. For example, they could develop a system in which program reimbursement is tied to worker health outcomes or undertake programs designed to eliminate wasteful spending.

5. **Right innovation.** Employers and employees as well as other stakeholders must focus on identifying new health promotion programs and approaches to health care delivery. They need to try to improve the innovation engines themselves—for instance, by advancing the offerings of workplace health promotion programs.

One of the characteristics of big data is that new data is continually becoming available, creating a feedback loop. The concept of right care, for instance, could change if new data suggest that the standard protocol for a particular health promotion intervention does not produce optimal results. And a change in one pathway could spur changes in others, since they are interdependent. An evaluation, for example, could reveal that workers are most likely to suffer costly complications after back surgery, thereby encouraging more effective and less costly alternative treatments. This finding could influence opinions not only about value but also about the health professionals selected to address musculoskeletal pain and injuries among employees.

Workplace Health Promotion Big Data Evaluation Challenges

Although the potential value of big data to evaluate workplace health promotion programs is large, challenges do exist (Institute for Health

Technology Transformation, 2013; Savel & Foldy, 2012). These include integration of disparate sources, consistency/standardization (defined similarly throughout organization), data fragmentation, trustworthiness (confidence in the data), and protection (security of the data). The challenges highlight a critical need for workplace health promotion program staff and evaluators to understand the data's provenance (i.e., to know the data's origin and purpose) so as to understand its potential contribution and role in any big data processing and analysis.

Integration of Disparate Sources

The sources of big data vary in a number of ways. For example, some data will come from systems that use older technology and software that may or may not be compatible with newer technologies and techniques. In many cases, organizations don't have easy options to upgrade or otherwise adapt their technologies to growing data demands. Frequently data is stored in databases and the organization's vendor has only certain mechanisms in place to exchange data, limiting the organization's ability to roll out new tools. Likewise health care organizations are collecting and storing so much data that improved data governance measures are urgently needed to identify, enter, and leverage the most useful data. Organizations are struggling with such questions as how best to determine the value of their data, how to store their data, and how and when to delete and/or archive their data. Related to this is the timeliness or freshness of data at point of it being used as part of the evaluation. If employee turnover is high then it is possible to be making programmatic decisions based on employees who are no longer part of the organization. Finally, understanding how the data can be simplified and reduced is important to be able to draw meaningful conclusions and make recommendations.

Consistency/Standardization

Often data is not defined similarly across organizations and even throughout the same organization. For example, it might be coded (transformed) for a particular purpose, such as billing. Inaccurate or incomplete data require having to have data checked and rechecked before use, which is labor and time intensive. Data can exhibit the statistical phenomenon of censoring. For example, the first instance of a health concern in a record may not be when it was first manifested (left censoring) or the data source may not cover a sufficiently long time interval (right censoring). Data may also incompletely adhere to well-known standards, which makes combining it from different sources more difficult (Hersh et al., 2013).

Data Fragmentation

The separation, or fragmentation, of data among medical offices, health systems, human resources, and EHRs is another significant obstacle to leveraging big data in health promotion program evaluations. Each entity serves as a single repository, or silo, for information whose purpose is to provide programs, clinical care, scheduling or billing information, or operational information. This continues to be problematic for organizations seeking to get individual systems to communicate with each other easily. It remains especially challenging in smaller organizations with multiple systems and taxonomies that make extracting useful information difficult. The overall result is that organizations end up with little pieces of data from various sources that make it hard to understand how everything fits together.

Trustworthiness

Data trustworthiness or confidence in the data is a major challenge especially with respect to making program and clinical decision. Most clinical data is stored in "unstructured" form, especially within EHRs, making it difficult to access for effective analytics. For example, individual providers can read narrative text within a record or report, but most current analytics applications cannot effectively utilize this unstructured data. Currently, most program analytics rely on claims or administrative data. These data consist largely of more structured data, but are of limited value in evaluating the efficacy of care and program outcomes (Amarasingham et al., 2010). Emerging big data technology and techniques show promise in helping organizations to process and evaluate data from records, clinic equipment, telehealth devices, and home health monitors.

Protection

Health care organizations and employers in general and workplace health promotion programs in particular need to diligently focus on protecting and securing four types of data (Ascenzo, 2013; Institute for Health Technology Transformation, 2013).

1. Personally identifiable information. The loss of personally identifiable information such as dates of birth, driver's license numbers, and social security numbers is among the greatest of privacy threats. While external threats dominate top-of-mind discussions, information breaches are growing, presenting the potential for significant loss of customers, incurrence of high compensation claims lawsuits, and permanent damage to reputation.

2. Clinical data. Electronic health records contain a wide range of employee-specific information, including prescription data, treatment details, and other data. Combined with a policy number, a hacker can use it to receive unauthorized medical care or bill for services never received. The leakage and/or corruption of such information can even result in irrevocable harm to one's personal and professional life.

3. Financial data. With banks and individuals getting more proactive about protecting their financial information, the medical industry is becoming an easy target for hackers. The outsourcing of billing activities and increased Internet and mobile involvement in health care create more avenues for potential data theft; the resulting legal consequences and loss of patient trust can taint an organization's brand for life.

4. Behavioral data. Behavioral data are the newest and possibly fastest-growing in health care, thanks to monitoring devices, GPS tracking, Internet site visits, social media, purchasing habits, exercise activity, and self-reporting. Behavioral data is increasingly becoming the "hot favorite" for cyber thieves as it helps to draw up startlingly accurate representations of human behavior that are of great demand among marketing companies (and also others with illicit intentions). With growing usage of tablets, smartphones, and other mobile devices, this data is becoming more vulnerable to theft.

Big Data Applications and Services for Workplace Health Promotion

The use of big data for workplace health promotion programs hinges on the development of advanced data management platforms, data storage solutions, and frameworks. A platform refers to a software or hardware architecture that serves as a foundation or base for computing to be done. Data storage refers to the action of a computer or database holding data or values in one place, and it can be done via multiple means. A data storage framework is the infrastructure in which the data storage solutions are achieved, such as a network. Two main types of databases should be considered when working with large data sets such as those existing in health promotion programs, health care industries, and the like. The two types are relational databases (SQL) and nonrelational (NoSQL) databases. The databases differ in the way in which they store the data and how the developer calls upon the information. The choice to use either type depends on the nature of the data and how they are being used. Although traditional relational databases work well with big data sets of some types and uses, due to the continuous nature of health information and records, health information and records fit well into the NoSQL database model. For this reason, NoSQL databases have become the good option in the health care industry for dealing with big data sets. By using a NoSQL database in the health industry, users are able to experience easier and faster development and greater flexibility in the data model. In addition to these advantages, NoSQL databases have greater scalability to different types of data sets such as data sets across different organizations with specific needs (Date, 2004; He, Fan, & Li, 2013).

The following sample indicates the diverse range of big data solutions and the databases in the health industry. Their immediate application and use in workplace evaluations differ in that some are research focused while others are health care industry (including health promotion) focused. Together they provide an overview of future directions for the potential use and impact of big data to promote the health of individuals (employees).

The National Institutes of Health (NIH)—Big Data to Knowledge (BD2K; http://www.bd2k.nih.gov): With the BD2K, NIH aims to develop the new approaches, standards, methods, tools, software, and competencies that will enhance the use of biomedical big data by supporting research, implementation, and training in data science and other relevant fields. With this, the mission is to enable biomedical scientists in using big data sets that they and the research community are generating.

The tranSMART Foundation (http://www.transmartfoundation.org): The tranSMART foundation is a global nonprofit organization with a mission aimed at creating a homogeneous and open-source data community that allows open sharing and collaboration across researchers. The vision of tranSMART is a knowledge base built by and for the translational research community—a repository of open-access, open-source data designed to enable collaboration across disciplines, specialties, and geography. This will allow scientists and researchers access to the massive amount of global data and increase productivity, understanding, and usability.

IBM Watson Foundation (http://www-01.ibm.com/software/data /bigdata/): The IBM Watson Foundation provides a platform of big data and analytics capabilities that can be leveraged to the specific big data needs of an organization. The capabilities of the Watson Foundation include data management and warehousing, Hadoop system (an Apache programming framework), stream computing, content management, and information integration and governance.

Institute for Health Metrics & Evaluation (IHME; www .healthmetricsandevaluation.org): IMHE, an independent global health research center at the University of Washington, provides rigorous and comparable measurement of the world's most important health problems and evaluates the strategies used to address them. IHME makes this information freely available so that policymakers have the evidence they need to make informed decisions about how to allocate resources to best improve population health. The IHME gathers large distributed data sets globally for data analysis and health measurement data from disparate sources including censuses, surveys, vital statistics, disease registries, and hospital records. Its aim is to support policy decisions in order to improve population health.

University of California, Santa Cruz Cancer Genome Initiative (http://news.ucsc.edu/2012/05/cancer-genomics.htm): In this $10.5 million project, which is the world's largest repository for cancer genomes, a huge database with biomedical information is structured, which will allow to get a complete molecular characterization of cancer. These programs are laying the foundation for personalized cancer care by creating a database that scientists around the world can use to connect specific genomic changes with clinical outcomes.

Healthx (http://www.healthx.com): Healthx provides self-service web-based solutions for their members and providers resulting in 16 million logins by health plan members and over 9 million logins by providers. It develops and manages online cloud-based portals for health care companies, with a focus on enrollments, claims management, and business intelligence. It uses databases including but not limited to benefits, physician, and prescription information. http://www.healthx.com

Sickweather LLC (http://www.sickweather.com): Scans social media (Facebook, Twitter) to track outbreaks of disease and then offers forecasts to users, similar to weather forecasting, to keep individuals aware of outbreaks in their area. Just as Doppler radar scans the skies for indicators of bad weather, Sickweather scans social networks for indicators of illness, allowing a user to check for the chance of sickness as easily as checking for the chance of rain. Sickweather can be used to track illnesses, compare symptoms, and see which viruses are going around in a given area.

Humedica Inc. (http://www.humedica.com): Humedica is a medical informatics company that connects clinical and patient information across varied settings and time periods to generate longitudinal and comprehensive views of patient care. It provides accurate and detailed predictive models by the normalizing data to produce more accurate and precise inputs over longer periods of time.

Practice Fusion (http://www.practicefusion.com): This cloud-based EMR platform for medical practices also aggregates population data across multiple sites to improve clinical research and public health analysis. The platform includes ePrescribing, labs, meaningful use, charting and scheduling. Recent projects of Practice Fusion are on cancer and heart disease. Practice Fusion analyzes aggregated data from the EMR and public health to monitor health on a population level. These data include:

- Health population surveillance and education (e.g., flu, asthma)
- Drug surveillance
- Public health research
- Care plan
- Best practices

(http://www.practicefusion.com)

Summary

Big data is used in the evaluation of workplace health promotion programs. Big data refers to a set of information and data so large and complex that it becomes difficult to process using conventional database management tools. In program evaluation, data mining is used for processing and modeling of large amounts of data to discover previously unknown patterns or relationships. The professionals who work with big data in the evaluation of workplace health promotion programs are individuals trained the fields of health information management and health informatics. Three levels of analytics are used for workplace health promotion program evaluation, each with increasing functionality and value: descriptive, predictive, and prescriptive. Increasingly, big data analyses for program evaluation focus on predictive and prescriptive analytics as a way to maximize resources and outcomes. And although the potential value of big data to evaluate workplace health promotion programs is large, challenges do exist. Finally, the development of advanced data management platforms, data storage solutions, and frameworks, with their promise to lower cost and improve employee health, will increase the demand for knowledge and expertise in the use of big data to evaluate workplace health promotion programs and to create continuous feedback loops to improve program quality and efficiencies.

For Practice and Discussion

1. Big data plays a role in the evaluation of workplace health promotion programs. How does the role differ based on the size of an organization (large, midsized, small)? Compare and contrast the four data attributes

(volume, velocity, variety, veracity) of big data for different sized organizations.

2. Algorithms are key in big data for analyzing the health information. In plain language, what is an algorithm? What is the relationship between algorithms and data mining?

3. Select a workplace health promotion program implementation health priority area (e.g., physical, nutrition, physical activity, or another). Propose evaluation questions for that priority using the five pathways (right living, right care, right provider, right value, right innovation) suggested by Kayyali et al. (2013), which could be used to guide data mining as part of a workplace health promotion program evaluation.

4. Five challenges exist for using big data in workplace health promotion programs: integration of disparate sources, consistency /standardization (defined similarly throughout organization), data fragmentation, trustworthiness (confidence in the data), and protection (security of the data). The challenges cause employers to mistrust and resist using the results generated from big data analyses. How do you expect health information management and health informatics professionals to address the challenges and overcome employer mistrust and resistance?

5. The chapter lists several advanced data management platforms, data storage solutions, and frameworks. Which ones do you believe hold the most promise for using big data in health promotion programs?

Case Study: Getting the Data You Need and Can Use—What Would You Do?

Elmar Mursaliyev, the human resource director for a large food franchise operator in the Midwest, is overwhelmed by reports from the company's health insurance provider. He feels like data is growing and moving faster than he and his work colleagues can consume it. He knows that getting access to and using data to factor into the design of the company work-place health promotion program is critical to promoting employee health. However, Mr. Mursaliyev recently received eight e-mailed reports covering employee pharmacy claims, workers' compensation records, health risks appraisal results, worker health promotion program satisfaction and interest surveys, employee attendance, and benefits selections. Each report was at least 40 pages long. A few were closer to 80 pages long. He asked for executive summaries and was e-mailed eight one-page summaries. Mr. Mursaliyev has a dilemma. The long reports were too much whereas the executive summaries were too little. If you were Mr. Mursaliyev what would you do? What would you request from the health insurance company?

KEY TERMS

Big data

Data mining

Healthcare Effectiveness Data and Information Set (HEDIS)

Health information management

Health informatics

Algorithm

Clinical data system

Clinical decision tool

Consumer health informatics

Decision support system (Computer decision aid)

Decision tree

Individual health record

Primary record

Secondary record

Descriptive analytics

Predictive analytics

Prescriptive analytics

Big data evaluation challenges

Advanced data management platforms

Data storage solutions

Frameworks

References

Adams, J., & Klein, J. (2011). *Business intelligence and analytics in health care—A primer*. Washington, DC: The Advisory Board Company.

Amarasingham, R., Moore, B. J., Tabak, Y. P., Drazner, M. H., Clark, C. A., Zhang, S., . . . Halm, E. A. (2010). An automated model to identify heart failure patients at risk for 30-day readmission or death using electronic medical record data. *Medical Care, 48*(11), 981–988.

Ascenzo, C. (2012, September 20). *4 big data threats health org's are socially obligated to safeguard against*. Retrieved from http://www.govhealthit.com/blog /4-big-data-threats-health-org%E2%80%99s-are-socially-obligated-safeguard-against

Bellazzi, R., & Zupan, B. (2008). Predictive data mining in clinical medicine: Current issues and guidelines. *International Journal of Medical Informatics, 77*(2), 81–97.

Date, C. J. (2004). *An introduction to database systems* (8th ed.). New York, NY: Pearson.

He, C., Fan, X., & Li, Y. (2013). Toward ubiquitous healthcare services with a novel efficient cloud platform. *IEEE Transactions on Biomedical Engineering, 60*(1), 230–234.

Hersh, W. R., Weiner, M. G., Embi, P. J., Logan, J. R., Payne, P. R., Bernstam, E. V., . . . Cimino, J. J. (2013). Caveats for the use of operational electronic health record data in comparative effectiveness research. *Medical Care, 51*, S30–S37.

Institute for Health Technology Transformation. (2013). *Transforming health care through big data strategies for leveraging big data in the health care industry*. Retrieved from http://ihealthtran.com/wordpress/2013/03/iht2-releases-big-data-research-report-download-today/

Kayyali, B., Knott, D., & Van Kuiken, S. (2013, April). *The big-data revolution in US health care: Accelerating value and innovation*. Retrieved from http://www.mckinsey.com/insights/health_systems_and_services/the_big-data_revolution_in_us_health_care

Kirby, M., Kersting, M., & Flick, E. (2010). The benefits of digging deeper: Using data mining to improve employee health and reduce employer costs. *Perspectives, 18*(2). Retrieved from http://www.sibson.com/publications/perspectives/volume_18_issue_2/digging-deeper.html

Savel, T. G., & Foldy, S. (2012). The role of public health informatics in enhancing public health surveillance. *Morbidity and Mortality Weekly Report Surveillance Summary, 61*, 20–24.

TechAmerica Foundation. (2012). *Demystifying big data: A practical guide to transforming the business of government*. Retrieved May 27, 2015 from http://www.techamerica.org/Docs/fileManager.cfm?f=techamerica-bigdatareport-final.pdf

Zikopoulos, P. C., Eaton, C., DeRoos, D., Deutsch, T., & Lapis, G. (2012). *Understanding big data*. New York, NY: McGraw-Hill.

PART FIVE

WORKPLACES

CHAPTER 17

SMALL AND MIDSIZED EMPLOYERS AND HEALTH PROMOTION

How Small and Midsized Employers Promote Employee Health

Small and midsized employers occupy a substantial position within the U.S. economy, annually employing more than 50% of the private-sector workers (McDowell, 2009). And over the past decade, the number of health promotion programs in small and midsized workplaces has increased significantly. The employers are paying more attention to the relationship between preventive health practices and productive employees.

How small and midsized employers plan, implement, and evaluate workplace health promotion programs is to balance their (employers') value of the well-being of employees with their (employers') concerns about workplace health promotion programs. Employers are amenable to employee health promotion programs and most already have some experience with them. Often small businesses employ family members and personal acquaintances. And, if they don't know an employee before being hired, then chances are that the very size of the workplace will promote the closeness and concern for one another that small businesses value. At the same time employer concerns drive workplace health promotion program implementation (Muchnick-Baku & Warshaw, 2011). Seven factors shape how small and midsized employers promote their employees' health and safety: health insurance, cost, time, complexity, effectiveness, expertise, and space.

LEARNING OBJECTIVES

- Describe how small and midsized employers promote employee health

- Discuss how to work with small and midsized employers to promote health

- Discuss the challenges and opportunities for small and midsized employer health promotion programs

- Describe small and midsized employer health promotion tools and resources

1. **Health insurance:** In 2005, 62% of small businesses (those with fewer than 50 employees) purchased health insurance for their employees, compared with 96% of large employers (Sommers & Crimmel, 2007). And when they provide health benefits, smaller employers paid larger amounts for administering and underwriting those benefits (Stanton & Rutherford, 2004). Furthermore small and midsized businesses have witnessed greater growth of health care costs relative to payroll, compared with their larger counterparts (National Small Business Association, 2014; Office of Advocacy, 2011).

With the full implementation of the Affordable Care Act (ACA) employers face an obligation to provide health insurance for their employees. The ACA stipulates the number of employees employed by an organization (e.g., 50, 100, or less) that obligates an employer to offer employee health insurance coverage. With the implementation of the ACA, interest among small and midsized employers to lower employee-related health care costs (i.e., insurance premiums) has soared given this new obligation. To assist small and midsized employers, the Small Business Health Options Program (SHOP) Marketplace was created as part of the ACA, to help businesses provide health coverage for their employees (https://www.healthcare.gov/small-businesses/).

In 2014, the SHOP Marketplace was open to employers with 50 or fewer full-time-equivalent employees (FTEs). Employers with fewer than 25 employees can qualify for tax credits when purchasing insurance through SHOP. In 2017 employers with up to 100 employees are eligible to participate in SHOP. Another option for employees in small and midsized organizations is to purchase individual health care coverage for them and their families through the Individual Health Exchanges operated by the state or federal government (depending on the state where they live). With this option an employer might reimburse employees a set amount allowing individuals to select the coverage best matched to their (i.e., the employees') needs.

2. **Cost:** Small and midsized employers consider costs to promote employee health from two points of view. The first point of view is that addressing employee health and safety concerns is a cost of doing business. It is part of the overhead (or operating expense) that must be factored into making or delivering the product or service, and it ultimately impacts the price of the product or service to its consumer, client, or customer. In a competitive marketplace employers compete for workers. An attractive benefit package (e.g., health insurance, vision, dental, sick days, pharmacy plan, short- and long-term disability, health promotion, and reasonable copays and premiums) is necessary to attract and retain workers, but it can

be expensive. Furthermore a safe work environment requires attention and costs money (e.g., safety equipment, ergonomic work stations). Therefore a tension exists regarding how much of employee health care expense can be factored into the product's price without making the price so high that consumers, clients, and customers look elsewhere (i.e., to a competitor's product). The second point of view is that employee health and health promotion costs come after the product and service is delivered. The expense is deducted from any earnings (profits). In many situations this means the employers (owners) are getting less money from their business (if any) or incurring more debt. In this latter point of view the health and health promotion expenses are not part of the organizational overhead. A modest approach for an employer with this point of view, who wants to promote employee health but does not have resources, is to give employees a set amount of money (e.g., $100.00) a month to purchase insurance on the ACA Individual Health Exchange.

Simply considering costs, the smaller the firm, the less likely it is to provide group health insurance to employees and their dependents. It is difficult for an employer to claim concern for employees' health as a basis for offering health promotion activities when basic health insurance is not made available. Even when it is made accessible, exigencies of cost restrict many small businesses to "bare bones" health insurance programs with very limited coverage.

On the other hand, many of the "bare bones" plans do cover periodic medical examinations, mammography, Pap smears, immunizations, and well baby/child care. Unfortunately, the out-of-pocket cost of covering the deductible fees and copayments required before insured benefits are payable often acts as a deterrent for the small and midsized organization employees to use these preventive services. To overcome this, some employers have arranged to reimburse employees for all or part of these expenditures; others find it less troublesome and costly simply to pay for them as an operating expense.

3. **Time:** Small and midsized employers are busy. The demands on their time to complete what seems to be endless lists of things to do, conflicts with having time to first plan programs and second to implement programs. The employers know that employee programs require attention. Employers are most concerned that poorly planned and implemented programs will hurt production and waste employee time in a way that ultimately impacts employee engagement and adds costs. Frequently employers report that it is best to wait until they have time to plan a high-quality program rather than a plan and implement a low-quality program.

4. **Complexity:** Employers are concerned that health promotion programs are too elaborate to fit into the structure of the average small and midsized business. The large organization health promotion model, with programming in each of the six program priorities areas, is too much for small and midsized employers. The employers need to reframe the complexity in terms of choosing a model, but given the organization size their choices need to be strategic and selective.

5. **Effectiveness:** Small and midsized businesses simply do not have the resources to do formal program effectiveness and cost-benefit analyses of their health promotion programs. They are forced to rely on anecdotal experience (which may often be misleading) or on inference from the research done in large organizations. They try to learn from the bigger companies and extrapolate the information to fit their situation (Pelletier, 2009).

6. **Expertise:** Small and midsized employers have experience with workplace health promotion but generally lack expertise. They have to rely on individuals who are external to their organizations for the expertise and guidance on what works best for small and midsized employers when it comes to promoting employee health. And the question is always who is the best external person to talk with. Who has the expertise and knows exactly what the organization needs and actions to take? Furthermore for the small and midsized business person it is a matter of trust, as he or she will be spending limited company resources (money) to pay for the expertise and will want to make sure the advice is correct.

7. **Space:** Small and midsized employers often are concerned about space for workplace health promotion program. It is true that most would not have space (or the money) for an onsite fitness facility including changing rooms and showers. However, the majority of the program activities and interventions do not require space. And if space is required the employers typically look to share facilities with other groups or use existing community facilities.

Small and Midsized Employer Health Promotion Coalitions, Partnerships, and Collaborations

Coalitions, partnerships, and collaborations play a role in how employers promote employees' health. For example many small and midsized organizations are associated with the National Business Group on Health (https://www.businessgrouphealth.org/). In Pittsburgh the Business Group on Health (PBGH) is an employer-led, coalition of organizations representing various business segments including private-sector and public employers (e.g., government and education). Representing over 90 organizations, PBGH offers group-purchasing, leveraging the collective power of employers, employee engagement programs, supporting employers' health and wellness efforts, networking, benchmarking and education opportunities, and health care and benefit analyses and other industry information.

Business groups on health are found in many communities. They typically use a similar approach that includes creating a health mission, data collection, benefit design, supporting environment, programming, and evaluation. Figure 17.1 is an example of a tool to plan and implement programs commonly used by these groups; it was developed by the Partnership for Prevention/The WorkCare Group. The groups do not need to be only small employers. In fact the membership of most groups spans small, midsized, and large employers, providing a mix of expertise and power in the number of employees and a potential risk pool for group purchasing initiatives.

In Kansas City a partnership was formed by 16 large and small businesses in the Coalition on Health Care with the National Business Coalition on Health and Pfizer Inc., which used existing data to support corporate health strategies and drive decision making around workforce health and wellness, promoting prevention, eliminating barriers to healthy behaviors, and encouraging use of evidence-based health care (Partnership for Prevention, 2011a). This initiative focused on aligning health benefits and utilizing high-value intervention programs to improve employee health and wellness and manage health care costs for the employees and employers. The four core principles of this initiative are a strong health management team, actionable data, the fostering of healthier and more productive employees, and achieving higher value for investments.

The Healthy Workplace Recognition Program is an initiative of the San Antonio Business Group on Health (SABGH) and the San Antonio Mayor's Fitness Council. The program was created to recognize local employers for their workplace wellness efforts. The Mayor's Fitness Council and the SABGH recognize local employers in the following categories—Small Workplaces (up to 200 employees) and Medium to Large Workplaces (200 employees) (FitCitySA, 2014).

Small and midsized business health collaborations are also led by non-business groups interested in workplace health promotion. For example, Health Links Colorado is a nonprofit initiative spearheaded by health and safety experts at the Center for Worker Health and Environment within the Colorado School of Public Health. It works in partnerships with the Colorado Small Business Development Center Network. The initiative focuses on employers with fewer than 500 employees, using a Health Business Certification to implement workplace health promotion programs that provide

Health Management Initiative Assessment for Small and Medium-Sized Employers

	Strongly Agree	Agree	Undecided	Disagree	Strongly Disagree
Mission					
1) Our management and supervisory staff are committed to health promotion as an important investment in our employees and our business goals.	☐	☐	☐	☐	☐
2) All employees including managers/supervisors are educated on the link between personal health and the health of the company (total economic impact) including direct medical and indirect costs such as sick days, disability, and on-the-job productivity.	☐	☐	☐	☐	☐
Data Collection					
3) We use a Health Risk Assessment (HRA) to identify aggregate risks and track improvements	☐	☐	☐	☐	☐
4) We measure participation rates among our employees for care program offerings, such as HRA participation, health screenings, and wellness events.	☐	☐	☐	☐	☐
5) We measure employee satisfaction of our health promotion efforts.	☐	☐	☐	☐	☐
Supportive Environment					
6) We encourage regular physical activity through such initiatives as subsidizing gym memberships and/or providing changing rooms/showers, promoting walking clubs, pedometer challenges, walking during meetings, cycling to work, using the stairs, and/or periodic stretching breaks.	☐	☐	☐	☐	☐
7) We provide healthful food selections in our vending machines/cafeteria and at company meetings/functions.	☐	☐	☐	☐	☐
8) An employee volunteer team promotes our health promotion programs.	☐	☐	☐	☐	☐
9) We provide a clean and safe work environment.	☐	☐	☐	☐	☐
Programming					
10) We offer annual HRAs with appropriate follow-up and resources to all employees.	☐	☐	☐	☐	☐
11) We attempt to provide a variety of core initiatives that support primary prevention (e.g. health screenings, immunizations), lifestyle management (e.g., physical activity, nutrition) and risk reduction (e.g., weight control, tobacco cessation).	☐	☐	☐	☐	☐
12) We encourage employees/family members to use resources provided by our health plan for managing chronic health conditions (e.g., asthma, diabetes).	☐	☐	☐	☐	☐
Evaluation					
13) Within the past three years, 86 percent of our workforce has participated in six company-sponsored health promotion programs including an HRA, plus three or more coaching sessions (e.g., online, telephone), plus two other programs..	☐	☐	☐	☐	☐
14) At least 70percent of our workforce is considered low risk (e.g.,0-2 risk factors).	☐	☐	☐	☐	☐

Figure 17.1   Partnership for Prevention/The WorkCare Group Small and Midsized Employer Tool

resources and onsite support; connect businesses with local resources; improve business, local, and state economies; and identify and promote the best business practices. Health Links provides support for businesses new to workplace wellness programs through the Kick-Start Program, which provides one-on-one coaching and funding for businesses (Health Links Colorado, 2014). Hospital systems work directly with small employers. For example, Kaiser Permanente in California has a small business plan that includes built-in workforce health tools to improve employee health.

They offer a comprehensive approach to workforce health or an employer do-it-yourself approach with activities tailored to the particular employer population. Both emphasize step-by-step program guides to assess, plan, engage, and measure program activities (Kaiser Permanente, n.d.).

How to Work With Small and Midsized Employers to Promote Worker Health

Most small and midsized employers will have a point person for human resources. In small businesses it can be one of the owners, who simply adds the human resource responsibilities and task to his or her already busy list of tasks and responsibilities. As organizations grow, the human resource function and responsibilities grow. And depending on the size of the organization's human resource function a person employed by the organization may be assigned the employees' health promotion activities within the overall human resources activities. An internal person would most likely have a number of human resource responsibilities (e.g., benefits, payroll) with one of which would be employee health promotion. Potentially the individual is the employee health promotion champion and advocate, actively engaging the employer and employees in the overall organization's employee health promotion activities. Working with small and midsized employers on employee health requires finding the point person in the organization. That is the person to work with.

Working Directly With Decision Maker(s) to Manage Time and Energy

Small and midsized organizations do not have large infrastructure and complex systems. Workplace health promotion advocates work directly with the people who have the authority and responsibility to make decisions that impact the people they work with each day. This is different from working with large organizations where decision making requires a series of reviews and approvals prior to a final decision, often by individuals removed from the daily operation of the workplace health promotion program.

Provide information, education, and support to the person facilitating the program about how to promote employee health, given the reality of the particular business (organization), by connecting them with local and regional coalitions, partnerships, and collaborations. The business coalitions and groups (e.g., Business Groups on Health, Councils of Smaller Enterprises, Manufacturing and Small Business Associations) provide connections with the health and safety vendors that have small and midsized business account representatives and specialists who work on product design and implementation for the small and midsized employers. Health insurance broker account representatives and specialists may also be involved with the marketing and sales of the vendor products, as well as with delivery of the products. Working with small and midsized employers to promote worker health requires networking and interacting with many groups and organizations.

Building small and midsized employers' capacity for creating a healthy and safe workplace requires helping the individuals who are charged with employee health to manage their time making critical human resource decisions (e.g., hiring staff) and delegating to others discrete human resource tasks and responsibilities. These later tasks and responsibilities include payroll and benefit management functions as well as OSHA compliance. These tasks are time consuming and require a fair amount of attention to detail. Paying employees is complicated and takes a significant amount of time if you are not a professional in the field. Each employee must complete a W-4 for federal withholding, the employer must match the employee's Social Security/Medicare payments, and this money must be deposited weekly, monthly, or quarterly with the IRS. If the deposits are made one day late or are for an incorrect amount, hefty penalties are assessed. Unemployment returns must be paid, and states and localities that have income tax also require regular deposits and filings. W-2 and W-3 forms must be filed with the Social Security Administration annually, too.

Using the strength of the coalitions, partnerships, and collaborations, smaller and midsized employers can select and contract with vendors that specialize in the above areas (e.g., payroll). For example, companies such as Paychex, ADP, and Paylocity work extensively with small and midsized employers on managing the payroll and benefit management functions. Workplace health and safety vendors include companies such as Cintas, JKeller, Thompsons HR Compliance Expert, East Coast Risk Management, and Pomaybo, Inc. To help the employers keep up to date on the changing health care laws and requirements, consultants beyond the payroll and benefits management companies are also used. The insurance carriers are active in this arena as well as the National Association of Health Underwriters.

Employee Engagement

Employees influence programming directly through their level of program engagement. Employee engagement is a barrier to program implementation for small and midsized employers. Components of employee engagement are employees' interest, their initial and ongoing participation, and their active resistance. Companies with the most sustained programming and strongest traditions of workplace wellness consciously build employee engagement through multiple levels, including employee membership on a wellness team (supervisors and rank-and-file workers) and surveying and using employee feedback on desired programs and satisfaction. Where there is a labor union, its leadership and shop stewards should be similarly involved. Often an invitation to cosponsor the program will defuse a union's latent opposition to company programs intended to enhance employee welfare if that exists; it may also serve to stimulate the union to work for replication of the program by other companies in the same industry or area. Finally, employers are increasingly communicating with employees about how the program can affect personal finances (e.g., effect on the bottom line as far as the cost of the health insurance) to support employees deciding to participate.

Engaging employees means building on the advantages of small and midsized employers. Although these employers do face significant challenges related to financial and administrative resources, they also have advantages. These include (Muchnick-Baku & Orrick, 1992):

- Family orientation. The smaller the organization, the more likely it is that employers know their employees and their families. This can facilitate health promotion becoming a corporate-family affair building bonds while promoting health.

- Common work cultures. Small organizations have less diversity among employees than do larger organizations, making it easier to develop more cohesive programs.

- Interdependency of employees. Members of small units are more dependent on each other. An employee absent because of illness, particularly if prolonged, means a significant loss of productivity and imposes a burden on coworkers. At the same time, the closeness of members of the unit makes peer pressure a more effective stimulant to participation in health promotion activities.

- Approachability of top management. In a smaller organization, management is more accessible, more familiar with the employees, and more likely to be aware of their personal problems and needs. Furthermore the smaller the organization, the more promptly the owner/chief operating officer is likely to become directly involved in making decisions about new program activities, without the often stultifying effects of the bureaucracy found in most large organizations. In a small firm, that key person is more apt to provide the top-level support so vital to the success of workplace health promotion programs.

- Effective use of resources. Because they are usually so limited, small businesses tend to be more efficient in the use of their resources. They are more likely to turn to community resources such as voluntary, government, and entrepreneurial health and social agencies, as well as hospitals and schools, for inexpensive means of providing information and education to employees and their families.

Challenges and Opportunities for Small and Midsized Employer Health Promotion Programs

Working with the small and midsized employers to promote the health of their employees presents challenges and opportunities that need to be considered prior to initiating contact with employers. Creative problem solving and decision making within the economic and time realities of the employers are required to address the challenges and build on the opportunities.

Employers' (i.e., Organization Executives and Business Owners) Interest and Personal Health Experiences Influence Initial Program Implementation

Initially small and midsized employer programs struggle with how to address the seven concerns of health insurance, cost, time, complexity, effectiveness, expertise, and space. Programs start small, adding components and improving program quality and employee satisfaction over time. As program parts are added they may reflect the employers' (i.e., organization executives and business owners) interest and personal health experiences (including those of family members, relatives, and close friends). Examples are organizations supporting local 5K runs, public health campaigns, community safety programs, and charity bike rides that are personally connected to the organizational leadership. The workplace programs become an extension of the leaderships' experience and interest. Care is needed to not disregard or marginalize the program planning process along with a needs assessment of the organization and the employees. However, it is important to recognize and validate the leaderships' health experience and interest. It provides the organization leaders an opportunity to build on what they know and learn practical details about implementing programs in the areas. They can then use this knowledge and experience to expand programs and add new policies, innovation, and activities. Such validation and the resulting outcomes provide the foundation upon which a program first develops and then grows.

Small Actions Are Building Blocks

Employers interacting with their peers and colleagues through the coalitions, partnerships, and collaborations share programs and ideas about what works best. They learn small actions can have positive effects on employee health that represent the building blocks of a positive health culture within an organization. Big programmatic actions and initiatives can generate a lot of attention, energy, and support but may be hard to sustain. Often employers find the small actions more acceptable and easier to do. For example: enacting and enforcing a no-smoking policy at the workplace, laying out a walking route at the workplace or in the surrounding area, allowing employees a little longer lunch or break to exercise, providing sunscreen to employees working outside, and encouraging employees to use their personal protective equipment (Bowen, Smith, Wilson, & DeJoy, 2009). Being positive, making it easy to be involved, and offering incentives and rewards are often used by small and midsized employers. Many employers adopt program templates and structures suggested professional organizations. For example, the Wellness Council of America (WELCOA) recommends health screening, physical activity campaigns, Lunch and Learns, wellness library, and health promotion newsletter (Hunnicutt, 2007). The small actions build toward a larger sustainable health promotion program.

Small actions for workplace health promotion with small and midsized employers (Muchnick-Baku & Warshaw, 2011):

- *Give the program a positive theme and keep changing it.* Give the program a high profile and publicize its objectives widely. Without dropping any useful activities, change the program's emphasis to generate new interest and to avoid appearing stagnant. One way to accomplish this is to piggyback on national and community programs such as National Heart Month and Diabetes Week.

- *Make it easy to be involved.* Activities that cannot be accommodated at the workplace should be located at convenient locations nearby in the community. When it is not feasible to schedule them during working hours, they may be held during the lunch hour or at the end of a work shift; for some activities, evenings or weekends may be more convenient.

- *Consider offering incentives and awards.* Commonly used incentives to encourage program participation and recognize achievements include released time, partial or 100% rebates of any fees, reduction in employees' contribution to group health insurance plan premiums ("risk-rated" health insurance), gift certificates from local merchants, modest prizes such as T-shirts, inexpensive watches, or jewelry, use of a preferred parking space, and recognition in company newsletters or on worksite bulletin boards.

Focus on Small and Midsized Employer Advantages

Small and midsized employers have fewer resources for workplace health promotion programs. The organization's leaders are at a disadvantage with having little flexibility to address their concerns and comply with the OSHA requirements. Furthermore some small and midsized business owners may have a distorted perception of their firm's problems and wrongly believe that the status quo is acceptable (Antonsson, 1997; Eakin et al., 2001). However, small and midsized employers do provide a highly advantageous context for promoting employee health (Mercer & U.S. Department of Health and Human Services, 2000). Although the impression can be gained that small and midsized employers are not able to offer workplace health promotion, these organizations often show the most creative and innovative workplace health promotion interventions (Kirsten, 2006). Stokols, McMahan, and Phillips (2001) outlined a number of advantages that small businesses have in relation to workplace health promotion:

- Visible, accessible, and approachable top management

- Fewer people to accommodate

- Fewer administrative costs

- Less time and money required for communicating with employees about health and safety issues

- Easier to integrate and link health promotion objectives with business outcomes

- Interdependency among employees

- Supportive environment conducive to group participation

- Higher rates of employee participation

- Employee health improvements are more visible

- Simpler, less expensive data gathering for program evaluation

- Large and locally accessible marketplace towards which community health agencies and organizations can direct free and low-cost services.

Monitoring and Evaluating Small and Midsized Employer Health Promotion Programs

Small and midsized workplace health promotion program evaluation is important. Typically the employers will not have access to the health informatics data found as part of large employer health insurance benefit packages. Data on service utilization, absentee management, and pharmacy and medication benefits may not be available, however, and for small and midsized employers this data may not be as valuable as programmatic data related to employee program participation. For example, the numbers of employees participating in a program and their drop-out rates will demonstrate the acceptability of particular activities. Measurable changes, such as smoking cessation, loss or gain of weight, lower levels of blood pressure or cholesterol, indices of physical fitness, for instance, can be used to appraise their effectiveness. Periodic employee surveys can be used to assess attitudes toward the program and elicit suggestions for improvement. And review of such data as absenteeism, turnover, appraisal of changes in quantity and quality of production, and utilization of health care benefits may demonstrate the value of the program to the small and midsized employer. Similar to evaluations of large employers, small and midsized employers need to make a point of keeping personal information about employees health problems, test results, and even participation in particular activities out of personnel files and obviate potential stigmatization by keeping it confidential.

Small and Midsized Employer Workplace Health Promotion Tools and Resources

Small and midsized employers are working with business coalitions, community resources, public and voluntary health agencies—and adopting creative, modest strategies designed to meet their specific needs—to successfully implement low-cost workplace health promotion programs that yield significant benefits. Furthermore the ACA creates opportunities for the small and midsized employer to promote employee health and safety. Increasingly the availability of models, resources, and support for small and midsized employers allows and encourages partnerships and collaborations to promote worker health.

Partnership for Prevention (http://www.prevent.org/)
Partnership for Prevention is a nonprofit organization that works to create a healthier nation through disease prevention

and health promotion throughout the country. The partnership is made up of many organizations, including corporations, trade associations, nongovernmental organizations, patient groups, associations for health professionals, health care delivery organizations, and government agencies. Three small and midsized health publications are:

1. *Leading by Example: Creating a Corporate Health Strategy— The Kansas City Collaborative Experience* (Partnership for Prevention, 2011a)

2. *Leading by Example: Creating a Corporate Health Strategy—The American Health Strategy Project Early Adopter Experience* (Partnership for Prevention, 2014)

3. *Leading by Example: The Value of Worksite Health Promotion to Small and Medium Sized Employers* (Partnership for Prevention, 2011b)

How to Find the Right Workplace Wellness Vendor: A Toolkit for Organizations (http://depts.washington.edu/hprc/workplace-wellness-toolkit)

The toolkit was developed by the partnership of The Puget Sound Health Alliance, Communities Putting Prevention to Work, and the Health Promotion Research Center to assist small business to select health and health promotion vendors. A chosen vendor should meet the specific needs of the employer and of the employees, the workplace culture, and the budget. The toolkit provides vendor questions regarding general information, promotion strategies, evidence, accessibility, data measurement and evaluation, collaboration, customer support, pricing, and medical credentials about the vendor and its programs. This guide can then be sent to various vendors for answering and justification of their programs. Once returned, the employer can review the answers and justifications to choose the best fitting vendor for their organization. Using the guide an employer can know what potential vendors offer and identify the employer's specific needs and wants.

Work@Health CDC program (http://www.cdc.gov/workathealth/)

The Work@Health Program is a CDC initiative to develop comprehensive workplace health training for employers of various sizes, industries, and geographic areas. The training will assist in an employer's ability to implement evidence-based workplace wellness programs effectively to their employees. The goal of the training is to teach employers to address chronic health conditions—specifically, heart disease, stroke, cancer, diabetes, arthritis, and obesity—through workplace wellness programs and prevention.

National Business Group on Health (https://www .businessgrouphealth.org/)

The National Business Group on Health (NBGH) is a non-profit organization devoted exclusively to representing employers' perspective on national health policy issues and providing practical solutions to its members' most important health care problems. The NBGH is devoted to controlling health care costs, improving patient safety and quality of care, and sharing best practices in health benefits management with member organizations. The member organizations include Fortune 500 companies small, midsize and large public sector employers. The list below highlights three different initiatives that can help small and midsized businesses.

- **National Committee on Evidence-Based Benefit Design** seeks to improve quality of care and promote value by using benefit design to encourage and reward effective care and discourage ineffective care. By linking benefit design to medical practices with demonstrated effectiveness, the committee seeks to enhance the health and quality of life of employees and their dependents and improve employers' return on benefits investment.

- **National Leadership Committee on Consumerism and Engagement (NLCCE)** provides a forum for business leaders to focus on:
  - Finding and evaluating effective solutions to the health care benefits challenges of employers
  - Identifying and disseminating best practices and innovative ideas for empowering and engaging employees and their dependents in the health care process
  - Identifying gaps in effective programs and practices and influencing businesses to fill the gaps
  - Promoting effective public policies
  - Promoting individual accountability and consumerism in all types of plans and financing methods.

- **Institute on Innovation in Workforce Well-Being** actively involves employers in thought leadership, problem solving, and the identification and development of best approaches to motivate employee/family engagement in improving health and well-being, with measurable results.

Small Business Administration (https://www.healthcare.gov/small-businesses/)

The United States Small Business Administration (SBA) is an independent agency of the federal government that provides assistance to small businesses around the country in the form of loans, loan guarantees, contracts, counseling sessions, and other forms of assistance. SBA's goal is to preserve free competitive enterprise and to maintain and strengthen the overall economy of our nation. Through an extensive network of field offices and partnerships with public and private organizations, recent initiatives that the SBA has sponsored and developed include SBA Emerging Leaders Initiative, Startup America, the Cluster's Initiative, Small Business Saturday 2013, the Small Business Jobs Act of 2010, and more.

Small Business Majority (http://www.smallbusinessmajority.org/)

The Small Business Majority is a national organization focusing on helping small businesses and finding solutions for problems among small businesses. The organization actively engages small business owners and policymakers to support solutions that promote small business growth and drive a strong economy. This support includes advocacy for policies that create jobs and maximize business opportunities and cost savings in health care reform, clean energy, access to capital, and other areas. In addition to policy, the Small Business Majority, in collaboration with many strategic partners, focuses on the education of small business owners and employees around the country about important issues affecting their businesses.

Indiana Healthy Worksites Toolkit for Small Businesses (http://www.inhealthyweight.org/files/Toolkit_with_Cover.pdf)

A small business health promotion guide outlines strategic policies, environmental supports, and activities to provide your employees with opportunities for healthy eating and physical activity. This guide is divided into five sections:

1. Assess your worksite—Identify and determine the best opportunities for physical activity and healthy eating in your worksite.

2. Enhance your environment—Use strategies and tools to implement policies, environmental supports, and activities in your

worksite to provide your employees with opportunities to make the healthy choice the easy choice.

3. Promote your efforts—Ensure employees are aware of your efforts to create more opportunities for healthy eating and physical activity; create opportunities for employees to participate.

4. Reassess your efforts—Measure the effectiveness of your efforts.

5. Useful tools and information.

Wellness Council of America (WELCOA) (https://www.welcoa.org/)
The Wellness Council of America (WELCOA) is a nonprofit organization dedicated to workplace wellness. Its core beliefs include that a healthy workforce is essential to America's continued growth and prosperity, that much of the illness in the United States is directly preventable, that the workplace is an ideal setting to address health and well-being, and that workplace wellness programs can transform corporate culture and change lives. WELCOA conducts workshops to help workplace wellness practitioners create and sustain results-oriented wellness programs.

Summary

How small and midsized employers plan, implement, and evaluate workplace health promotion programs is to balance their (employers') value on the well-being of employees with their (employers') concerns about workplace health promotion programs. Working with coalitions, partnerships, and collaborations, small and midsized employers together can leverage resources, and with public and voluntary health agencies as well, to create modest strategies designed to meet their specific employee health needs. These employers can and do implement successful yet low-cost programs that yield significant benefits. Health promotion programs may be no less, and sometimes even more, valuable in small and midsized employers than in larger organizations. Although valid data are difficult to come by, it may be expected that they will yield similar returns of improvement with regard to employee health, well-being, morale, and productivity. To achieve these outcomes with resources that are often limited requires careful planning and implementation to address employer concerns, endorsement and support of executives, involvement of employees, integration of the health promotion program with the organization's health and safety policies and practices, coordination with a health care insurance plan, and building on the advantages of small and midsized employers.

For Practice and Discussion

1. Deriving greater value from workplace health promotion programs for small and midsized organizations raises several important questions for employers. What bottom-line results can be expected from investments in the implementation of the different health priority areas? For small and midsized employers, what is the connection between the priority areas and improved employee health and productivity? Does one priority area take priority over other areas? For small and midsized employers how can improved employee health be measured? Does it make economic sense for small and midsized employers with more limited resources and staff to invest in employee health promotion and wellness?

2. In your community and state find the coalitions, partnerships, and collaborations that work with small and midsized employers to address employee health promotion programs. Who are the members and what activities are planned for the upcoming year? What are examples of past and current projects and initiatives? Prepare a brief report on your experience with the small and midsized employers active with the groups. What are the benefits to the employers for participating?

3. Research small and midsized vendors who provide payroll and benefits management and workplace health and safety services to small and midsized employers. What are the services and their costs? What are the pros and cons of the different vendors? How are the services marketed? How would you help a small employer decide which vendor to select to work with their organization?

4. The owners of a successful small manufacturing company operate five workplaces employing 35 factory workers and five office staff at each location within your state. The company is active with the local Business Group on Health. The owners are recreational riders. They frequently participate in local 5K and 10K fundraising events for local community organizations. After a thorough planning process and needs assessment the owners decide that they want an employee physical activity health promotion program at each workplace. What questions would you ask the owners about their decision and decision-making process? What questions do you recommend the owners ask other members of the Business Group on Health?

Case Study: Small Business Exhaustion—What Would You Do?

Susan Washington is the owner and operator of the small business Coffee by Design (four coffee shop locations with 65 employees). When asked about what her life is like being a small business owner, her response was, "I am exhausted. Starting a small business doesn't come easy. We're squeezed with a hectic life involving family and day jobs to help pay the bills. Managing the ongoing success of a small business created more stress for me than any other aspect of our lives—spouses, children, and personal finances included. The key to managing the stress and exhaustion was to get organized and recruit the workers I needed. Now I am trying to figure out health benefits for the staff. I am talking with a broker and a local business association. With the ACA there is the Individual Exchange for our staff to get health insurance. Also there is the SHOP. I have to figure that out." If you were Susan Washington what would you do about promoting the health of your employees?

KEY TERMS

Small and midsized employers	Space
Small Business Health Options Program (SHOP) Marketplace	Coalitions
	Partnerships
Individual Health Exchange	Collaborations
Cost	National Business Group on Health
Time	Decision making
Complexity	Employee engagement
Effectiveness	Selective and strategic decision making
Expertise	Small and midsized employer advantages

References

Antonsson, A. (1997). Small companies. In D. Brune, G. Gerhardsson, G. W. Crockford, & D. D'Auria (Eds.), *The workplace* (Vol. 2, part 5.3, pp. 466–477). Geneva, Switzerland: International Labour Office.

Bowen, H., Smith, T. D., Wilson, M. G., & DeJoy, D. M. (2009). Company size and health promotion program design. In N. P. Pronk (Ed.), *ACSM's worksite health handbook: A guide to building healthy and productive companies.* Champaign, IL: Human Kinetics.

Eakin, J. M., Cava, M., & Smith, T. F. (2001). From theory to practice: A determinants approach to workplace health promotion in small business. *Health Promotion Practice, 2,* 172–181.

FitCitySA. (2014). *Healthy Workplace Recognition Program.* Retrieved from http://fitcitysa.com/at-work/san-antonio-business-group-on-health-sabghHealthy/111-healthy-workplace-recognition-program

Health Links Colorado. (2014). *Bring wellness to work.* Retrieved May 8, 2015, from https://www.healthlinkscolorado.org/

Occupational Safety and Health Administration. (2015). *Help.* Retrieved from https://www.osha.gov/SLTC/workplaceviolence/

Kaiser Permanente. (n.d.). Retrieved May 12, 2015, from https://businessnet .kaiserpermanente.org/health/plans/ca/home

Kirsten, W. (2006). Internationale perspektiven des betrieblichen gesundheitsmanagements. *B&G Bewegungstherapie und Gesundheitssport, 22*(4), 126–129.

McDowell, M. (2009). Small business economy provides details of struggling 2008 economy. *The Small Business Advocate, 28*(7), 1–4.

Mercer, W. M., Inc., & U.S. Department of Human Health and Services. (2000). *1999 National worksite health promotion survey: Report of survey findings.* Northbrook, IL: Association for Worksite Health Promotion.

Muchnick-Baku, S., & Orrick, S. (1992). *Working for good health: Health promotion and small businesses.* Washington, DC: Washington Business Group on Health and the U.S. Department of Health and Human Services.

Muchnick-Baku, S., & Warshaw, L. J. (2011). Health promotion in small organizations: The US experience. In J. Messite & L. J. Warshaw (Eds.), *Encyclopedia of Occupational Health and Safety.* Geneva, Switzerland: International Labor Organization. Retrieved from http://www.ilo.org/iloenc/part-ii/health-protection-a-promotion/item/100-health-promotion-in-small-organizations-the-us-experience

National Small Business Association. (2014). *2014 Small Business Health Care Survey.* Retrieved from http://www.nsba.biz/wp-content/uploads/2014/02/Health-Care-Survey-2014.pdf

Office of Advocacy. (2011). *Health insurance in the small business market: Availability, coverage, and the effect of tax incentives.* Retrieved from https://www.sba.gov/sites/default/files/files/386tot.pdf

Partnership for Prevention. (2011a). *Leading by example: Creating a corporate health strategy: The Kansas City collaborative experience.* Retrieved from http://www.prevent.org/data/files/initiatives/lbe%20kc2_final.pdf

Partnership for Prevention. (2011b). *Leading by example: The value of worksite health promotion to small and medium sized employers.* Retrieved from http://www.prevent.org/data/files/initiatives/lbe_smse_2011_final.pdf

Partnership for Prevention. (2014). *Leading by example: Creating a corporate health strategy: The American Health Strategy Project Early Adopter Experience.* Retrieved from http://www.dfwbgh.org/documents/Leading_by_Example

Pelletier, K. R. (2009). A review and analysis of the clinical and cost-effectiveness studies of comprehensive health promotion and disease management programs at the worksite: Update VII 2004–2008. *Journal of Occupational and Environmental Medicine, 51*(7), 822–837.

Sommers, J. P., & Crimmel, B. L. (2007). *Employer-sponsored health insurance for large employers in the private sector, by industry classification: 2005* (Statistical Briefs No. 174). Retrieved from http://meps.ahrq.gov/mepsweb/data_files/publications/st174/stat174.pdf

Stanton, M., & Rutherford, M. (2004). Employer-sponsored health insurance: Trends in cost and access. *Research in Action.* (Issue 17, ARHQ Pub. No. 04-0085). Rockville, MD: Agency for Healthcare Research and Quality.

Stokols, D., McMahan, S., & Phillips, K. (2001). Workplace health promotion in small businesses. *Health promotion in the workplace* (3rd ed., pp. 493–518). Albany, NY: Delmar.

CHAPTER 18

HOSPITAL EMPLOYEE HEALTH PROMOTION PROGRAMS

How Hospitals Promote Employee Health

Hospitals and the health care industry are significant employers of health and medical professionals, administrators, and staff. The health service industry employs nearly 1 of every 10 workers in the United States (Health Resources and Services Administration, 2013). And hospitals employ one of every four health care professionals and are generally among their communities' largest employers (Bureau of Labor Statistics, 2014a, 2014b).

Health promotion is integral to the role of hospitals. Health promotion is part of the hospitals' core services focused on improving patients' (individuals') health status and quality of life. It reflects the merging of the fields of health and medicine (Fertman, Allensworth, & Auld, 2010; Johnson, 2000). Hospitals provide health promotion programs to the community, including workplace health promotion programs to small, midsized, and large employers in the community. And finally, hospitals provide workplace health promotion programs for their own employees. According to the American Hospital Association (AHA), most hospitals currently employ some type of employee health or wellness plan but they are all widely varied. Flu shots or other immunizations are offered at nearly every hospital. A large majority of hospitals also offer EAP/mental health services, healthy food options in cafeterias and vending machines, a tobacco-free campus, safety programs to reduce workplace accidents, health

LEARNING OBJECTIVES

- Describe how hospitals promote employee health

- Discuss how to work with hospitals to promote employee health

- Discuss the challenges and opportunities for hospital employee health promotion programs

- Describe hospital employee health promotion tools and resources

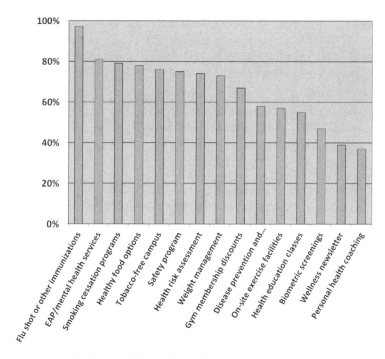

Figure 18.1   Hospital Employee Health and Wellness Offerings

risk assessments, weight loss programs, and gym membership discounts. About half of hospitals offer disease prevention and management programs, onsite exercise facilities, classes in nutrition or healthy living and stress management, web-based resources for healthy living, and biometric screenings (Figure 18.1). The number one motivator for hospitals to promote employee health is to set a good example for health throughout the community in which they serve (AHA, 2011).

Hospitals typically have robust employee workplace health promotion programs focused on wellness. For example the Saint Elizabeth's Medical Center, part of Ministry Health Care, is a critical access hospital in Wabasha, Minnesota (Saint Elizabeth's Medical Center, 2015). The hospital's employee health promotion program, Wellness Works, serves employees and their families. The program objective is to create a culture of wellness. The program started in 2003 to encourage employee participation in activities that promote physical exertion and improve nutrition. This later expanded to a larger initiative that includes an onsite family wellness center, biometric screening/health risk assessment, clinical consultation/coaching, tobacco cessation and nicotine replacement products, LEARN Healthy Lifestyle series, medication therapy management, chronic disease management programs, healthy cafeteria options, and an abundance of wellness education, activities, and resources. In transforming the culture of health at Saint Elizabeth's Medical Center, the comprehensive wellness program catered to the needs of both high- and low-risk employees, offering varying levels of participation based on health status and physical ability, ensuring a broad range of engagement in the workplace.

Many offerings of Wellness Works are either free or discounted. The program provides monetary incentives to further encourage staff and family participation. For example, employees receive a $50 reward for completing an annual physical, a yearly dental checkup, a flu shot and a biometric screening/consultation. They may also earn up to $200 for completing tiered exercise and nutritional requirements. Over time, the employees' program participation rates have grown and health status improved. Early in 2011, Saint Elizabeth's Medical Center reported that more than 60% of its workforce is participating in onsite wellness programs and activities. Many employees are also adopting healthy habits and reducing risk factors. Over a 5-year period, participants experienced 67% reduction in high-risk total cholesterol, 36% reduction in high-risk LDL cholesterol, and 56% reduction in prediabetes (AHA, 2013).

Hospitals have made worker health promotion a prominent part of their strategic resource human management. For example the U.S. Department of Veteran Affairs (VA) created the *Employee Health Promotion Disease Prevention Guidebook* (U.S. Department of Veterans Affairs, 2011). The VA operates the nation's largest integrated health care system, with more than 1,700 hospitals, clinics, community living centers, counseling centers, and other facilities. As part of the VA strategic human resource management the guidebook was written to improve and standardize the development, implementation, and evaluation of employee health promotion programs within the VA medical system. The guidebook provides VA health professionals, hospital workers, and administrators with information and references for developing employee health promotion programs at individual VA facilities. The guidebook includes best practices that were developed and evaluated at VA hospitals.

How to Work With Hospitals to Promote Employee Health

Working to promote hospital employee health requires navigating large, complex organizations that are safety and health focused. And at the same time, they are staffed with professionals who share a common purpose (patient health) but have different training, responsibilities, and expectations, which can result in conflicts and tension. Furthermore worker unions add a layer of complexity that while concerned about patients focus largely on worker rights and protections.

Large Complex Organizations

Promoting hospital employee health requires navigating large, complex organizations. Hospitals vary by purpose, size, location, and services. Furthermore the complexity of hospitals' organizational structure has grown with the increased complexities in the health care delivery system. Today, most hospitals have an internal personnel structure that consists of a board of directors or trustees, an executive management team, operations management, clinical staff including nursing and technical personnel, and administrative support staff. While some hospitals employ a limited number of physicians, most physicians working in a hospital are not employees of the hospital. Instead, they are granted privileges to admit patients to the hospital. This status provides physicians with considerable influence over hospital operations as they are one of two primary means by which patients flow into hospitals. Hospital employees report through managers to the hospital's executive team, which typically includes a chief executive officer, a medical director, and vice presidents responsible for various clinical and administrative areas (including human resources). The board of directors typically oversees strategic decisions for hospital organization and operation, has the power to approve or disapprove expenditures and plans, and is ultimately responsible for the hospital's services (State of Connecticut Department of Public Health (2014).

Hospitals by Purpose, Size, Location, and Services (AHA, 2014)

- **Critical access hospital:** Critical access hospitals are Medicare-participating hospitals located more than 35 miles from the nearest hospital or more than 15 miles from areas with mountainous terrain or secondary roads, or they were certified as a critical access hospital before January 1, 2006, based on state designation as a "necessary provider" of health care services to residents in the area. Critical access hospitals have no more than 25 beds for either inpatient or swing bed services. They provide 24/7 services with either onsite or on-call staff.

- **Small/rural hospital:** Small and rural hospitals have 100 or fewer beds, 4,000 or fewer admissions, or are located outside a metropolitan statistical area. Rural hospitals provide essential health care services to nearly 54 million people, including 9 million Medicare beneficiaries.

- **Safety-net health care system:** Safety-net health care systems provide care to low-income, uninsured, and vulnerable populations. They are not distinguished by ownership and may be publicly owned, operated by local or state governments or nonprofit entities. In some cases, they are for-profit organizations. These health care systems rely on Medicaid, and to a lesser extent Medicare, as well as state and local government grants as variable sources of revenue for most of their providers.

* **Independent community hospital:** Independent community hospitals are freestanding health care providers typically located in market areas with 50,000 or more residents. They operate between 100 and 350 beds.

* **Academic medical center:** An academic medical center is an accredited, degree-granting institution of higher education and can include hospitals with major or minor teaching programs.

* **Specialty hospital:** Specialty hospitals are centers of care that are built for certain patient populations, such as children, or that provide a particular set of services, such as rehabilitation or psychiatric services.

Hospitals have experienced vertical integration (an expansion in their range of services beyond acute care) and horizontal integration (mergers and affiliations between themselves and other health care institutions). Hospitals pursued integration strategies in order to increase their range of markets and to expand their geographic service areas. Many hospitals are part of corporations that own different types of providers along a continuum of care. These corporations also frequently own other holdings, such as real estate and other entities, which might be for-profit. The corporate health system organization chart depicted in Figure 18.2 is a model used by nearly all the acute care hospitals. It is now common for the health systems to have separate entities for foundations, auxiliary or fundraising, home health, real estate, and for-profit entities. Increasingly they form health insurance companies that provide them fiscal control and support for the systems (e.g., Kaiser Permanente). The systems have management services, billing and collection services, rehabilitation, physical therapy, ambulatory surgery centers, ambulatory (urgent) care centers, dialysis companies, laboratories, radiology centers, long-term care facilities, pharmacy, laboratory, radiology, long-term care, outpatient clinics, surgery centers, physician hospital organizations, behavioral health units, hospices, and community health or education entities. Likewise hospitals form multifacility health systems: networks of affiliations and partnerships with other hospitals. These care systems have two or more general acute care hospitals and are the most common organizational structure in the hospital

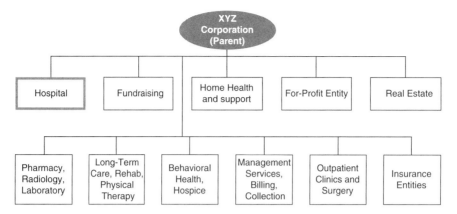

Figure 18.2   Hospitals as Part of Larger Health Care Systems in the 1990s
Source: State of Connecticut Department of Public Health (n.d.).

field; in fact, almost 200 hospital systems account for half of all hospitals and hospital admissions in the United States.

Worker Physical Safety in Hospitals

Worker physical safety is often overlooked as part of hospital worker health promotion, and needs to be attended to when working with hospitals. Back injuries and other repetitive stress and muscle disorders are among the most common injuries affecting hospital workers, from janitors and laundry machine operators to lab technicians—and of course, people who work with patients every day, including nursing assistants, orderlies, physical therapists, and patient attendants. In 2011, U.S. hospitals recorded 253,700 work-related injuries and illnesses, a rate of 6.8 work-related injuries and illnesses for every 100 full-time employees. This is almost twice the rate for private industry as a whole (Occupational Health and Safety Administration [OSHA], 2013). When an employee gets hurt on the job, hospitals pay the price in many ways, including: workers' compensation for lost wages and medical costs; temporary staffing, backfilling, and overtime when injured employees miss work; turnover costs when an injured employee quits; and decreased productivity and morale as employees become physically and emotionally fatigued. Worker safety also affects patient care. Manual lifting can injure workers and also put patients at risk of falls, fractures, bruises, and skin tears. Worker fatigue, injury, and stress are tied to a higher risk of medication errors and patient infections. Physical safety related to violence is a concern in hospitals (OSHA, n.d.). For example, Lanza, Shattell, and MacCulloch (2011) reported increasing concerns about assaults on nursing staff. And Spillane (2012) reported on high rates of aggression in Maine toward mental health care providers. In 2015 OSHA updated its guidelines for preventing workplace violence for health care and social service workers (OSHA, 2015).

The three hospital worker safety program components most often implemented are: understanding hospital safety, safety and management systems, and safe patient handling (OSHA, 2014a). Hospital programs need to develop and support a strong worker safety culture. Part of building a safety culture is employees gathering key information on how safe is the hospital and knowing how much a hospital spends on worker injuries and illnesses, what programs are in place to address the problem, and how the hospital compares with other hospitals nationwide (OSHA, 2014b). Safety and management systems focus on building systems with six core elements with strategies for implementing them in a hospital setting. These six elements can be adapted and implemented to fit the needs of a particular hospital. The elements are consistent with the recommendations for hospital safety from the OSHA Joint Commission Standard (OSHA, 2012).

Hospital Safety and Management Systems Core Elements (OSHA, 2013)

- **Management leadership:** Managers demonstrate their commitment to improved safety and health, communicate this commitment, and document safety and health performance. They make safety and health a top priority, establish goals and objectives, provide adequate resources and support, and set a good example.

- **Employee participation:** Employees, with their distinct knowledge of the workplace, ideally are involved in all aspects of the program. They are encouraged to communicate openly with management and report safety and health concerns.

- **Hazard identification and assessment:** Processes and procedures are in place to continually identify workplace hazards and evaluate risks. There is an initial assessment of hazards and controls and regular reassessments.

- **Hazard prevention and control:** Processes, procedures, and programs are implemented to eliminate or control workplace hazards and achieve safety and health goals and objectives. Progress in implementing controls is tracked.

- **Education and training:** All employees have education or training on hazard recognition and control and their responsibilities under the program.

- **System evaluation and improvement:** Processes are established to monitor the system's performance, verify its implementation, identify deficiencies and opportunities for improvement, and take actions needed to improve the system and overall safety and health performance.

The third hospital worker safety program component is safe patient handling with a minimal lift policy. The policy directs the use of mechanical lifting or other patient assist devices (instead of manual) to lift, transfer, and reposition patients, but it acknowledges there may be circumstances in which mechanical devices cannot be used. Hospital strategies to encourage workers to use the lifts include lift operation demonstrations, continuing education credits, inclusion as an annual review competency, and reminding staff that pulling "an extra pair of hands" for a manual lift means one less employee helping patients (OSHA, 2014a).

Worker Psychological Safety in Hospitals

A strong and just hospital safety culture is recognized as a key element to accurate reporting of quality and patient safety outcomes and concerns. However, as attention to creating a culture of safety in health care organizations has increased, so have concomitant reports of retaliation and intimidation targeting staff members who voice concern about safety and quality deficiencies.

Some health care workers acknowledge that they fear reporting events or conditions that could endanger quality and patient safety. Some workers whose direct responsibilities include the monitoring and reporting of quality and patient safety outcomes have experienced pressure, outright harassment, or even serious legal and licensure challenges when they recognize and report events of concern. Only with integrity in reporting can health care organizations identify and eliminate the root causes of systemic problems that threaten patient safety.

The accelerating implementation of new financial models that tie quality outcomes to payment increase the stakes associated with quality results. The need is increasing for a protective infrastructure to safeguard accurate reporting of quality data and patient safety concerns.

In any given situation where quality or patient safety is called into question, the process by which an issue is reported is as important as the query itself. Not every question of concern about patient safety or quality of patient care will ultimately be deemed valid, but every reported concern deserves consideration. A culture that encourages such disclosures is critical to improved patient care. So is the process by which concerns are examined, investigated, and ultimately determined to be valid or not.

Psychological worker harm in hospitals is not only limited to pressures related to patient safety and medical errors. Hospitals are high-pressure and emotional environments. In many situations in hospitals, staff members are not treated with respect or, worse yet, they are routinely treated with disrespect. Emotional abuse, bullying, and even threats of physical assault and learning by humiliation are all often accepted as "normal" conditions of the health care workplace, creating a culture of fear and intimidation that saps joy and meaning from work. The absence of cultural norms that create the preconditions of psychological safety obscures the meaning of work and drains motivation. The costs of burnout, litigation, lost work hours, employee turnover, and the inability to attract newcomers to caring professions are wasteful and add to the burden of illness. Disrespectful treatment of workers increases the risk of patient injury.

The National Patient Safety Foundation (NPSF) and National Association for Healthcare Quality (NAHQ) have worked to create psychologically safe hospital worker environments. The NPSF report, *Through the Eye of the Workforce: Creating Joy, Meaning, and Safer Health Care* (NPSF, 2013), recommends seven strategies around which hospitals develop and embody shared core values of mutual respect and civility. The core values include: transparency and truth telling, safety of all workers and patients, and alignment and accountability from the boardroom through the front lines.

The NAHQ report, *Call to Action Safeguarding the Integrity of Healthcare Quality and Safety Systems* (NAHQ, 2012) proposed hospitals implement four protective structures to assure accountability for integrity in quality and safety evaluation and comprehensive, transparent, accurate data collection, and reporting to internal and external oversight bodies. The four protective structures are believed to create a psychologically safe environment for hospital workers, in order to protect against bullying, emotional abuse and physical threats. NAHQ proposed the four structures to promote accountability for the integrity of hospital safety systems, accurate quality and safety data reporting, protection for those who report injustices in the workplace, and robustly addressing all safety concerns and improvements.

The four protective structures of the National Association for Healthcare Quality report (NAHQ, 2012) are:

1. Create a focus on accountability for quality and safety as part of a strong and just culture. Help clinicians recognize their responsibility for quality and safety.

   • Educate every employee on the expectations for timely reporting of quality and safety concerns.

- Publicize ethical responses to error and "good catches" through management praise, peer recognition, and other techniques. Benchmark regularly.

- Engage patients and families to report their concerns and ideas, participate on committees and councils to drive the quality and safety agenda, and maintain a focus on integrity and patient outcomes.

2. Ensure that protective structures are in place to encourage reporting of quality and safety concerns.

   - Set clear expectations for identifying and reporting errors

   - Educate every employee on the reporting of quality and safety concerns and the penalties for behaviors that restrict unfettered reporting.

   - Respond, counsel, and discipline as needed to ensure that egregious violators of the policies regarding error reporting will not be permitted to work or practice at the organization.

   - Engage hospital counsel to provide the necessary guidance for addressing situations of conflicting interests or intimidation.

3. Ensure comprehensive, transparent, accurate data collection and reporting to internal and external oversight bodies.

   - Establish quality improvement plans to ensure that the primary goal of data collection is true improvement in patient outcomes, not the attainment of performance metrics or compliance with external mandates.

   - Establish policies that protect data integrity.

   - Model internal transparency of performance data, ensuring that data and associated improvement opportunities are openly discussed.

   - Communicate to clinicians any identified gaps in the patient care process.

4. Ensure an effective response to quality and safety concerns.

   - Demonstrate a just response to quality and safety concerns with immediate investigation and respond to any adverse event, complaint, or concern.

   - Establish and enforce policies for responding to a quality or safety concern, including adverse events, errors, and incidents that result in unsafe conditions for staff and patients.

   - Implement effective action plans at the systems level to address vulnerabilities and gaps in quality and safety processes.

Unions and Hospitals

Many hospital employees including nurses, nursing assistants, food service workers, housekeeping staff, custodians, technicians, and physicians are members of unions. Separate unions often represent nurses, physicians, and allied health professionals. There are several national and international unions that represent many of these workers. These notable unions are detailed below. Worker safety and health promotion are among the hospital unions' priorities, but worker wages and benefits are chief among the unions' priorities. As with educational organizations unions are part of working with hospitals. They need to be included in each step of the process, and at times it is a balancing act between getting hospital leadership and unions to agree on hospital worker health promotion programs

Nursing Unions

American Nurses Association (http://www.nursingworld.org): The American Nurses Association (ANA) represents over 3.1 million nurses including its state associations and affiliate organizations. ANA advances the nursing profession by fostering high standards of nursing practice, promoting the rights of nurses in the workplace, projecting a positive and realistic view of nursing, and by lobbying congress and regulatory agencies on health care issues affecting nurses and the public.

California Nurses Association (http://www.nationalnursesunited.org /affiliates/entry/california-nurses-association): The California Nurses Association (CNA) is an affiliate of National Nurses United that represents 86,000 members throughout the country. CNA works to promote safety and advocacy for patients, giving voice to nurses to effect policy regarding working conditions and safety, and providing protection for nurses and patients.

National Nurses United (http://www.nationalnursesunited.org): National Nurses United (NNU) is the largest nursing union in the country, representing almost 185,000 members across the country. NNU works toward negotiating many of the best collective bargaining contracts for RNs in the nation, and toward establishment of innovative legislation and regulatory protections for patients and nurses.

Nursing Assistants, Food Service Workers, Housekeeping Staff, Custodians, Technicians Service Employees International Union (http://www.seiu.org): The Service Employees International Union (SEIU) is the fastest growing union in the country. Its members include health care workers, property services workers, and public services workers. The SEIU works to promote the dignity and worth of workers and the services they provide, and is dedicated to improving the lives of workers and their families and creating a more just and humane society.

National Union of Hospital and Health Care Employees (http://www.nuhhce.org/mission.html): The National Union of Hospital and Health Care Employees (NUHNCE) was established in November of 1973. The mission of this union is to represent and protect all professional, technical, clerical and service and maintenance employees, and all employees in health care institutions such as medical centers, hospital, nursing homes, pharmacies and other related services.

Physicians Unions Committee of Interns and Residents (http://www .cirseiu.org): The Committee of Interns and Residents is part of the National Doctors Alliance (NDA). It was founded in 1957 and is the largest house staff union in the country, representing 13,000 residents, interns, and fellows in several states. The committee works to improve their salary and working conditions, their education and training, and the quality of care they provide to patients.

Allied Health Professionals Unions The Health Professionals and Allied Employees Union (http://www.hpae.org): The Health Professionals and Allied Employees Union (HPAE) represents the largest health care union in New Jersey, representing over 12,000 employees. The HPAE represents nurses, social workers, therapists, technicians, medical researchers, and other health care professionals in hospitals, nursing homes, home care agencies, and more. The mission of HPAE is to advance and improve patient care and professional practices and working conditions in their health care facilities.

Challenges and Opportunities for Hospital Employee Health Promotion Programs

Health care is changing in the United States. The ability of hospitals to provide high-quality care depends in a large part on the health of its workers. However, hospitals are now part of the evolving U.S. health care system. One example of the evolution is the formation of integrated delivery systems (I.D.S). Likewise, hospitals continue to be challenged by technological, financial and social changes.

Integrated Delivery Systems

An integrated delivery system (IDS) is a network of organizations that provides or arranges to provide a coordinated continuum of services to a defined population and is held accountable for the health outcomes, health status, and financial risk of the population served (Shortell, Gillies, Anderson, Erickson, & Mitchell, 1996). With the passage of the Affordable Care Act (ACA), hospitals are pressured and encouraged to innovate and redefine payment and care delivery. Hospitals' response to the ACA is to form integrated delivery systems (AHA, 2014). The American Hospital Association presents five pathways hospitals will need to do as IDSs are formed. Employee health promotion programs in hospital will be impacted by the influence of strategic human resource management ability to blend professional cultures and increased cooperation, teamwork, and communication across systems.

Five Future Paths for Hospitals and Care Systems to Form IDSs (AHA, 2014)

1. *Redefine* to a different care delivery system (i.e., either more ambulatory or oriented toward long-term care)

2. *Partner* with a care delivery system or health plan for greater horizontal or vertical reach, efficiency, and resources for at-risk contacting (i.e., through a strategic alliance, merger or acquisition)

3. *Integrate* by developing a health insurance function and/or services across the continuum of care (e.g., behavioral health, home health, post-acute care, long-term care, ambulatory care)

4. *Experiment* with new payment and care delivery models (e.g., bundled payment, accountable care organization, medical home)

5. *Specialize* to become a high-performing and essential provider (e.g., children's hospital, rehabilitation center)

Technological, Financial, and Social Change

Three kinds of changes are faced by a modern health care organization and therefore faced by hospital employee health promotion programs: technological, financial, and social. Not only are the three interrelated, but these major areas of change have resulted in many specific modifications of the ways in which health care is organized and delivered, and impacted hospital workers and programming including worker health promotion programs (Fallon & McConnell, 2007).

Technological change encompasses advances being made in methods of diagnosis and treatment, including all new or improved equipment, new procedures, and new or improved drugs. In short, this encompasses most advances made in any dimension of restoring health and preserving life. But technological changes collide with considerations of finance because the cost of having the benefits of the latest and best equipment and the information that such resources generate can produce conflict with the pressures experienced to stem the rapid increase of health care costs. Social change becomes a strong influence as the population ages and society experiences the changing attitudes of contemporary generations.

As a result of the changes, hospital staff also needs to change. Change within a hospital occurs in one of two ways. Change is either intentional, that is, planned and executed for some specific purpose, or it is forced, coming about in response to circumstances beyond the control of an organization. Hospitals experience far more reactionary changes than planned changes, a situation that can create stress and a psychologically unhealthy environment.

Hospital employee health promotion programs need to be agents of change. However, few hospitals engage in planning that creates change. Because of workload and other continuing problems, hospital leaders and staff have little time to focus on change. Resistance to change is often prevalent throughout many organizations (including hospitals). Middle managers and department managers do not view themselves as agents of change. Finally, few managers are skilled or effective at creating and managing change.

Employee health promotion programs as part of hospital human resource management can foster a climate that is conducive to constructive change. Hospitals benefit from a culture of change that encourages innovation, rewards risk taking, and which values employee participation and input. Work is needed to implement up-to-date policies and procedures that convey respect for the capabilities of every employee. Job descriptions should be flexible and should allow room for innovation and employee participation and input. A modern performance appraisal process should permit employees to set objectives for themselves and participate in their own growth and development fosters change. Opportunities for promotion and transfer from within should reinforce employees' personal growth and development. A compensation structure, which includes the opportunity to influence earnings through performance, and a flexible benefits structure that recognizes the divergence of individual needs, also support change.

Hospital Employee Health Promotion Tools and Resources

The tools and resources available to promote the health of hospital employees span both health and safety concerns. They are from professional organizations and federal government, including the Hospital Corporation of America and the U.S. Department of Veterans Affairs, respectively. The materials take an ecological approach to hospital employee health promotion within large and complex systems that are transforming as well to reflect and keep up with changes in how health care is delivered in the United States.

American Hospital Association—*Your Hospital's Path to the Second Curve: Integration and Transformation* (http://www.aha .org/research/cor/paths/index.shtml)

To navigate the evolving health care environment, the 2013 American Hospital Association (AHA) Committee on Research developed the report *Your Hospital's Path to the Second Curve: Integration and Transformation* (AHA, 2104). This report outlines must-do strategies, organizational capabilities to master, and 10 strategic questions that every organization should answer to begin a transformational journey. The report's "guiding questions" help hospitals and care systems reflect and gain new perspectives on the benefits and value of integration. Case studies of hospital employee health promotion programs are included.

The American Society for Healthcare Human Resources Administration (http://www.ashhra.org/about/index.shtml)

Founded in 1964, the American Society for Healthcare Human Resources Administration (ASHHRA) is a personal membership group of the American Hospital Association (AHA) and has more than 3,500 members nationwide. It encourages members to be effective, valued, and credible leaders in health care human resources. It provides timely and critical support through research, learning and knowledge sharing, professional development, and products and resources, and provides opportunities for networking and collaboration.

National Patient Safety Foundation (NPSF) (http://www.npsf.org/ about-us/)

The National Patient Safety Foundation's vision is to create a world where patients and those who care for them are free from harm. A voice for patient safety since 1997, NPSF partners with patients and families, the health care community, and key stakeholders to advance patient safety and health care workforce safety and disseminate strategies to prevent harm. According to NPSF, patient safety is the prevention of health care errors, and the elimination or mitigation of patient injury caused by health care errors; a health care error is an unintended health care outcome caused by a defect in the delivery of care to a patient.

Healthy Hospital Practice to Practice Series (http://www.cdc.gov /nccdphp/dnpao/hwi/resources/hospital_p2p.htm#)

The Centers for Disease Control and Prevention (CDC) Practice to Practice (P2P) Series presents case studies of hospitals improving their environments to better support the health of their employees and embody the mission of their organization. Materials include concise one page briefs and posters. Case studies include:

Issue #1: Improving Hospital Food and Beverage Environments: Find out how Cleveland Clinic and Good Shepherd Hospital are leading the way by offering a healthier food and beverage environment.

Issue #3: Improving Hospital Food and Beverage Environments: Saint Vincent Healthcare and University Health Systems of Eastern Carolina describe the steps they are taking to help employees make healthy choices.

Issue #5: Improving Hospital Physical Activity Environments: Kaiser Permanente and Logansport Memorial Hospital talk about creating environments in and around their hospitals that encourage active living.

Issue #6: Improving Hospital Physical Activity Environments: Learn how Penrose–St. Francis and Fresno VA Medical Center encourage their employees to stay active.

Issue #8: Improving Support for Breastfeeding Employees: Find out how University Medical Center and The Children's Hospital of Philadelphia provide support for breastfeeding employees.

Issue #9: Improving Support for Breastfeeding Employees: Learn how Davis Memorial and Georgetown University Hospitals are improving access to private spaces for employee lactation.

Issue #10: Improving Support for Tobacco-Free Hospital Environments: Read how LSU Health Systems and University of Kansas Medical Center improve support for tobacco-free hospital campuses.

Department of Veteran Affairs—*Employee Health Promotion Disease Prevention Guidebook* (http://www.publichealth.va.gov /employeehealth/wellness/guidebook.asp)

This guidebook was written to improve and standardize the development, implementation, and evaluation of employee health promotion programs within the U.S. Veterans Health

Administration (VHA) medical (hospital) system. The guidebook provides health professionals and administrators with information and references for developing employee health promotion programs at individual facilities. Many of the guidebook examples are from programs that have been developed in VHA's pilot Employee Health Promotion Department Programs in the Veterans Integrated Service Network 23 (one of 21 Veteran Integrated Service Networks within the Department of Veterans Affairs) and elsewhere in the VHA network.

Hospital Corporation of America—*Your Guide to Healthy Work Environment* (English and Spanish versions) (https://hcahwe .ehr.com/Pages/mission.aspx)

The Hospital Corporation of America (HCA) is a large health care services company comprising locally managed facilities that includes about 165 hospitals and 115 freestanding surgery centers in 20 states and England and employing approximately 204,000 people. The HCA guide book is designed to support HCA employees (hospital workers) to provide high quality, medical-error-free hospital care. The book connects healthy hospital environment to high quality hospital care. Discussed are five key areas: culture, leadership, voice, rewards, and staffing. Each area is defined along with standard operating procedures and best practices.

Summary

Promoting the health of hospital employees is consistent with the mission of hospitals. It is what hospitals do for its patients, community members (including employers) as well as its employees and their families. In general hospitals have large, well supported, active employee health promotion programs with a strong focus on employee and family wellness. What often is overlooked as part of hospital worker health promotion is the need to attend to hospital workers' physical and psychological safety. In 2011, U.S. hospitals recorded work-related injuries and illnesses at a rate of almost twice the rate for private industry as a whole. Hospital worker health directly impacts medical errors and patient safety. In a hospital a measure of worker health is the quality of the health care provided to patients in the hospital. Working with hospitals to promote worker health requires particular attention to the delivery of high quality health care. Likewise, similar to educational institutions, unions are also important partners in hospital employee health promotion.

For Practice and Discussion

1. Select a local hospital. What type of hospital is it? Is it part of a hospital system? Does the system include a health insurance plan? What are the health insurance benefit plan offerings? What employee health promotion programs and services are offered to the hospital workers? What actions would the hospital need to take to be recognized as an American Heart Association fit-friendly worksite? (American Heart Association, 2014).

2. You are being requested to prepare training for new hospital workers on the topic of hospital employee safety and quality patient care. As part of your training design, prepare activities to introduce the workers to the OSHA hospital worker safety program components, "Safe Patient Handling" (OSHA, 2014a) and "Understanding the Problem" (OSHA, 2014b). Design hands-on activities that have the employees learn about the multiple tools and resources in each OSHA hospital component. As part of the training planning design 30 minutes is allotted for the new employees to explore each component.

3. The Baylor Health Care System in Dallas, Texas, health promotion program for Baylor employees and their partners has five main focus areas: Weight Management, Stress Management, Fitness, Tobacco Cessation, and Nutrition (http://media.baylorhealth.com/pages/thrive-wellness-program). As part of the stress management program area they want you to create a program that hospital employees can use to interrupt and stop psychologically harmful blaming that occurs in the hospitals as a result of medical errors and poor patient outcomes. Suggest strategies and program models.

4. Consider how hospitals are now part of vast health care systems. Discuss how a hospital employee health promotion program can be the cornerstone and platform for a system-wide initiative to create a psychologically and physically safe health care worker environment across a range of health care professionals and sites?

5. Using the Centers for Disease Control and Prevention (CDC) P2P Series as a model, select a hospital worker health and safety concern and create a one-page employee health promotion brief and poster (http://www.cdc.gov/nccdphp/dnpao/hwi/resources/hospital_p2p.htm#).

Case Study: Hospital Worker Sleep Hygiene Program—What Would You Do?

If you're a nurse, physician, physical therapist or any other allied health care professional, you know that your work demands a lot of energy. When your shift supervisor gives you an 8-hour shift (or maybe a 10-, 12-, 15-, or 24-hour assignment), it means hours of pure work with potentially no downtime. You're up on your feet almost 100% of the time. You're assigned critical tasks that will directly affect your patient's life. Once you step into a hospital, your environment drastically changes. From here on out, you will fully comprehend the meaning of the phrase "every second counts." And suddenly there is no time for you, your life, and your health. One consequence of working in a hospital is sleep deprivation. Staff members are tired.

Harvey Chester, Coordinator, Hospital Employee Health Promotion, is asking you to design a hospital worker sleep hygiene program. Mr. Chester is clear that what he does not want is a program that has workers keeping logs of their sleep. He already knows staff members are not getting enough sleep. He wants a program that on one hand is all about sleep and on the other hand never mentions sleep. What would you do?

KEY TERMS

Hospital	Health care industry unions
Vertical integration	American Hospital Association
Horizontal integration	Integrated delivery systems
Hospital systems	Technological, financial, and social changes
Saint Elizabeth's Medical Center Wellness Works	Cleveland Clinic Employee Health Plan Total Care
Physically safe hospital environment	Veteran Affairs Employee Health Promotion Disease Prevention Guidebook
OSHA	
Psychologically safe hospital environment	American Heart Association Fit-Friendly Worksite Program
Medical error and patient safety	

References

American Heart Association. (2014). *Fit-friendly worksites.* Retrieved from http://www.startwalkingnow.org/start_workplace_fit_friendly.jsp

American Hospital Association. (2011). *A call to action: Creating a culture of health.* Retrieved from http://www.aha.org/research/cor/creating-culture/index.shtml

American Hospital Association. (2013). *Engaging health care users: A framework for healthy individuals and communities.* Retrieved from http://www.aha.org/research/cor/content/engaging_health_care_users.pdf

American Hospital Association. (2014). *Your hospital's path to the second curve: Integration and transformation.* Retrieved from http://www.aha.org/research/cor/paths/index.shtml

Bureau of Labor Statistics. (2014a). *Healthcare and social assistance workforce statistics.* Retrieved from http://www.bls.gov/iag/tgs/iag62.htm#workforce

Bureau of Labor Statistics. (2014b). *Hospitals workforce statistics.* Retrieved from http://www.bls.gov/iag/tgs/iag622.htm

Fallon, L. F., Jr., & McConnell, C. R. (2007). *Human resource management in health care: Principles and practice.* Sudbury, MA: Jones & Bartlett Learning.

Fertman, C., Allensworth, D., & Auld, E. (2010). What are health promotion programs? In C. Fertman & D. Allensworth (Eds.), *Health promotion programs: From theory to practice* (pp. 3–27). San Francisco, CA: Jossey-Bass/Wiley.

Health Resources and Services Administration. (2013). *The U.S. health work-force chartbook—In brief.* Retrieved from http://bhpr.hrsa.gov/healthworkforce /supplydemand/usworkforce/chartbook/chartbookbrief.pdf

Johnson, J. L. (2000). *The health care institution as a setting for health promotion.* Thousand Oaks, CA: Sage.

Lanza, M. L., Shattell, M. M., & MacCulloch, T. (2011). Assault on nursing staff: Blaming the victim, then and now. *Issues in Mental Health Nursing, 32*(8), 547–548.

National Association for Healthcare Quality. (2012). *Call to action safeguard-ing the integrity of healthcare quality and safety systems.* Retrieved from http://www.nahq.org/uploads/NAHQ_call_to_action_FINAL.pdf

National Patient Safety Foundation. (2013). *Through the eyes of the workforce: Creat-ing joy, meaning, and safer health care.* Retrieved from http://www.npsf.org/wp-content/uploads/2013/03/Through-Eyes-of-the-Workforce_online.pdf

Occupational Safety and Health Administration. (n.d.). *Workplace violence.* Retrieved May 8, 2015, from https://www.osha.gov/SLTC/healthcarefacilities /violence.html

Occupational Safety and Health Administration. (2012). *Safety and health management systems and Joint Commission standards.* Retrieved from https://www.osha.gov/dsg/hospitals/documents/2.2_SHMS-JCAHO _comparison_508.pdf

Occupational Safety and Health Administration. (2013). *Safety and health man-agement systems: A road map for hospitals.* Retrieved from https://www .osha.gov/dsg/hospitals/documents/2.4_SHMS_roadmap_508.pdf

Occupational Safety and Health Administration. (2014a). *Safe patient handling.* Retrieved from https://www.osha.gov/dsg/hospitals/patient_handling.html

Occupational Safety and Health Administration. (2014b). *Understanding the problem.* Retrieved from https://www.osha.gov/dsg/hospitals/understanding _problem.html

Occupational Safety and Health Administration. (2015). *Guidelines for preventing workplace violence for healthcare and social service workers.* Retrieved from. https://www.osha.gov/Publications/osha3148.pdf

Saint Elizabeth's Medical Center. (2015). *Wellness pays off for Saint Elizabeth's medical center employees.* Retrieved from http://ministryhealth.org/SEMC /News/WellnessPaysOffforSaintElizabethsMedicalCenterEmployees.nws

Shortell, S. M., Gillies, R. R., Anderson, D. A., Erickson, K. M., & Mitchell, J. B. (1996). Remaking health care in America. *Hospitals & Health Networks/AHA, 70*(6), 43–44, 46, 48.

Spillane, B. (2012). *Maine's caregivers, social assistance and disability rehabilitation workers injured by violence and aggression in the workplace in 2011.* Maine State Department of Labor. Retrieved from http://www.maine .gov/labor/labor_stats/publications/patient_violence_report_2012.pdf

State of Connecticut Department of Public Health. (2014). *The health of Connecticut's hospitals.* Retrieved from http://www.ct.gov/dph/cwp /view.asp?a=3902&q=277046

State of Connecticut Department of Public Health. (n.d.). *Hospitals today.* Retrieved from http://www.ct.gov/dph/lib/dph/ohca/hospitalstudy/HospToday.pdf

U.S. Department of Veterans Affairs. (2011). *Employee health promotion disease prevention guidebook.* Retrieved from http://www.publichealth .va.gov/docs/employeehealth/health-promotion-guidebook.pdf

CHAPTER 19

FEDERAL GOVERNMENT EMPLOYEE HEALTH PROMOTION

How the Federal Government Promotes Employee Health

Health programs and services including health promotion for federal employees are authorized by Public Law 79-658 (Cornell University Law School, 1986). These services promote the physical and mental fitness of federal employees. Several legislative initiatives have shaped the guidance and implementation of health and wellness programs in the federal government. The U.S. Office of Personnel Management (OPM) is the federal agency charged with these legislative initiatives. OPM provides overall guidance to federal agencies and helps agencies implement programs as part of its overall mission to manage the civil service of the federal government, coordinate recruiting of new government employees, and manage their health insurance (including health promotion programs) and retirement benefits programs. OPM is classified as an independent establishment and government corporation that interacts with all of the federal branches and departments (Table 19.1).

As of July 2015 there are approximately 2.8 million civil servants employed by the U.S. government (this includes executive, legislative, and judicial branches of government and more than 600,000 U.S. postal workers). The federal government is the nation's single largest employer. Although most federal agencies are based in the Washington, DC, region, only about 16% (or about 288,000) of the federal government workforce is employed in this region. There are over 1,300 federal government agencies.

LEARNING OBJECTIVES

- Describe how the federal government promotes employee health

- Discuss how to work with the federal government to promote health

- Discuss the challenges and opportunities for federal employee workplace health promotion programs

- Describe federal government employee workplace health tools and resources

Table 19.1   Office of Personnel Management Five Broad Areas With Activity Listings (OPM, 2014a)

Policy	Insurance	Retirement	Agency Services
Assessment & Selection	Life Events	My Annuity and Benefits	Classification & Job Design
Classification & Qualifications	Health Care	CSRS Information	Workforce Restructuring
Data, Analysis, & Documentation	Dental & Vision	FERS Information	Workforce & Succession Planning
Disability Employment	Life Insurance	Special Notices	Recruiting & Staffing Solutions
Diversity & Inclusion	Flexible Spending Accounts	Calculators	Assessment & Evaluation
Employee Relations	Long Term Care	Publications & Forms	Nationwide Testing
Hiring Authorities	Multi-State Plan Program	Benefits Officers Center	Leadership Development
Human Capital Management	Indian Tribes	Retirement FAQs	Federal Executive Institute
Labor-Management Relations	Special Initiatives	Contact Retirement	Performance Management
Oversight Activities	Insurance Glossary		Telework Management
Pandemic Information	Insurance FAQs	**Investigations**	Technology Systems
Pay & Leave	Contact Health Care & Insurance	e-QIP Application	Training-Management Assistance
Performance Management		Background Investigations	HR Line of Business
Senior Executive Service		Requesting Investigation Copies	Administrative Law Judges
Settlement Guidelines		Contact Investigations	Federal Executive Boards
Snow & Dismissal Procedures			Contact Agency Services
Training & Development			
Veterans Services			
Work/Life			
Workforce Restructuring			
Policy FAQs			
Contact Policymakers			

The U.S. civil service includes the Competitive Service and the Excepted Service. The majority of civil service appointments in the United States are made under the Competitive Service, but certain categories in the Diplomatic Service, the FBI, and other National Security positions are made under the Excepted Service. U.S. state and local government entities often have competitive civil service systems that are modeled on the national system, in varying degrees.

In addition to departments (e.g., Department of Health and Human Services, State, Education), a number of agencies are grouped into each of the federal branches (Table 19.1). For example, the Executive Branch includes the White House staff, the National Security Council, the Office of Management and Budget, the Council of Economic Advisers, the Office of the U.S. Trade Representative, the Office of National Drug Control Policy, and the Office of Science and Technology Policy. The Legislative Branch includes the Congress as well as its supporting agencies. The Judicial Branch is the Supreme Court and its supporting agencies.

There are also independent establishments and government corporations such as the United States Postal Service, the National Aeronautics and Space Administration (NASA), the Central Intelligence Agency (CIA), the Environmental Protection Agency (EPA), and the United States Agency for International Development (USAID). In addition, there are government-owned corporations such as the Federal Deposit Insurance Corporation (FDIC) and the National Railroad Passenger Corporation. The OPM is another example of such an entity (Figure 19.1).

The OPM works in several broad categories. Its mission is to "Recruit, Retain, and Honor a World-Class Workforce to Serve the American People." OPM supports U.S. agencies with personnel services and policy leadership including staffing tools, guidance on labor-management relations, and programs to improve workforce performance. Its federal mandate includes:

* Manage federal job announcement postings at USAJOBS.gov, and set policy on government-wide hiring procedures.

* Conduct background investigations for prospective employees and security clearances across government, with hundreds of thousands of cases each year.

* Uphold and defend the merit systems in federal civil service, making sure that the federal workforce uses fair practices in all aspects of personnel management.

* Manage pension benefits for retired federal employees and their families. Administer health and other insurance programs for federal employees and retirees including health promotion programs and services.

* Training and development programs and other management tools for federal employees and agencies.

* Developing, testing, and implementing new government-wide policies that relate to personnel issues.

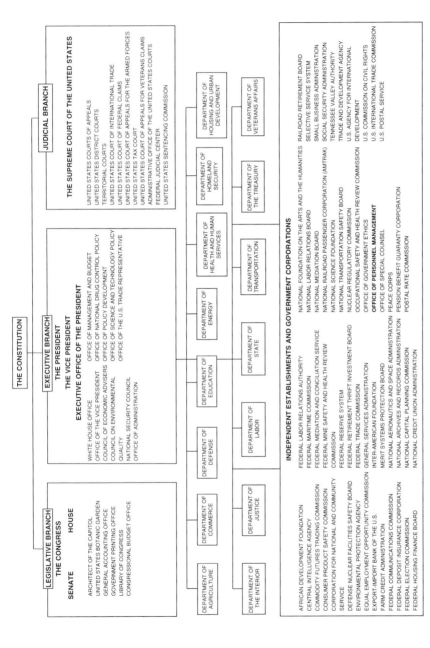

Figure 19.1 Federal Government Organizational Chart

Source: U.S. Government, 2010.

The breadth of OPM activities is shown in Table 19.1 spanning five broad areas: policy, insurance, retirement, investigations, and agency services. And while within each area several activities are clearly linked to health promotion programs, no single activity in any area is designated as health promotion.

To support federal employee health throughout the employment life-cycle, OPM employs a chief medical officer, program and policy analysts, health economists, work-life wellness specialists, research psychologists, data analysts, and others to work synergistically in four distinct crosscutting areas: (1) Health Care and Insurance, (2) Planning and Policy Analysis, (3) Work/Life, and (4) National Prevention Council.

Health Care and Insurance is responsible for the government-wide administration of health benefits and insurance programs and services for federal employees, retirees, and their families, through the Federal Employees Health Benefits Program (FEHBP; OPM, 2014c). These programs and services offer employees choice, value, and quality, and help maintain the government's position as a competitive employer. OPM contracts and manages around 40 health insurance carriers.

Health Insurance Plans Serving Federal Employees

Aetna, Inc.

Altius Health Plans

Anthem Blue Cross Select HMO

APWU Health Plan

APWU Health Plan CDHP

AvMed Health Plans, Inc.

Blue Cross and Blue Shield

Blue Preferred Plus POS

Capital Health Plan, Inc.

CareFirst BCBS

CDPHP Universal Benefits Inc.

Coventry Health Care

Fallon Community Health Plan

Foreign Service Benefit Plan

Geisinger Health Plan

GHI

Government Employees Health Association (GEHA)

Hawaii Medical Service Association

Health Net of California

HealthAmerica

HealthPartners

HealthPlus of Michigan

HIP Health plan of New York

Humana

Kaiser

KPS Health Plans

M.D. IPA

Mail Handlers Benefit Plan (MHBP)

NALC Health Benefit Plan

Optima Health Plan

Physicians Health Plan of Northern Indiana

Rural Carrier Benefit Plan

Special Agents Mutual Benefit Association (SAMBA)

UnitedHealthcare Benefits of Texas, Inc.

UnitedHealthcare of California

UnitedHealthcare of the Midwest

UnitedHealthcare of the River Valley

UPMC Health Plan

Annually the OPM issues the Federal Employee Health Benefits (FEHB) Program Carrier Letter (OPM, 2014b). OPM considers applications only from comprehensive, prepaid medical plans. The FEHB Program contracts only with health benefits carriers that offer a complete line of medical services, such as doctor's office visits, hospitalization, emergency care, prescription drug coverage, and treatment of mental conditions and substance abuse. They do not have the authority to contract with companies that offer limited services, such as dental and/or vision plans, prescription drug plans, supplemental insurance, and disability insurance. Examples of current carriers are listed above.

In 2012 the carrier letter stated the expectation for insurance carriers to offer programs that promote health and wellness and which are aimed at improving employee productivity, enhancing healthy lifestyles, and lowering long-term health costs. This included incentives for enrollees who complete a health risk assessment, are compliant with disease management programs, or who participate in wellness activities or treatment plans aimed at managing and improving health status. As part of the negotiations with the federal department or agency, part of the department and agency budget is allocated the health promotion program offered to the workers.

Planning and Policy Analysis (PPA) assesses program trends and policy issues that affect OPM. The scope of PPA analysis spans the full range of human resource management issues facing federal agencies (such as workforce supply, pay, benefits, diversity) and involves a variety of analytical tools (including actuarial analysis, surveys, economic analysis, and policy analysis). A particular area of responsibility is the analysis of policy options, legislative changes, and trends that affect OPM's management of health and insurance benefits for federal employees.

As the nation's largest employer, the federal government recognizes that great work/life policies, programs, and practices make good business sense. Work/life programs and policies are designed to create more flexible, responsive work environments supportive of commitments to community, home, and loved ones. OPM provides work/life leadership to the federal government by:

*   Partnering with federal agencies to help them develop and manage excellent work/life programs that meet the needs of the federal workforce

*   Providing the policies, guidance, and research tools that form the foundation of these programs

Finally, OPM is part of the National Prevention Council, mandated by the Affordable Care Act to implement the National Prevention Strategy U.S. Surgeon General, n.d.). As the primary department responsible for the federal workforce, OPM oversees functions related to the National Prevention Council Commitments, including procurement, management of federal employee health benefit plans, and promotion of wellness within the federal workforce.

Federal Employee Health Programs and Services are Most Commonly Provided to Employees Through Their Agencies

Following the legislative directives and using the OPM guidance, federal agencies implement programs and services through agencies at the employees' workplaces. Agencies offer a wide variety of health services choosing the services that best meet employees' needs. The level of services will vary from agency to agency. The basic programs include preventive services such as immunizations, physical examinations, and medical screening tests.

Federal employee health programs are widely established and accepted as a valuable resource for enhancing work force effectiveness. Over the past few decades, many agencies have expanded the traditional scope of services and established more comprehensive programs. These programs place more emphasis on physical fitness, health education, intervention activities, and preventive health screenings. Table 19.2 lists programs and services authorized under the Health Services, 5 U.S.C. §7901.

How to Work With the Federal Government to Promote Employee Health

Each federal agency (Figure 19.1) determines how to provide employee health promotion programs and services based on the scope of the desired program and services and available resources. The level and methods for

Table 19.2   Programs and Services Authorized Under 5 U.S.C. §7901 (Cornell University Law School, 1986)

Administration of Treatments and Medications: Qualified agency medical staff may administer treatment/medication during working hours when prescribed by employee's personal physician.

Emergency Response/First Aid: Qualified agency medical staff may provide first response and Cardiopulmonary Resuscitation (CPR) for emergencies as well as assessment and initial treatment/first aid to employees who are injured, or become ill during work hours.

Health Education: Agency health education encourages employees to maintain a healthy lifestyle, to understand their risk for disease, and to become aware of appropriate preventive practices. Examples of agency health education include health questionnaires, health fairs, newsletters, brochures, and presentations.

Physical Examinations: Qualified agency medical staff may administer properly authorized preplacement and periodic physical examinations to assess an employee's health status.

Disease Screening Examinations and Immunizations: Specific preventive health screenings or examinations may be sponsored at the workplace to detect the presence or risk of disease. Common workplace screenings include exams for blood pressure, mammography, blood lipids, glucose, vision and hearing. Medical staff may provide employees with immunizations, such as influenza and tetanus.

Environmental Health Hazards Appraisals: Agency may appraise and report work environment health hazards to department management as an aid in preventing and controlling health risks.

Physical Fitness Programs and Facilities: Agency can establish and operate physical fitness programs and facilities designed to promote and maintain employee health. Facilities may establish on-site or use the services of a community facility. Fitness programs include activities such as walking clubs/events, aerobic exercise classes, weight lifting instruction, stretching classes, fun runs, lectures on safe participation, and fitness assessments.

Health Intervention Services and Programs: Agency can offer health intervention services programs to promote and maintain physical and mental fitness and to help prevent illness and disease. Interventions are designed to encourage and enable employees to initiate healthy behavior changes. Agency may offer group activities and classes, individual counseling, demonstrations, and self-help materials. Health intervention areas include smoking cessation, diet and nutrition, cholesterol management, hypertension control, substance abuse, HIV/AIDS prevention, back care, and weight control.

Public Access Defibrillation Programs: Agency may establish a public access defibrillation program in a federal facility following the guidelines contained in "Guidelines for Public Access Defibrillation Programs in Federal Facilities," a product collaboratively produced by the General Services Administration and the Department of Health and Human Services.

administering programs and services will be particular to an agency. The availability of resources (funding, space, and staff) will define the type of programs and services agency can offer. Across the federal government it is possible to find programs and services fully funded by agencies, funded by a combination of employee fees and agency funding, and entirely funded by employee contributions. Budgets vary.

Agencies may choose to staff and manage employee health programs from a variety of options and ensure that the staff persons delivering health services are qualified and trained. For example, agencies may hire employees or use existing agency personnel to develop, manage, and deliver programs and services. The staff may be employed full-time or part-time, or assigned the duties on a collateral basis. Many agencies organize all of their employee health staff and programs into one division for more efficient coordination. Sometimes agencies form employee health committees with representatives from various offices to integrate services, coordinate, and promote programs. Many departments and agencies contract with qualified (federally qualified) vendors to develop, manage, and deliver programs. Federally qualified vendors need to verify compliance with federal regulations and procedures as well as approval prior to any contracting process (i.e., General Services Administration regulations contained in Title 41 of the Code of Federal Regulations). Examples of such vendors include hospitals, nonprofit organizations, private consultants and universities.

Federal Occupational Health

Each federal agency (Figure 19.1) is allowed to determine its own employee health promotion program. However, Federal Occupational Health (FOH), a nonappropriated agency within the U.S. Department of Health and Human Services (DHHS), increasingly provides federal agency employees with their occupational health and wellness services. FOH works in partnership with federal agencies nationally and internationally to design and deliver comprehensive solutions to meet their occupational health including health promotion needs. FOH programs and services include (1) automated external defibrillators; (2) employee assistance program; (3) environmental health; (4) health clinics; (5) organizational development and leadership; (6) wellness/fitness; (7) work/life program; and (8) workers' compensation management.

FOH is the largest provider of occupational health services in the federal government, serving more than 360 federal agencies and reaching 1.8 million federal employees. It was created in 1946 by an amendment to the Public Health Service Act (42 U.S.C.). In 1984, FOH became fully reimbursable, operating free of congressional appropriations. This means that FOH operates like a business within the government and charges fellow government agencies for the services it provides them. Over the years, FOH has created numerous programs to:

* Improve the health and fitness of federal employees.
* Prevent and reduce workplace illnesses and injuries.
* Improve employee/employer relationships.

- Decrease absenteeism and employee turnover.

- Decrease costs associated with workers' compensation claims.

- Help agencies comply with OSHA regulatory requirements.

FOH works in partnership with managers and workers alike to design and deliver comprehensive solutions to meet their occupational health needs. FOH helps build a healthier and more productive federal workforce and safer workplaces for employees. Agencies have the freedom to decide the type and mix of programs they want to offer. The following list shows the commonly requested health promotion programs. FOH customizes programs that are tailored to agency goals and budgets, as well as employee risk profiles.

Commonly Requested FOH's Health Promotion Programs

- Health Education Programs

- Smoking Cessation

- AED Programs

- Employee Assistance Programs (EAPs)

- Environmental Health Services

- Worksite Health Center

- Wellness/Fitness Center

- Medical Surveillance

- Ergonomics

- Hearing Conservation

- Financial Services

- Legal Services

- Medical Employability Program

- Work/Life Services

- Training and Education

Starting in 2009, FOH organized and consolidated federal worker health promotion into one program: FedStrive (FOH, n.d.). FOH launched FedStrive in response to President Obama's challenge to improve federal employee health with programs modeled after best practices in the private sector. Since its inception, participation has significantly increased in all programs, but especially in the health assessment (HA). Between FY 2010 and FY 2011, 60.7% (1,822) of the population completed the HA at least once, up from .1% prior to the program launch, and 14.8% (444) of the population have completed HAs in two consecutive years (Delowery, Lindsay, Hochberg, Price, & Spencer, 2012).

FedStrive offers four types of programs: clinical, wellness/fitness, EAP, and environmental health and safety. Clinical programs, including emergency response, physical exams, immunizations, vision and health screenings, and health risk appraisals are available at FOH's 298 health and wellness centers located in federal buildings throughout the United States and through a large network of more than 15,000 private-provider physicians and nurses. Wellness/fitness programs focus on healthy lifestyle and behavior choices offering health education, activities, and support in health areas such as diet, exercise, stress management, and tobacco cessation. EAP programs are provided by staff counselors located in 75 counseling offices in federal buildings as well as through a vast network of affiliate counselors in approximately 17,000 locations across the country and overseas. The environmental health and safety programs help agencies identify and resolve environmental health issues by addressing them early through assessments, abatement programs, and ongoing monitoring, as well as specialized training for employees and managers.

Agencies receive services through an agreement process. Authorized representatives from FOH and the requesting agency sign an Interagency or Interservice Agreement (IAA/ISSA, or IAA). The IAA serves to outline the goods or services to be furnished, reporting requirements, method for the transfer of funds, and if appropriate, acquisition authority for any contracts to be awarded pursuant to the IAA. In addition, agencies can be assured that FOH will comply with all Federal Acquisition Regulation (FAR) requirements via full and open competition when FOH procures any additional services for our customers.

The FOH staff is made up of a broad range of occupational health and wellness professionals. The administration of the FOH is public health service commissioned officers, general schedule federal employees (civil servants), and independently contracted consultants. FOH program staff members generally are not federal employees but rather part of organizations that are subcontract to develop the programs: vendors. The use of vendors is consistent with other large U.S. business practices that organizations subcontract with the FOH to deliver programs to government agencies and departments. The model is consistent with the U.S. economic model of capitalism, which directs commerce (i.e., business) to compete to deliver products (i.e., services) at lowest price and highest quality. Furthermore it is the basis for one of the distinguishing characteristics of federal contracts with private sector (i.e., business) organizations. Government contracts are subject to myriad statutes, regulations, and policies that encourage competition to the maximum extent practicable, ensure proper spending of taxpayer money, and advance U.S. socioeconomic goals (Cornell University Law School, n.d.).

Challenges and Opportunities for Federal Employee Workplace Health Promotion Programs

Working with the federal government to promote federal worker health presents challenges and opportunities that need to be considered prior to initiating contact with the OPM, FOH, or an individual agency. The size and breadth of the federal government present the ever present danger of frustrations and potential burnout that accompany working within the government bureaucracy with the federal regulations governing programs, funding cycles, contracting procedures, and employee work rules.

Understanding the Federal Government Approach

The OPM, as an independent establishment and government corporation, provides the federal health promotion program regulations, policies, and framework. In other words, the OPM provides the big picture while also providing each department and agency the authority and responsibility to address the needs of its workers. As part of giving the agencies the authority and responsibility for health promotion, the federal government created the FOH as part of the Department of Health and Human Services as a resource and technical assistance organization for federal employee health promotion programs and services. Federal agencies work with FOH; however, not all do. For, although the Economy Act facilitates and supports using FOH, federal departments and agencies at times operate their employee health promotion programs with minority- and women-owned businesses to fulfill the federal government's mandate for social and business equity.

Disconnections occur in the federal approach with the separation of the OPM, FOH, and vendors. For example, department personnel budgets may or may not be impacted by employee absences due to workers' compensation claims as well as FLMA, since they are funded from different sources within the government. Furthermore a FOH vendor contracted to provide absent management, and which is working with the health insurance carriers to provide workers' compensation insurance coverage, might be separated from OPM. Pharmacy benefit management is a second area in which disconnections occur, with services spanning the OPM, FOH, and departments and agencies contracting independently with vendors.

Finally, confusion occurs between OPM, FOH, and other federal government initiatives to address workplace employee health promotion. Within the Department of Health and Human Services (DHHS) is the Centers for Disease Control and Prevention (CDC) with the Workplace Health Promotion Program and the National Institute for Occupational Safety and Health (NIOSH). Both are involved with research and evaluation of workplace health promotion and focus on the total U.S. workforce and all workplaces. Neither is involved with federal employee health promotion service provision.

OPM Health Insurance Providers and FOH FedStrive Coordination and Collaboration

FOH through FedStrive provides health promotion programs for the majority of the federal employees. Likewise the federal employees' health insurance providers working to lower health care costs and improve federal employee health. The 2012 OPM carrier letter directed carriers to include as part of federal employee coverage incentives for enrollees who complete a health assessment, are compliant with disease management programs, or who participate in wellness activities or treatment plans aimed at managing and improving health status. To standardize operations, maximize worker engagement, and eliminate duplication of services, OPM and FOH will in the future need to collaborate and coordinate efforts.

FedStrive Workers Versus Vendor Employees

The majority of FedStrive workers are employed by the vendor organizations. In an era of smaller government operations and higher efficiency, governments have over the past several decades contracted programs and services. For each of the FedStrive program areas the workers are employees of the vendor organizations: wellness/fitness, EAP, health clinic, environment service. The workers receive their salary and benefits from the vendor (not from the federal government). However, to make for seamless services and encourage federal worker engagement, the contracted employees are all presented and considered as FedStrive employees. This is a disincentive for departments and agencies contracting directly with vendors who have the extra expense (costs) to engage federal employees in their services.

Interagency Agreements and Consortia

A vast diversity and scale of FOH programs now exist. This can create opportunities but at times seem overwhelming. Adding to the challenge is the structure of the contract for the programs. Increasingly departments and agencies are electing to coordinate health promotion programs. Depending on its size and mission, a department or agency determines whether to create its own program or share services with other departments and agencies. Sometimes it is more cost effective to share employee health services and facilities in the same building or geographic location. This can be done through interagency agreements or consortia.

Interagency agreements: To share services, agencies may enter into an interagency agreement on a reimbursable basis with another federal agency. This process offers a convenient alternative to contracting and is often quicker and less cumbersome than the contracting process. As with contracting, an agency may choose to use one agreement to provide either all of its employee health services or just specific services such as periodic examinations. The Economy Act, 31 U.S.C. §1535, gives agencies authority to enter into interagency agreements with other federal agencies.

Consortia: When no single agency can serve as a workplace health promotion service provider for similarly situated agencies, the combined employee population may pool resources and establish a workplace health promotion consortium. A lead agency enters into a contract or agreement with a service provider. An interagency agreement links participating agencies to the contract, and the combined employee population enjoys access to workplace health promotion services. The lead agency must have authority to provide the services to other agencies.

Employee Financial Needs a Priority for FOH

Federal employees' financial needs are a priority for FOH, although they are not traditionally thought of as a health promotion area but rather related to benefits and retirement planning. FOH Financial Service Program is offered along with its EAP services and provides the employees objective, tailored information on a wide range of issues such as retirement planning, education funding, estate planning, savings, and investment strategies. To access the program, employees call a toll-free telephone number to speak with a financial counselor to identify employee needs and explore options on a variety of topics including:

+ Buying or leasing a car
+ Selecting which credit card to pay off first
+ Family budgeting
+ The basics of financial planning
+ Savings and investment strategies

⬩   Determining how much to save to retire comfortably

⬩   How to identify a financial planner in the community

Monitoring and Evaluating Federal Health Promotion Programs

Monitoring and evaluating the federal health promotion program requires that systems are created to measure and help understand the program performance. And while traditionally the federal Office of Management and Budget (OMB) is charged with the evaluation of federal programs (including OPM and FOH), OMB's priorities are evaluations linked to national political objectives. For example the most recent collaboration of OPM and OMB was the new Senior Executive Service (SES) appraisal system to provide a consistent and uniform framework for agencies to communicate expectations and evaluate the performance of SES members, particularly centering on the role and responsibility of SES employees to provide executive leadership. The burden to evaluate the federal health promotion efforts has fallen to OPM and FOH.

Within OPM the policy review system evaluates and updates policies related to federal worker health. OPM through the contracting process monitors health insurance carrier compliance and service delivery as specified in the contract. FOH's strategic plan for integration outlines a framework for achieving data integration and use of the National Committee for Quality Assurance (NCQA) Wellness and Health Promotion (WHP) performance standards and measures to evaluate FedStrive. One of the critical components in measuring success of FedStrive is to standardize reported metrics across programs. Health analytics and standard performance measures have been developed in four categories: culture, values and satisfaction, health impact, and economic impact. Table 19.3 lists examples of the FOH health analytics and performance measures in each category. A link between the OPM health insurance carriers' data and the FOH FedStrive data will in the future allow the evaluation of health care costs and service utilization linked to the four types of FedStrive programs: clinical, wellness/fitness, EAP, and environmental health and safety.

Federal Government Employee Workplace Health Promotion Tools and Resources

The federal government through both the OPM and FOH provide a range of tools and resources. These are publically available through their websites both for federal employees as well as the general public. Access to some

Table 19.3 Selected FOH Health Analytics and Performance Measures

Performance measure by category	Definition
Culture metrics	
Leadership engagement	Assessment of leadership's participation and support of WHP program
Resources	Assessment of current resources including budget and staff
Organizational culture	Assessment of workplace culture, including working in groups and employee attitudes.
Ergonomics	Assessment of the work station ergonomics of employees
Values and satisfaction metrics	
Brand awareness	Assessment of employees awareness of the WHP offerings
Web analytics	Assessment of use of website and web portal utilization including login totals, total of unique users, total hits, etc.
Health impact metrics	
Health risk appraisal (HRA)	Percentage of adults who have completed HRA
Risk stratification	Percentage of adults who have competed a HRA and who have been identified within the following risk categories, Low (0–2), Moderate (3–4), and High (>5)
Risk reduction—Overall	The percentage of adults who had at least one of the three core risk factors as identified by a baseline HRA and who reduced their risk as identified buy a follow-up HRA
Economic impact metrics	
Cost —Absenteeism	The average cost of missed days of work per person for specific health condition
Return on Investment	A financial measure representing how much is saved compared to how much is spent on WHP programs

materials and resources is restricted and require contacting the particular agency material sponsor.

WellCheck

WellCheck is a survey based on Healthy People 2010's Elements of a Comprehensive Worksite Wellness Program. Implemented in 2009 by OPM's Work/Life/Wellness Group, the web-based tool collects information on federal agencies' health promotion programs at specific work locations. WellCheck is sent electronically via a web link to agencies each fall. The electronic survey results are analyzed and reported to the agency. WellCheck reports on health promotion programs, services, policies, and costs. Based on the results agencies submit an annual Wellness Implementation Plans to OPM's Work/Life and Performance Culture staff. Feedback is provided to agencies to support program efforts and suggest ways to improve programs and to identify relative strengths. OPM's Work/Life and Performance Culture staff uses the results to provide feedback to the Office of Management and Budget (OMB) and to identify areas of need, such as training, programs, and resources. Once multiple years are reported, agencies can track progress and adjust strategic plans and programs accordingly.

OPM Health Regulations, Guides, Policies and Procedures (http://www.opm.gov/about-us/)

OPM promotes and supports balanced, effective combinations of workplace health promotion programs and insurance benefits for employee health. To provide consistent and high-quality programs, OPM develops regulations, guides, policies, and procedures to address employee health. Their program guides are widely used. One example of a recent guide is the OPM *Guide for Establishing a Federal Nursing Mother's Program* to provide information on developing a program at the workplace to support mothers and their families. Released in January 2013, the guide details the legislative requirements according to the Patient Protection and Affordable Care Act that Federal agencies must meet in support of nursing mothers. The guide includes benefits of breastfeeding to agencies, mothers, and their nursing infants. In the guide are the steps to develop a program from the ground up as well as specific information on how an agency can improve and sustain an existing program. Examples of federal agencies with outstanding nursing mother's programs are included for benchmarking purposes.

FOH FedStrive (https://fedstrive.foh.hhs.gov/)

The entry portal to the FedStrive provides a program overview while directing employees to program services at their workplace. It is password protected for employee confidentiality.

FOH EAP Monthly Campaigns (http://www.foh.dhhs.gov/default.asp)

The EAP offers monthly campaigns to raise awareness of various mental and emotional well-being and work-life issues. Among the campaigns resources are the *Your Source* newsletter and a poster with a new theme for each monthly campaign.

Army Wellness Center: U.S. Army Public Health Command (http://phc.amedd.army.mil)

The Army Wellness Centers of the U.S. Army Public Health Command advocates for global force fitness through strategically developing, integrating, standardizing, and evaluating health promotion and wellness services within the army public health system. The Army Wellness Centers are an example of a federal employee health promotion program not operated by FOH but within the OPM guidelines. The centers use a health risk assessment with feedback approach to encourage positive health behavior change.

Summary

The federal government is the nation's single largest employer. As of July 2015 there were approximately 2.8 million civil servants (civilian, i.e., nonuniformed persons) employed by the U.S. government. Although most federal agencies are based in the Washington, DC, region, only about 16% (or about 288,000) of the federal government workforce is employed in this region. There are over 1,300 federal government agencies. The U.S. Office of Personnel Management (OPM) is the federal agency charged with the legislative initiatives to provide overall guidance to federal agencies and help agencies implement health promotion programs. OPM's overall mission is to manage the civil service of the federal government, coordinate recruiting of new government employees, and manage their health insurance and retirement benefits programs. Following the legislative directives and using the OPM guidance, federal agencies implement programs and services through agencies at the employees' workplaces. Agencies offer a wide variety of health services, choosing the services that best meet its employees' needs. The level of services will vary from agency to agency. Each federal agency determines how to provide employee health promotion programs and services based on the scope of the desired program and services and available resources. Many federal agencies use the services of Federal Occupational Health. FOH is the largest provider of occupational health services in the federal government, serving more than 360 federal agencies and reaching 1.8 million federal employees. Starting in 2009, FOH organized and consolidated federal worker health promotion into one program. FedStrive. FOH provides clinical services, on-site health clinics, wellness/fitness centers, employee assistance programs, and environmental health services to federal agencies via interagency agreements.

For Practice and Discussion

1. The majority of the OPM health-related professional positions are represented by the civil servants, armed forces, and Public Health Service Corp professionals. Likewise the FOH professionals include

these same career paths (civil service, armed forces, etc.). Compare and contrast health promotion positions that exist within each career path. How will their professional preparation and experience be the same and different? What are the advantages and disadvantages of having the three different career paths within OPM and FOH health promotion efforts?

2. Explain the pros and cons of the federal approach to federal employee health promotion with OPM, FOH, the use of vendors, and federal government contracts being subject to myriad statutes, regulations, and policies that encourage competition to the maximum extent practicable, ensure proper spending of taxpayer money, and advance U.S. socioeconomic goals (Cornell University Law School, n.d.).

3. Select a federal agency to explore its current employee health promotion services. How do you propose to conduct the exploration? Prepare a plan including potential contact people (including telephone and e-mail information), questions to ask as part of an informational interview, website content reviews, and desired examples of current program offerings. How will you determine if the agency contracts with FOH or directly with vendors? How will you identify the vendors serving the agency? Include background information on the agency workplace sites and employees. Compare and contrast health promotion programs across agency workplace sites.

4. Research and discuss how vendors contract with the FOH. Investigate the role of the Federal Register in the process (https://www.federalregister.gov/). Identify current federal request for proposals (RFPs) for health promotion services and products.

5. Select a federal department or agency and research its staffing and workplaces. Based on your research propose and design a FOH EAP monthly campaign for the federal employees (http://foh.hhs.gov/whatwedo/eap/EAPInformation.asp).

Case Study: Getting a Job Working at FedStrive—What Would You Do?

Sofia Casillas is a recent college graduate. She has the ACSM Certified Health Fitness Specialist and ACSM Certified Clinical Exercise Specialist certificates. She recently became a Certified Health Education Specialist (CHES). She completed two college health promotion internships. One was for health coaching, the second for fitness center management and supervision. She has experience working in corporate wellness. Ms. Casillas wants to get a job working with FedStrive. If you were Ms. Casillas what would you do to get a job with FedStrive?

KEY TERMS

Office of Personnel Management (OPM)

Independent establishments and government corporations

Federal Civil Service

OPM chief medical officer

Health Care and Insurance

Federal Employee Health Benefits (FEHB) Program Carrier Letter

Planning and Policy Analysis (PPA)

Work/life

Federal Occupational Health (FOH)

Nonappropriated federal agency

HHS Program Support Center

Health promotion program vendors

Interagency or Interservice Agreement (IAA/ISSA, IAA)

FedStrive

Health programs

Wellness/fitness

Clinical health

Behavioral health

Environmental health

Interagency agreements

Consortia

FOH Financial Service Program

National Committee for Quality Assurance (NCQA) Wellness and Health Promotion (WHP) performance standards and measures

Culture metrics

Values and satisfaction metrics

Health impact metrics

Economic impact metrics

References

Cornell University Law School. (n.d.). *Government contracts.* Retrieved from http://www.law.cornell.edu/wex/government_contracts

Cornell University Law School. (1986). *5 U.S. Code § 7901—Health service programs.* Retrieved from http://www.law.cornell.edu/uscode/text/5/7901

Delowery, M., Lindsay, G., Hochberg, M., Price, J., & Spencer, K. (2012). *FedStrive progress report 2009 to 2011.* Washington, DC: Federal Occupational Health, U.S. Department of Health and Human Services.

Federal Occupational Health. (n.d.). *FedStrive.* Retrieved from http://www.foh.hhs.gov/fedstrive/fedstrive.html

Office of Personnel Management. (2014a). *About us.* Retrieved from http://www.opm.gov/about-us/

Office of Personnel Management. (2014b). *Carriers.* Retrieved from http://www.opm.gov/healthcare-insurance/healthcare/carriers/

Office of Personnel Management. (2014c). *Healthcare.* Retrieved from http://www .opm.gov/healthcare-insurance/healthcare/

U.S. Government. (2010). U.S. Government Organization Chart—Constitution level. Retrieved from http://www.netage.com/economics/gov/Gov-chart-top.html

U.S. Surgeon General. (n.d.). *National prevention strategy.* Retrieved May 8, 2015 from http://www.surgeongeneral.gov/initiatives/prevention/strategy/

CHAPTER 20

SCHOOL AND UNIVERSITY WORKPLACE EMPLOYEE HEALTH PROMOTION

How Schools and Universities Promote Employee Health

Universities, colleges, and schools have been slower than many workplaces to establish workplace health promotion programs for employees. In the past, when they addressed disease prevention and health promotion, they focused on student health problems. Historically, primary and secondary schools (K–12) were identified as places for motivating students to lead healthy lifestyles, and teachers and staff were identified as the agents for showing them how to adopt and maintain healthy behavior. Likewise, colleges and universities until recently mainly focused on students, with university student health centers traditionally providing physical health services, counseling, and health education activities (e.g., drug and alcohol problem prevention) within a student affairs department operated as part of the university administration.

Different from K–12 staff and faculty being role models of healthy lifestyles, university and college faculty and staff were presented as role models for academic achievement and success. Preschool education programs including day care providers are perhaps the most health-conscious organizations focused on healthy child development and disease prevention. However, since many are community-based organizations, budget constraints frequently limit employee health promotion programs and services.

Recently the commercialization of education at all levels has transformed education from primarily publicly

LEARNING OBJECTIVES

- Describe how schools and universities promote employee health

- Discuss how to work with schools and universities to promote health

- Discuss the challenges and opportunities for schools and university workplace health promotion programs

- Describe schools and university workplace health tools and resources

supported and operated institutions and organizations into private for-profit businesses that include large corporation (e.g., University of Phoenix, Career Education Corporation, KinderCare/Knowledge Universe) whose stock is publicly traded on the New York Stock Exchange. Many of these organizations focus on career education for young adults as well as adults reentering the job market and changing careers. With these education "business" organizations, employee health promotion programs are largely separate from any organizational focus on students' health. Furthermore these organizations in general may have less emphasis on students' health and health promotion than the previously discussed educational organizations.

The roots of the recent efforts to promote faculty and staff health in schools, colleges, and universities, including as well preschools, child care centers and commercial- and business-operated schools, can be traced to the Centers for Disease Control and Prevention (CDC)'s eight-component model that was originally labeled and defined as comprehensive school health programs (Allensworth & Kolbe, 1987; Allensworth, Lawson, Nicholson, & Wyche; Kolbe, 1986) but now as coordinated health programs. What was important about this particular model was its inclusion of staff health promotion as one of the model's eight components. The model reflects a growing recognition at the time for the need of school staff health promotion. For example, in 1977 the Oregon Department of Education launched the Seaside Health Education Conference. This week-long conference, later called the Seaside Health Promotion Conference, aimed to build awareness of the importance of school health education, including the promotion of health among faculty and staff. The conference brought together teams of school administrators, counselors, health and physical education teachers, school nurses, and school board members. The success of this conference prompted the U.S. Department of Health and Human Services to provide funding for teams from other states to attend the conference, provided that the teams made a commitment to replicate the conference in their own states. By 1990, more than 25 states had duplicated Seaside-style conferences. Nearly 60% of these replication conferences addressed the establishment and improvement of school workplace wellness programs.

In the mid-1980s, several nationwide organizations developed documents endorsing school workplace programs for health promotion. The American School Health Association passed a resolution promoting the design and implementation of school health promotion programs. The American Association of School Administrators published *Promoting Health Education in America*, which devotes a chapter to developing employee wellness programs, and the Health Insurance Association of America developed and distributed a manual titled *Wellness at the School Worksite.*

In 2000, the School Health Policies and Programs Study conducted by the CDC found that 41.7% of districts and 93.5% of schools provided some type of health-promotion activities or services for employees. Activities ranged from making announcements or posting flyers about health-related topics to offering health-promoting activities such as sponsoring competitions between groups, giving release time, awarding prizes, and providing financial incentives for employees to participate. The potential benefits of such programs were publicized to help generate support for school employee health promotion programs.

Benefits of School Employee Health Promotion Program
http://www.schoolempwell.org/

*   Decreased employee absenteeism

*   Lower health care and insurance costs

*   Increased employee retention

*   Improved employee morale

*   Fewer work-related injuries

*   Fewer worker compensation and disability claims

*   Attractiveness to prospective employees

*   Positive community image

*   Increased productivity

*   Increased motivation to teach about health

*   Increased motivation to practice healthy behaviors

*   Healthy role models for students

College and university employee health promotion programs have benefitted from the K–12 movement as well as efforts by the World Health Organization (WHO). In particular, the WHO promoted the concept of both Health-Promoting Schools (WHO, 1997) and Health-Promoting Universities (Tsouros, Dowding, Thompson, & Dooris, 1998). The goals of a Health-Promoting University are similar to those for coordinated health programs. These goals include improving the health of students, university personnel, and the wider community as well as integrating health into the university's culture, structure, and processes (Tsouros et al., 1998). Elements that have been found to be important in starting and sustaining a Health-Promoting University initiative include: a senior-level advocate who will argue for the initiative and make funding available for start-up; funding for a coordinator to facilitate the formation and implementation of the initiative; early successes and securing long-term funding for the initiative; formation of a steering committee and continued networking by the coordinator and the committee in order to establish broad-based legitimacy, ownership, and accountability for the initiative; and an initiative that responds dynamically to the context in which it is developed and implemented (Dooris & Martin, 2002).

Recently the American College Health Association's (ACHA) Healthy Campus Coalition provided leadership on the research, planning and writing of Healthy Campus 2020. The document is often referred to as the "sister document" to Healthy People 2020, and much of the development process for Healthy Campus 2020 was guided by the Healthy People 2020 framework (Office of Disease Prevention and Health Promotion, 2010.)

Healthy Campus 2020 is a result of a multiyear process that reflects the thoughts and perspectives of 600-plus diverse higher education professionals representing multiple professional organizations and disciplines. And while the Healthy Campus mission is for students, staff, and faculty, it provides national objectives for faculty and staff. The objectives and recommendations mirror Healthy People 2020.

Healthy Campus 2020 Mission

* Identify current and ongoing nationwide health improvement priorities in higher education

* Increase campus community awareness and understanding of determinants of health, disease, and disability, and the opportunities for progress

* Provide measurable objectives and goals that can be used at institutions of higher education

* Engage multiple constituents to take actions to strengthen policies, improve practices, and empower behavior change that are driven by the best available evidence and knowledge

* Identify and promote relevant assessment, research, and data collection needs

The framework for serving faculty and staff as part of Healthy Campus 2020 is built upon a framework titled 3FOUR50. According to 3FOUR50, there are three risk factors—tobacco use, poor diet (including the harmful use of alcohol), and lack of physical activity—which contribute to four chronic diseases: heart disease, type 2 diabetes, lung disease, and some cancers. Those diseases, in turn, contribute to more than 50% of preventable

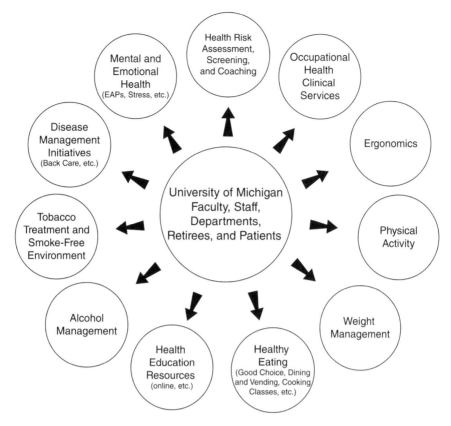

Figure 20.1 University of Michigan Employee Health Promotion Program
Source: Palma-Davis, 2014.

deaths in the United States. The University of Michigan used the framework to create its program Mhealthy (Figure 20.1). A unique aspect of Mhealthy is its engagement and development of a campus wide network of health champions (University of Michigan employees). The champions serve 2-year volunteer terms raising awareness and motivating coworkers to participate in the program. The champions are trained to work with their supervisors and managers to tailor and fit Mhealthy to the health needs of coworkers and colleagues in their units (e.g., department, school, office).

How to Work With Schools and Universities to Promote Employee Health

Educational institutions and organizations broadly share the same priority populations: students. And educational institutions by their missions and purpose are dedicated to the development of competent and healthy individuals. Either implicitly or explicitly health is part of all of education. At the same time each organization educates a unique and different population of students. Therefore, employees of preschool, K–12, college, career and professional preparation, and adult education institutions all reflect the people they educate and how they do it. At first glance schools all seem to be the same regardless of the students. And in many ways they are. However, just stepping inside a school building (or logging onto a school website) reveals that the differences are concrete and visible.

The implication of the contradiction that schools seems to be the same but in fact are very different highlights the need to take time to know the preschool and child care centers, school districts, colleges and universities, career educational, and adult education programs when working to promote the health of school employees. Successful efforts require navigating the complexity of schools and building relationships with teacher unions. And beyond unions there are many organizations that partner and collaborate with schools and educational professionals in the promotion of employee health.

Schools Are Complex

Schools are complex organization. School districts have complicated structures and many different types of jobs. Figure 20.2 shows a large district organization chart that illustrates such complexity. Districts have a school board that maintains authority over the school district operation. In addition to choosing and hiring a superintendent (in most, but not all, school districts), school board members make decisions about the school district's budget, curriculum, and policies within the framework established by state laws and policies. School boards comprise five to eight community members who are elected by fellow residents in the district to serve for a set number of years (term length varies by district). Some school districts elect a board representative from designated regions of the district, while others allow residents from any part of the district to serve. There are cases where school boards are appointed by and respond to another municipal authority (e.g., School District of Philadelphia) or where state legislatures delegate authority to other entities.

School district superintendents provide leadership to all schools within a school district and to district administrators. Superintendents serve as chief executive officers of their district and are charged with managing personnel, providing educational leadership, developing operating procedures based on policy, and acting as a district spokesperson. In most school districts in the United States, the superintendent is appointed by the district

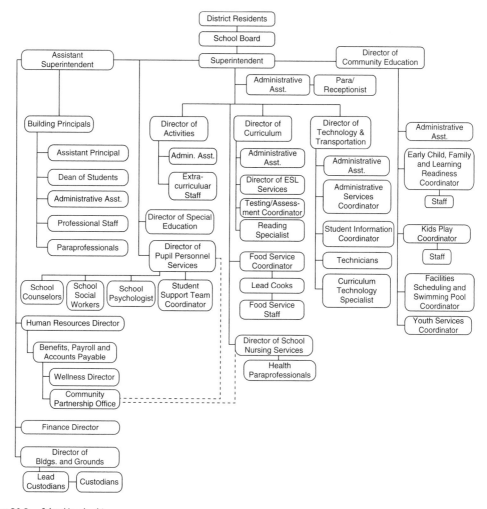

Figure 20.2   School Leadership

school board. In some school districts in Florida, Alabama, and Mississippi, the superintendent is elected by school district residents (National School Boards Association, 2015).

A school district also will often employ assistant superintendents who support the work of the superintendent and focus on a particular element of the school district, such as curriculum and instruction. Other school support personnel who work in administration may include directors of activities, curriculum, community education, special education, technology, communications, and school health. Staff members who work with the superintendent, responsible for school operations across all of the school buildings, are referred to as central office administrative staff (or just central office staff). Staffs in school buildings are building staff.

School buildings are led by a school principal. The principal supervises instruction and discipline; enforces rules, policies, and laws; supervises and evaluates teachers; and represents the school to parents and the community. Many schools have assistant principals who support the work of the principal (Bogden, 2003).

Looking at Figure 20.2, the individuals most involved with the employee health promotion program decisions are the school board members, superintendents, central office, and building-level staff. In particular, the individuals in the district's central administrative office, such as the human resource coordinator, are the most involved.

College and universities are equally complex as K–12 schools with a central administration, board of trustees (directors), staff charged with the schools' operations and student affairs (e.g., activities, health services) and academic faculty. Schools vary in their mission and scope ranging from large public research institutions (e.g., Penn State, UCLA, Ohio State, University of Texas, Florida State), Ivy League colleges (Princeton, Yale, Harvard), to small liberal arts colleges (e.g., Oberlin, Evergreen College, Reed College). Community colleges with 2-year academic and training programs serve many students across the country.

Understanding how schools are structured and operate is necessary for the implementation of school employee health promotion programs. On one hand, schools are large organizations that like other larger employees offer health insurance coverage that probably includes health promotion services and products. On the other hand, the complex school structure and varieties at the primary and secondary levels (K–12) mean that each school workplace (i.e., school building) implementation even within a district can have unique characteristics and needs that require a program implementation to be tailored and fitted to the particular building. At the post-secondary level (e.g., university, college, community college, career education), programs, departments, and university colleges (e.g., art and sciences, engineering, health sciences) and schools (e.g., business, social work, medicine) can have unique characteristics and needs that frequently require the tailoring and fitting of the program implementation.

Teacher Unions

Teacher unions are active in the field of education and in particular in K–12 school settings. They are also active at community colleges and 4-year colleges. The unions are the National Education Association and the American Federation of Teachers. The National Education Association is the largest union in the United States, and one of the most powerful

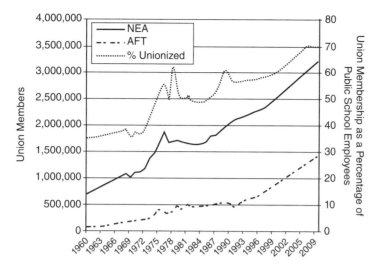

Figure 20.3 Union Membership and Union Share of the Total Public School Workforce
Source: Dillow, Hoffman, and Snyder, 2009.

political forces in the nation. The smaller of the two national education unions, the American Federation of Teachers is an affiliate of the AFL-CIO. In the past half century, public school union membership has sextupled, and the share of union members within the public school sector has doubled (Figure 20.3). This is in contrast to the private sector, where union membership has fallen substantially since the 1960s, and now stands at barely 6% in the service sector.

Peterson (1999) proposed three different models of teacher unionism: industrial-style, professional, and social justice. The distinctions are most useful in helping to frame discussion of teacher unions. In practice, the models are rarely so purely implemented and often overlap, blending into one another depending on circumstances.

The industrial unionism model focuses on defending the working conditions and rights of teachers. The professional model incorporates yet moves beyond an industrial model and suggests that unions also play a leading role in professional issues, such as teacher accountability and quality of school programs. The social justice model embraces concepts of industrial and professional unionism, but also is linked to a tradition that views unions as part of a broader movement for social progress. It calls for participatory union membership; education reform focused on serving all children, with special attention to collaboration with parents and community organizations; and a concern for broader issues of equity throughout society.

Health promotion programs are included as part of the employee benefit package union negotiation. As part of the negotiation process the union is engaged with the health promotion program planning, implementation, and evaluation and encouraged to make employee health a priority. Frankly discussed are barriers faced by the school organization and union to implement the program and engage union members (employees). Labor negotiations between school districts and their employee groups may be equated to a contest. While many issues may be resolved using "win-win" or "interest-based bargaining" tactics, distributive issues (wages, benefits, work hours and other work conditions) usually result in two opposing forces trying to exert their will upon the other. The consequence is that unions are an organization within school buildings, as well as spanning school building and districts, which can be both collaborative and mission driven (regarding students' education) as well as adversarial and conflictual (in terms of salary, retirement, and health benefit, including health promotion program negotiations). Union leadership (president and negotiation team members) as well as building-level leaders (union stewards) all play a role in the shape and implementation of health promotion programs in school buildings and districts. Part of any school health promotion program and team are union representatives. To be effective, school programs collaborate and work with unions as well as the district leadership. At times it can be a balancing act.

Union Engagement With Workplace Health Promotion Programs (Moss, Kincl, & O'Neill, 2008; State of California, 2008)

Message to Unions: Workplace health promotion programs require employees AND management engagement early in planning a workplace health promotion program, and they must continue joint participation in the program implementation and evaluation.

Why Should Unions Add Employee Health Promotion to Their List of Priorities?

Current staff and faculty have increased risk for chronic health issues (i.e., # smokers, poor diets). Current double-digit health care cost keeps increasing.

Aging labor force (faculty and staff postpone retirement).

Could shape as a positive intervention instead of discipline.

Way to offer programs to faculty and staff who value wellness.

Way to work with schools and universities to address health and safety issues in the workplace.

Barriers Schools, Universities, and Unions Face

Lack of interest by employees. (This could be due to some workplace culture factors such as poor program advertising, additional cost for participating in programs, not being able to access programs easily, because other stressful/hazardous working conditions are not being addressed so workers are skeptical, and privacy issues).

Lack of staff resources.

Lack of funding. (It is hard to show the cost payoff of reducing injuries and illnesses without good evaluation and data gathering efforts).

Beyond Unions: A Variety of Professional Organizations Support School Employees

Beyond unions a variety of professional organizations have emerged to support employees who work in schools. All of the organizations are potential allies in promoting the health of educational staff and faculty by providing alternative routes into schools and universities to promote employee health. For example, teachers often are members of discipline-based organizations (e.g., English teachers, arts education, health educators, science and math education, career education, foreign languages) that interact and support education professions. Likewise, professions and professional organizations that are dedicated to promoting the health and well-being of children (e.g., health educators, school nurses, physicians, physical educators, counselors, psychologists, social workers, dieticians, and others) now also focus on promoting employee health. Partnerships and collaborations to promote employee health with these organizations are commonly implemented as part of continuing education and small grant programs. For example, many professional conferences offer programs on wellness, life and work balance, and fitness. Topics range from stress management, burnout prevention, physical activities, and healthy eating. Food provided as part of meetings and training will reflect healthy diets and food choices.

Professional health education organizations with an interest in promoting the health of K–12 employees include the American Public Health Association, the Society for Public Health Education, and the Society of State Directors of Health. The American College Health Association is the primary professional organization for working in college and university employee health promotion.

A variety of other national organizations represent school and university personnel as well as others involved in employee health promotion activities. Organizations that serve those interested in K–12 schools include, among others, the following groups: American Association for Health, Physical Education, Recreation, and Dance; National Association of School Nurses; National Athletic Training Association; American School Food Service Association; National Association for School Psychologists; American School Counselor Association; School Social Work Association of America; National Association of Social Workers; National School Transportation Association; Association for Supervision and Curriculum Development; American Association of School Administrators; National Association of Elementary School Principals; National Association of Secondary School Principals; Council of Chief State School Officers; National Association of State Boards of Education; National School Boards Association; and National Parent Teacher Association. Organizations that serve those interested in initiatives in colleges and universities include the National Association of Student Affairs Professionals and NASPA: Student Affairs Administrators in Higher Education.

School and University Workplace Employee Health Promotion Program Challenges and Opportunities

Each school, school district, college, and university is unique. And while each shares the mission of education, the particular organizational goals, resources, culture, climate, and surrounding communities can be quite different and reflective of how an educational institution promotes the health of its staff, faculty, and administrators. In spite of these differences, schools, school districts, colleges, and universities face very similar challenges and opportunities to promote the health of their staff, faculty, and administrators.

Increasing Accountability for Education Institutions

Schools and colleges are in an era of public accountability. For many years, education costs have been rising faster than family incomes. The expectations for accountability in the use of funds and for performance have reached a level never before seen in the United States (Polikoff, McEachin, Wrabel & Duque, 2014). Education institutions receive a significant amount of taxpayer support and, in this new era, schools and colleges are more accountable to the public for the rising costs of operations. Likewise students (and parents) who pay tuition to colleges and universities are now demanding accountability for rising fees and for the educational outcomes of their college experience. Finally, education has become the primary ladder of opportunity for individuals, adding pressure for schools

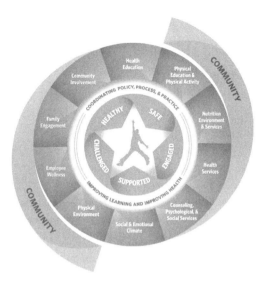

Figure 20.4   Whole School, Whole Community, Whole Child (With Employee Wellness Component)

to succeed with all students and to ensure that no qualified student is denied access to a college degree for financial reasons.

The impact of increased accountability of education institutions is competition for advocates and champions of employee health promotion programs to be seen and heard on the agenda of educational leaders and the public (i.e., parents and students). Most everyone would agree that the health of school employees is a priority, but in comparison to the needs of students it is a lower priority. Therefore creating and supporting an organizational culture and climate of health inclusive of students, families, staff, faculty, and administration that is linked to student learning outcomes and needs has gained urgency. The Whole School, Whole Community, Whole Child (Figure 20.4) developed by the Association for Supervision and Curriculum Development (ASCD) and the CDC combines and builds on elements of the traditional coordinated school health approach and the whole child framework that creates an educational institution that is accountable for both improving health and learning. Employee wellness is one of the model's core elements (ASCD, 2014).

Educational Finances

Financing education at the K–12 level is primarily through public tax dollars while colleges and universities rely on tuition revenues as well as grants and fund raising (e.g., endowments, alumna contributions, gifts). Knowing the fiscal reality of a school and college supports the individuals tasked

BOX 20.1   ABINGTON SCHOOL DISTRICT FACING FINANCIAL CHALLENGES

In 2011, Abington School District (Abington, Pennsylvania) faced a loss of $2.2 million in state funding for the year. The school board recognized that this loss could be detrimental to school programs but, being sensitive to the financial pressures taxpayers were facing, directed the School Superintendent to develop a school budget that resulted in no tax millage increase for residents. Also, the school board did not want to see the elimination of any educational programs or staff. The board's goal was: no increase in tax rates but maintenance of educational excellence. They were able to meet the challenges by forging agreements with 100% of the staff for a salary freeze for the school year. The human resources and business office staffs worked together to conserve costs by consolidating and reassigning job responsibilities of staff lost through attrition. With the savings the district was able to maintain its educational programs and advantageous class sizes, and even expand its foreign language programs at the junior and senior high schools, develop a new Cyber Education Program, and add a new Academic Adventures summer program (a free, summer remedial program for Title I students) within a budget that results in no tax millage increase, no furloughs of staff, and no student user fees. The direction, support, and teamwork of the school board were significant factors in successfully developing the budget.

with the employee health promotion program planning, implementation, and evaluation to make decisions that are consistent with the overall organizational fiscal goals. For example, Abington School District (Box 20.1) a suburban district north of Philadelphia, Pennsylvania, in 2011 faced a $2.2 million loss of state funding to the district. The Employee Health Program staff throughout the budget negotiations and subsequent district-wide budget reductions had to remain well informed and proactive in their decision making. New fee structures, community partnerships, public and private collaborations, and advocacy were all strategies that were employed to maintain and expand the program focused on promoting employee health. Program staff understand how the district is financed, which enables them to be viewed as a partner in financing and supporting the program, a key to being able to sustain the program.

Teacher Stress and Burnout

Public school teachers experience a large amount of stress, which can result in burnout and high turnover among new teachers. Teacher burnout is defined as "prolonged exposure to emotional and interpersonal stressors on the job, often accompanied by insufficient recovery, resulting in previously committed teachers disengaging from their work" (Steinhardt, Smith Jaggars, Faulk, & Gloria, 2011). Within the first three years of work, 40%–50% of teachers leave the profession, seemingly as a result of stress and burnout (Steinhardt et al., 2011). Teachers experiencing burnout feel dissatisfied and exhausted, alienate themselves from fellow teachers and their students, are less productive, and experience greater health problems. Stressors among teachers include role overload, disruptive students, nonsupportive parents, a lack of support from the administration, poor relationships with colleagues, being evaluated, and high-stakes student testing. These stressors and burnout attribute negatively toward a person's health status, specifically with increased mental illness, especially depression. Because depression in teachers is one of the primary causes for increased teacher absenteeism and high attrition rates, it threatens the quality of our educational system. Although not as correlated with burnout as stress, other factors seem to be related to teacher burnout as well. Age is highly correlated with burnout in teachers. Younger teachers report a higher level of burnout than older teachers (Steinhardt et al., 2011). In relation to job characteristics, high school teachers report a higher level of job burnout than lower grade level teachers (Beer & Beer, 1992). The most common measure of teacher burnout is by using the Maslach Burnout Inventory, which identifies three dimensions of burnout: emotional exhaustion, a sense of loss of personal accomplishment, and depersonalization where the student, patient, or client was at fault (Van Maele, Forsyth, & Van Houtte, 2014). This inventory can be used within a program to identify the current burnout status of teachers within a school or university.

Violence in Schools

Violence in its many manifestations, major or minor, has become such a part of the landscape in the United States that we are shocked momentarily by indescribable carnage and then continue to lead our daily lives without it having much impact on anything we do. That, unfortunately, is reflected in the values of our society in subtle ways and also permeates our schools, colleges, and universities. Workplace employee health promotion programs in educational settings cannot change the world, but programs can promote wellness in schools and communities so that conflicts do not turn into shoot outs. All types of violence in the school community, from chronic bullying to relational aggression, threaten the physical, psychological, and emotional well-being of students and school staff (Osher, Dwyer, & Jackson, 2004). These negative effects radiate to all members of the school.

Mass shootings are another kind of violence that occurs in schools. While deplorable and pointless, these shootings give Americans the false notion that dramatic increases in school-related violence are happening when, in fact, national surveys consistently find that school-associated homicides have stayed essentially stable or even decreased slightly over time. According to the CDC's School Associated Violent Death Study, less than 1% of all homicides among school-age children happen on school grounds or on the way to and from school. So the vast majority of school students and staff will never experience lethal violence at school (CDC, 2015).

An essential key to the prevention of violence is planning. Schools need to have policies, procedures, and comprehensive prevention plans in place to address school violence. The implementation of evidence-based prevention programs that teach social emotional skills, appropriate behaviors, conflict resolution, student support teams, and the fair application of discipline when infractions occur all contribute to reduction in violence. A caring and nurturing positive school climate and culture, where students and staff feel valued, also contribute to less violence. A crisis or emergency response plan that involves in its development the students, staff, local agencies and community-at-large, local law enforcement, local emergency management agencies, and first responders should be in place. There are many templates available on the web:

Facts About School Violence: CDC Youth Violence (http://www.cdc.gov/ViolencePrevention/youthviolence/schoolviolence/index.html)

Resources for Crisis Planning: U.S. Department of Education (USDE: http://www2.ed.gov/admins/lead/safety/emergencyplan/crisisplanning.pdf)

Resources for Responding to and Preventing School Violence and Suicide: Substance Abuse and Mental Health Services Administration (SAMHSA; http://www.sshs.samhsa.gov/resources/PreventingViolence.aspx)

Schools and University Workplace Employee Health Promotion Tools and Resources

Schools and university have only recently become more plentiful with the initiatives at the post-secondary level (colleges and universities) efforts to promote healthy campuses. Resources for primary and secondary schools are fewer with unions and independent organizations taking the lead to develop and disseminate the resources.

School Employee Wellness: *A Guide for Protecting the Assets of Our Nation's Schools* (http://www.schoolempwell.org/)

The guide covers the nine steps necessary for creating school employee wellness programs, and useful tools and resources (funding and publications) for implementing school employee wellness programs. It highlights the importance of school-site faculty/staff wellness programs as an essential component of a coordinated approach to school health and its significance in promoting health in schools.

Prevention and Intervention of Workplace Bullying in Schools: National Educational Association (http://www.nea.org/assets /docs/Workplace-Bullying-Report.pdf)

This NEA report summarizes the research on workplace bullying, as perpetrated by other educators, superiors, and students, and provides recommendations and behavior support plans to address workplace bullying. It argues that workplace bullying of educators impacts the students because their teachers, mentors, and staff are less prepared to do their jobs effectively.

Healthy Campus 2020 (http://www.acha.org/healthycampus/)

Healthy Campus 2020 provides a framework for improving the overall health status on campuses nationwide. Strategies suggested in Healthy Campus 2020 extend beyond traditional interventions of education, diagnosis, treatment, and health care at clinical levels. Through the collaborative efforts of health, academic, student affairs, and administrative colleagues, institutions of higher education can foster healthy environments and behaviors.

Healthy Campus 2020 has evolved to: include national health objectives for students and faculty/staff; promote an action model using an ecological approach; and provide a toolkit for implementation based on the MAP-IT (mobilize, assess, plan, implement and track) framework. These tools and resources help institutions of higher education determine which objectives are relevant, achievable, and a priority on their campus.

Tobacco-Free College Campus (http://tobaccofreecampus.org/) **and Smoke-Free College Campus** (http://www.no-smoke.org /goingsmokefree.php?id=447)

Tobacco-Free College Campus and Smoke-Free College Campus, a project of the American Nonsmokers' Rights Foundation, aims to have college or university campuses in the United States adopt 100% smoke-free campus policies that eliminate smoking in indoor and outdoor areas across the entire campus, including residences. According to the foundation, there are 1,127 100% smoke-free campuses in the United States, 758 of which are completely tobacco free. In addition to private mandates within the individual institutions, Alabama, Oklahoma, and Iowa have passed laws requiring 100% smoke-free college campuses within the state (Americans for Nonsmokers' Rights, 2014).

School Bus Drivers Safety Training (http://www.nhtsa.gov/Driving+ Safety/School+Buses/School+Bus+Driver+Training)

Although school buses are one of the safest forms of transportation on the road, accidents, injuries, and fatalities occur every year. To combat this reality, the National Highway Traffic Safety Administration has created a School Bus Driver Safety In-Service Series to promote and educate bus drivers on the importance of safe school bus driving. This program exists for current and experienced school bus drivers to enrich their knowledge on the subject. The series covers subjects such as route planning, loading and unloading, driver attitude, emergency procedures, proper railroad crossings, and more.

The Chronicle of Higher Education Great Colleges to Work for Annual Survey (http://chronicle.com/section/Great-Colleges-to- Work-For/156/)

The Great Colleges to Work For annual survey is based on responses from nearly 45,000 people at 300 institutions: 227 four-year colleges and universities (136 private and 91 public), and 73 two-year colleges. All accredited institutions in the United States with an enrollment of at least 500 were invited to participate, at no cost to them. The assessment had two components: a questionnaire about institutional characteristics and a faculty/staff questionnaire about individuals' evaluations of their colleges. The assessment also included an analysis of demographic data and workplace policies, including benefits, at each participating college. The questionnaires were administered online.

Summary

Schools and universities offer tremendous opportunities for employee workplace health promotion. The role of schools and universities in promoting and protecting the health of faculty and staff has gained importance over the past decade. Many initiatives have been put in place to support employee health promotion activities in schools and universities. Schools are complex organizations that require networking and building support across all of the school levels and units. Implementation requires the ability to tailor and fit program to employees needs in varied units (i.e., school, unit, discipline). Many school employees are union members, and in many school employee health promotion programs unions are active program partners. Unions are not the only potential professional organization that can partner with programs. A large number of professional education organizations are active in promoting school staff health. Challenges for employee health promotion programs include increased accountability for education institutions, concerns about school finances, teacher stress and burnout, and violence in schools.

For Practice and Discussion

1. Use the rationale for employee health promotion in school and university settings to create a brief three-minute presentation to justify the provision of employee health promotion programs in school or university settings.

2. Think about a specific elementary school, middle school, high school, or university. Identify and describe the programs, services, and policies that are designed to promote or protect employee health and safety in this school or university.

3. Use the Internet to explore three of the organizations that serve professionals who work in school or university settings to promote the health of employees. For each organization, identify its mission, the professionals that it serves, and its important initiatives.

4. Using the resources and tools described in this chapter, design a two-hour training session on promoting employee health for new community college staff members.

5. A school district is advertising a new job for an individual to plan, implement, and evaluate health promotion programs for its staff. Prepare a list of interview questions that the school district's human resource director can use to evaluate the job candidates.

Case Study: Innovative Teacher and Staff Health Promotion Program Recruitment—What Would You Do?

Melissa Venezia, a school district health promotion program director, wants to engage school district faculty and staff in a new health promotion program: Know Your Numbers Health Program. It is a collaborative effort among the district's health insurance providers, teacher union, and school district. The program goal is for teachers and staff to know and record, as part of a web-based program, key personal health indicators such as blood pressure, weight, height, BMI, cholesterol, date of last physical and vision examination and flu vaccination, and allergies. In the fall of 2015 the district enrollment is 105,650 students in 198 school buildings. The number of district employees (administrative, faculty, and staff) is 10,836. Ms. Venezia wants to do more than send e-mail blasts and school building flyers to engage the teachers and staff. If you were Ms. Venezia, what would you do?

KEY TERMS

Primary schools	3Four50
Secondary schools	Mhealthy
K–12	Complexity
Colleges and universities	Teacher unions
Coordinated school health programs	Professional organizations
Seaside Health Education Conference	Accountability
School Health Policies and Program Study	Educational finances
World Health Organization (WHO)	Teacher stress and burnout
Health-Promoting University	School violence
Healthy Campus 2020	

References

Allensworth, D., Lawson, E., Nicholson, L., & Wyche, J. (1997). *Schools and health, our nation's investment*. Washington, DC: Institute of Medicine.

Allensworth, D. D., & Kolbe, L. J. (1987). The comprehensive school health program: Exploring an expanded concept. *Journal of School Health, 57*(10), 409–412.

Americans for Nonsmokers' Rights. (2014). *Smokefree and tobacco-free U.S. and tribal colleges and universities*. Retrieved from http://no-smoke.org/pdf/smokefreecollegesuniversities.pdf

Association for Supervision and Curriculum Development. (2014). *Whole school, whole community, whole child*. Learning and health. Retrieved from http://www.ascd.org/programs/learning-and-health/wscc-model.aspx

Beer, J., & Beer, J. (1992). Burnout and stress, depression and self-esteem of teachers. *Psychological Reports, 71*(3f), 1331–1336.

Bogden, J. (2003). Cyber charter schools: A new breed in the education corral. *The State Education Standard, 4*(3), 33–37.

Centers for Disease Control and Prevention. (2015). *School-associated violent death study.* Retrieved from http://www.cdc.gov/violenceprevention /youthviolence/schoolviolence/SAVD.html

Dillow, S., Hoffman, C., & Snyder, T. (2009). *Digest of education statistics 2008.* Washington, DC: National Center for Education Statistics, Institute of Education Sciences, U.S. Department of Education.

Dooris, M., & Martin, E. (2002). The health promoting university—From idea to implementation. *Promotion & Education, 9*(Suppl. 1), 16–19.

Kolbe, L. (1986). Increasing the impact of school health promotion programs: Emerging research perspectives. *Health Education, 17*(5), 47.

Moss, H., Kincl, L., & O'Neill, C. (2008). *Health promotion programs and unions.* Retrieved from http://darkwing.uoregon.edu/~lerc/public/pdfs /healthpromotion.pdf

National School Boards Association. (2015). Retrieved from www.nsba.org

Office of Disease Prevention and Health Promotion. (2010). *Healthy People 2020.* Retrieved from http://www.healthypeople.gov/2020/default.aspx

Osher, D., Dwyer, K. P., & Jackson, S. (2004). *Safe, supportive and successful schools step by step.* Longmont, CO: Sopris West Educational Services.

Palma-Davis, L. (Producer). (2014, May 1, 2014). *Creating a culture of health at the University of Michigan.* [PowerPoint]

Peterson, B. (1999). Survival and justice: Rethinking teacher union strategy. In B. Peterson & M. Charney (Eds.), *Transforming teacher unions: Fighting for better schools and social justice* (pp. 11–19). Milwaukee, WI: Rethinking Schools.

Polikoff, M. S., McEachin, A. J., Wrabel, S. L., & Duque, M. (2014). The waive of the future? School accountability in the waiver era. *Educational Researcher, 43*(1), 45–54.

State of California. (2008). *The California Commission on Health and Safety and Workers' Compensation Summary of July 16, 2008, Workplace Wellness Roundtable.* C. Baker (Ed.). Retrieved from http://www.dir.ca.gov /chswc/Reports/CHSWC_SummaryWorkplaceWellnessRoundtable.pdf

Steinhardt, M. A., Smith Jaggars, S. E., Faulk, K. E., & Gloria, C. T. (2011). Chronic work stress and depressive symptoms: Assessing the mediating role of teacher burnout. *Stress and Health, 27*(5), 420-429.

Tsouros, A. D., Dowding, G., Thompson, J., & Dooris, M. (1998). *Health promoting universities.* Copenhagen, Denmark: WHO Regional Office for Europe.

Van Maele, D., Forsyth, P. B., & Van Houtte, M. (2014). *Trust and school life: The role of trust for learning, teaching, leading, and bridging.* Dordrecht, The Netherlands: Springer Science + Business Media.

World Health Organization. (1997). *Promoting health through schools: Report of a WHO expert committee on comprehensive school health education and promotion.* Geneva, Switzerland: Author.

INDEX

Page numbers followed by *e*, *f*, and *t* refer to exhibits, figures, and tables, respectively.